D1710659

GI Epidemiology

To the GI fellows and students of our GI Population Science course,
who inspired us to assemble this educational resource.

GI Epidemiology

EDITED BY

Nicholas J. Talley
MD MMedSc (ClinEpid) PhD

Chair, Department of Internal Medicine
Mayo Clinic College of Medicine
Jacksonville, Florida, USA

G. Richard Locke III
MD

Division of Gastroenterology and Hepatology
Mayo Clinic College of Medicine
Rochester, Minnesota, USA

Yuri A. Saito
MD MPH

Division of Gastroenterology and Hepatology
Mayo Clinic College of Medicine
Rochester, Minnesota, USA

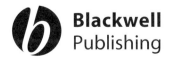

Blackwell
Publishing

© 2007 by Blackwell Publishing
Blackwell Publishing, Inc., 350 Main Street, Malden, Massachusetts 02148–5020, USA
Blackwell Publishing Ltd, 9600 Garsington Road, Oxford OX4 2DQ, UK
Blackwell Publishing Asia Pty Ltd, 550 Swanston Street, Carlton, Victoria 3053, Australia

First published 2007

1 2007

Library of Congress Cataloging-in-Publication Data
GI epidemiology / edited by Nicholas J. Talley, G. Richard Locke III, Yuri A. Saito.
    p. ; cm.
  Includes bibliographical references and index.
  ISBN 978-1-4051-4949-5 (alk. paper)
  1. Digestive organs--Diseases--Epidemiology. I. Talley, Nicholas Joseph. II. Locke, G.
Richard. III. Saito, Yuri A.
  [DNLM: 1. Gastrointestinal Diseases--epidemiology. 2. Epidemiologic Methods. WI
140 G428 2007]
  RA645.D54G53 2007
  614.5'93--dc22

                                                           2007002949

ISBN: 978–1–4051–4949–5

A catalogue record for this title is available from the British Library

Set in 9.25/11.5 pt Minion by Sparks, Oxford – www.sparks.co.uk
Printed and bound in Singapore by COS Printers Pte Ltd

Commissioning Editor: Alison Brown
Editorial Assistant: Jennifer Seward
Development Editor: Elisabeth Dodds
Production Controller: Debbie Wyer

For further information on Blackwell Publishing, visit our website:
http://www.blackwellpublishing.com

The publisher's policy is to use permanent paper from mills that operate a sustainable
forestry policy, and which has been manufactured from pulp processed using acid-free
and elementary chlorine-free practices. Furthermore, the publisher ensures that the text
paper and cover board used have met acceptable environmental accreditation standards.

R

Contents

List of Contributors

Paul Angulo, MD
Associate Professor of Medicine
GI Epidemiology/Outcomes Unit
Division of Gastroenterology and Hepatology
Mayo Clinic College of Medicine
Rochester, MN, USA

Adil E. Bharucha, MD
Professor of Medicine
Division of Gastroenterology and Hepatology
Mayo Clinic College of Medicine
Rochester, MN, USA

Suresh T. Chari, MD
Professor of Medicine
Division of Gastroenterology and Hepatology
Mayo Clinic College of Medicine
Rochester, MN, USA

Jessica A. Davila, PhD
Assistant Professor of Medicine
Sections of Gastroenterology and Health Services
    Research
Houston Department of Veterans Affairs Medical Center
Houston, TX, USA

Mary C. Dufour, MD MPH
Director, Division of Research and Analysis
CSR Inc
Arlington, VA, USA

Hashem B. El-Serag, MD MPH
Associate Professor of Medicine
Houston VA Medical Center
Baylor College of Medicine
Houston, TX, USA

James E. Everhart, MD MPH
Chief, Epidemiology and Clinical Trials Branch
Division of Digestive Diseases and Nutrition
National Institute of Diabetes and Digestive and Kidney
    Diseases
National Institutes of Health
Bethesda, MD, USA

Smita L.S. Halder, MBChB MRCP
Clinical Lecturer in Gastroenterology
Division of Medicine and Neurosciences
University of Manchester and Hope Hospital
Salford, UK

John M. Inadomi, MD
Dean M. Craig Endowed Chair in Gastrointestinal
    Medicine
Director, GI Outcomes and Health Services Research
University of California, San Francisco
Chief, Clinical Gastroenterology
San Francisco General Hospital
San Francisco, CA, USA

Steven B. Ingle, MD
Instructor in Medicine
Division of Gastroenterology and Hepatology
Mayo Clinic College of Medicine
Rochester, MN, USA

Steven J. Jacobsen, MD PhD
Director of Research
Research and Evaluation
Southern California Permanente Medical Group
Pasadena, CA, USA

John F. Johanson, MD MSc
University of Illinois College of Medicine at Rockford
Rockford, IL, USA

Torben Jørgensen, DMSci
Director and Associate Professor
Research Centre for Prevention and Health
Glostrup University Hospital
Glostrup, Denmark

Linda E. Kelemen, MSc ScD
Assistant Professor of Epidemiology
Department of Health Sciences Research
Mayo Clinic College of Medicine
Rochester, MN, USA

W. Ray Kim, MD
Associate Professor of Medicine
GI Epidemiology/Outcomes Unit
Division of Gastroenterology and Hepatology
Mayo Clinic College of Medicine
Rochester, MN, USA

James Lau, MD FRCS
Institute of Digestive Disease
Prince of Wales Hospital
The Chinese University of Hong Kong
Shatin, NT, Hong Kong

David Lieberman, MD
Chief, Division of Gastroenterology
Oregon Health and Science University
Portland, OR, USA

Paul J. Limburg, MD MPH
Director, Gastrointestinal Neoplasia Clinic
Associate Professor of Medicine
GI Epidemiology/Outcomes Unit
Division of Gastroenterology and Hepatology
Mayo Clinic College of Medicine
Rochester, MN, USA

Joseph Lipscomb, PhD
Professor of Public Health and
Georgia Cancer Coalition Distinguished Cancer Scholar
Department of Health Policy & Management
Rollins School of Public Health
Emory University
Atlanta, GA, USA

G. Richard Locke III, MD
Professor of Medicine
GI Epidemiology/Outcomes Unit
Division of Gastroenterology and Hepatology
Mayo Clinic College of Medicine
Rochester, MN, USA

Edward V. Loftus Jr, MD
Associate Director, Inflammatory Bowel Disease
Professor of Medicine
GI Epidemiology/Outcomes Unit
Division of Gastroenterology and Hepatology
Mayo Clinic College of Medicine
Rochester, MN, USA

L. Joseph Melton III, MD
Professor of Epidemiology
Department of Health Sciences Research
Mayo Clinic College of Medicine
Rochester, MN, USA

Paul Moayyedi, MB ChB PhD MPH FRCP (London), FRCPC
Professor of Gastroenterology
Department of Medicine, Division of Gastroenterology
McMaster University Medical Centre
Hamilton, Ontario, Canada

Joseph A. Murray, MD
Professor of Medicine
Division of Gastroenterology and Hepatology
Mayo Clinic College of Medicine
Rochester, MN, USA

Olof Nyrén, MD PhD
Professor of Clinical Epidemiology
Department of Medical Epidemiology and Biostatistics
Karolinska Institute
Stockholm, Sweden

Sarah J. O'Brien, MB BS FRCP FFPH
Professor of Health Sciences and Epidemiology
Section of GI Science
Division of Medicine and Neurosciences
University of Manchester
Hope Hospital
Salford, UK

Gloria M. Petersen, PhD
Professor of Epidemiology
Department of Health Sciences Research
Mayo Clinic College of Medicine
Rochester, MN, USA

Judith M. Podskalny, PhD
Director, Research Fellowship and Career Development
and Digestive Disease Centers Programs
Division of Digestive Diseases and Nutrition
National Institute of Diabetes and Digestive and Kidney Diseases
National Institutes of Health
Bethesda, MD, USA

Dawn Provenzale, MD MS
Associate Professor of Medicine
Director, Durham Epidemiologic Research and
    Information Center
Director, GI Outcomes Research
Duke University Medical Center
Durham, NC, USA

Linda Rabeneck, MD MPH
Regional Vice President, Cancer Care Ontario
Vice President, Regional Cancer Services
Sunnybrook Health Sciences Centre
Professor of Medicine, University of Toronto
Toronto, Ontario, Canada

Yvonne Romero, MD
Assistant Professor of Medicine
GI Epidemiology/Outcomes Unit
Division of Gastroenterology and Hepatology
Mayo Clinic College of Medicine
Rochester, MN, USA

Alberto Rubio-Tapia, MD
Division of Gastroenterology and Hepatology
Mayo Clinic College of Medicine
Rochester, MN, USA

Yuri A. Saito, MD MPH
Assistant Professor of Medicine
GI Epidemiology/Outcomes Unit
Division of Gastroenterology and Hepatology
Mayo Clinic College of Medicine
Rochester, MN, USA

William Sanchez, MD
Instructor of Medicine
Division of Gastroenterology and Hepatology
Mayo Clinic College of Medicine
Rochester, MN, USA

William J. Sandborn, MD
Vice Chair, Division of Gastroenterology and Hepatology
Professor of Medicine
Mayo Clinic College of Medicine
Rochester, MN, USA

Philip Schoenfeld, MD MSEd MSc (Epi)
Associate Professor of Medicine
University of Michigan School of Medicine
Anne Arbor, MI, USA

Nicholas J. Shaheen, MD MPH
Associate Professor of Medicine and Epidemiology
Director, Center for Esophageal Diseases and Swallowing
University of North Carolina School of Medicine
Chapel Hill, NC, USA

Crenguta Stepan, MD
University of Washington School of Medicine
Seattle, WA, USA

Joseph Sung, MD PhD
Chairman and Professor of Medicine
Department of Medicine and Therapeutics
Prince of Wales Hospital, Shatin
The Chinese University of Hong Kong
NT, Hong Kong

Christina M. Surawicz, MD
Professor of Medicine
Section Chief, Gastroenterology, Harborview Medical
    Center
Assistant Dean for Faculty Development
University of Washington School of Medicine
Seattle, WA, USA

**Nicholas J. Talley, MD MMedSc (ClinEpid) PhD
FRCP FRACP FAFPHM**
Professor of Medicine
Chair, Department of Internal Medicine
Mayo Clinic College of Medicine
Jacksonville, FL, USA
GI Epidemiology/Outcomes Unit
Division of Gastroenterology and Hepatology
Mayo Clinic College of Medicine
Rochester, MN, USA

Jayant A. Talwalkar, MD MPH
Associate Professor of Medicine
GI Epidemiology/Outcomes Unit
Division of Gastroenterology and Hepatology
Mayo Clinic College of Medicine
Rochester, MN, USA

Nimish B. Vakil, MD
Professor of Medicine
University of Wisconsin Medical School, Madison
College of Health Sciences, Marquette University
Milwaukee, WI, USA

Santhi Swaroop Vege, MD
Professor of Medicine
Division of Gastroenterology and Hepatology
Mayo Clinic College of Medicine
Rochester, MN, USA

Ingela Wiklund, PhD
Director, Patient Reported Outcomes
Global Health Outcomes
GlaxoSmithKline
Greenford, Middlesex, UK

Dhiraj Yadav, MD MPH
Assistant Professor of Medicine
Division of Gastroenterology, Hepatology and Nutrition
University of Pittsburgh School of Medicine
Pittsburgh, PA, USA

Foreword

Nearly 30 years ago, M.J.S. Langman, MD, then Professor of Therapeutics at the University of Nottingham Medical School, published *The Epidemiology of Chronic Digestive Disease* (Chicago: Year Book Medical Publishers, Inc, 1979). It was a thin book – only 139 pages. A general introduction described incidence, prevalence, death rates, official statistics and methods of population surveys. There were six disease chapters: peptic ulcer, gastrointestinal cancer, inflammatory bowel disease, diverticular disease and appendicitis, gallstones and pancreatitis. The book was a comprehensive, readable and authoritative overview of what was known about the epidemiology of digestive diseases at the time.

The book was remarkable in a number of ways. First, it was a single-authored text, something that is unusual today. Much of the epidemiology at that time was descriptive, and the book included comprehensive descriptions of disease prevalence across time and across area. The book was richly illustrated with graphs and figures. By summarizing the knowledge at the time, the book set the stage for the exciting work on the epidemiology of gastroenterologic diseases that followed.

In his preface, Professor Langman wrote "Chronic digestive disease is common, it is frequently disabling and, if due to cancer, is seldom curable. Knowledge of its root causes is fragmentary, but is increasing." The increasing knowledge noted by Langman has exploded, providing the motivation and the need for the present book.

Our improved understanding of digestive disease epidemiology was made possible by important gains in epidemiologic methods, advances in basic science, and the widespread availability of computers. In 1979 the statistical methods for case-control study, one of the foundations for etiologic epidemiology, had been developed but were not widely practiced. In fact, case-control methodology is not described in the introductory chapter of the Langman book. Multivariable statistics were tedious to perform on mainframe computers. Only a handful of gastroenterologists were trained in epidemiologic methods. Our understanding of genetics was rudimentary. When Langman speaks of genetics he is referring to family history, ABO blood groups and HLA typing.

The book in your hands provides the latest information about the epidemiology of digestive diseases. It includes a description of a number of methods and topics that were unknown in 1979 – health-related quality of life, health economics, systematic reviews, meta-analysis, health services research, decision analysis, and use of electronic administrative databases. There have been huge strides in our understanding of certain diseases. We now recognize *Helicobacter pylori* as a cause of peptic ulcer and gastric cancer. We have identified the viral agents for hepatitis B and C with implications for diagnosis and treatment. Optical endoscopes make it possible to examine, carefully and easily, the esophagus, stomach and colon. There are even capsule endoscopes that transmit images of the small bowel. We have discovered several genes that are associated with inflammatory bowel disease and hereditary non-polyposis colorectal cancer leading to hope that knowledge of these genes will translate into specific therapies. Irritable bowel syndrome and other functional disorders have now been organized and classified by the Rome criteria. Nonalcoholic fatty liver disease is recognized as an increasingly common cause of liver dysfunction. We have trained a large cadre of GI epidemiologists, many of whom have contributed chapters to this book. All of these gains have changed the face of GI epidemiology.

Despite the progress, summarized in the present volume, our understanding of many of these disorders remains nearly as primitive as when Langman wrote his landmark book. Diverticular disease is among the most common causes for GI hospitalization, and the prevalence in elderly Americans is very high. Although a low-fiber diet is often implicated, in truth we do not know the cause for diverticulosis or how to prevent it. We now understand the cascade of genes that are associated with colorectal cancer, but we don't know why the world's highest rates of colon cancer are now found in Japan, a country where colorectal cancer was previously unheard of. While we have made considerable strides in therapies for inflammatory bowel disease, we don't understand the interplay of genes and environment in its etiology.

Why is it important to understand the epidemiology of gastroenterological diseases? There are several reasons.

Prevalence – the number of individuals in the population who have a disease – is one measure of the burden of illness. Accurate information on prevalence of GI disorders is necessary for policy-makers appropriately to allocate healthcare dollars, for payers to estimate the costs of providing care, and for research agencies to prioritize funding. Prevalence is also of interest to pharmaceutical companies as they consider the development of new drugs. Practitioners need information on prevalence of disease in their patient population to estimate prior probability and thereby support the rational use of diagnostic testing. Understanding the incidence, prevalence and trends in disease provides clues to etiology and a benchmark against which purported etiologic agents can be judged. When we finally determine the causes of inflammatory bowel disease, for example, they must fit with what we know about the geography of the disease and the association with cigarette smoking. Understanding the principles of epidemiologic methods and study design make physicians more sophisticated consumers of the medical literature and permit them to practice evidence-based medicine.

We have come a long way since Langman's *The Epidemiology of Chronic Digestive Disease*. The current volume, GI Epidemiology, will appear equally quaint in 30 years, but for now it summarizes the state of our knowledge in this important field.

Robert S. Sandler

Preface

Several years ago we noticed that, despite a rich tradition of clinical epidemiological research in gastroenterology, few people, if any, recognized the existence of a distinct discipline called gastrointestinal (GI) epidemiology. When we decided to develop a gastrointestinal population sciences course at the Mayo Clinic as part of the Master's in Clinical Research degree program, this absence of recognition became even more apparent. This course was very well received, not only by gastroenterology trainees, but also by those people undertaking training in epidemiology. We noted that excellent textbooks of cardiovascular and neurological epidemiology were available, but when we searched for textbooks that focused on the epidemiology of GI diseases, there was a remarkable absence of any adequate resource. We therefore decided it was worth creating a new work with the aim of inspiring growth and interest in this important area. We view knowledge of GI epidemiology as key for designing and conducting outstanding clinical research in gastroenterology, and as important for guiding optimal decision making in clinical practice.

We have been fortunate to be able to recruit authors from around the world who are leaders in the discipline of GI epidemiology. The book focuses firstly on the public health impact of GI diseases. Next, we cover methodological issues from general epidemiology that are important in this field, including genetic epidemiology, nutrition, decision analysis, meta-analysis and clinical trial design; these areas are often ignored in comparable textbooks but have practical relevance to current, ongoing research in GI diseases. We also wished to strongly encourage the development of future leaders in the field with this book, and therefore included chapters on how to pursue a career in GI epidemiology and how to secure funding. The last half of the book deals with epidemiological knowledge of common and important gastrointestinal and liver diseases. The aim here is to summarize current knowledge of clinical epidemiology of specific GI disorders, in part to highlight areas for future study. We hope that readers will review this material critically, as there remain enormous gaps in knowledge which still need to be filled.

The authors have all worked hard to try and make the material both interesting and digestible. We hope that readers of this book will come to share our passion for the discipline of GI epidemiology as it emerges from the shadows of the past.

Nicholas J. Talley, MD, PhD
G. Richard Locke III, MD
Yuri A. Saito, MD MPH

Part 1

Gastrointestinal Diseases and Disorders: The Public Health Perspective

1

The Importance of GI Epidemiology

G. Richard Locke III and Nicholas J. Talley

Key points

- Gastrointestinal (GI) epidemiology is underestimated as a scientific discipline.
- GI epidemiologic insights have greatly improved the lives of patients.
- The current disease specificity of GI epidemiologic research may not provide the best milieu for advancement of the field.
- Great opportunity exists for a person interested in GI epidemiology.

Introduction

If one does a literature search and types in "epidemiology" over 76 000 references are cited; yet if one types in "GI epidemiology" the reference list is blank. Maybe the abbreviation is the problem. A search for "gastrointestinal epidemiology" yields just one paper that was published 10 years ago [1]. The combination of "gastrointestinal diseases" and "epidemiology" produces 200 citations. Yet, the combination of "cardiovascular diseases" and "epidemiology" produces 979 papers; and the combination of "neoplasm" and "epidemiology" provides 2413. The key word "epidemiology" has almost 6000 citations.

This exercise does not make GI epidemiology appear very important. However, the editors of this text strongly disagree. GI epidemiology is very important, but is underappreciated. Great work is being done in GI epidemiology, but is not recognized as GI epidemiology. By putting current work together in this book we hope to improve the understanding and recognition of this field.

Readers of this text will likely come from one of two backgrounds: (i) people who are trained and/or work in epidemiology and wish to learn more about gastroenterology, or (ii) people who are trained and/or work in gastroenterology and wish to learn more about epidemiology. GI epidemiology is of interest to both these groups of people but for different reasons. This chapter will highlight the importance of GI epidemiology from each perspective.

Why is GI epidemiology important to an epidemiologist?

The importance of GI epidemiology to the epidemiologist is nicely illustrated by the early work of Dr John Snow. The 150th anniversary of his work tracing a cholera epidemic was recently celebrated and an entire book has been written about this insightful use of epidemiologic methods to help save lives [2]. In 1851, people living in central London were suffering and dying from the acute onset of a fatal disease characterized by stomach cramps, vomiting and diarrhea. Snow examined the distribution of these cases and determined the source to be the water coming from the Broad Street pump. The handle was removed from the pump and the deaths stopped. Some consider this event to be the birth of the science of epidemiology.

Although this might be viewed as an example of infectious disease epidemiology, Snow did not know the organism. He studied the pattern of a gastrointestinal illness that was later shown to be cholera. Since that time, epidemiologists have worked diligently on eradicating infectious diseases and improving the health of the public. Infectious disease epidemiology is a well-established field and mysterious epidemics continue to fascinate both epidemiologists and the general public. Often these involve digestive diseases. For example, the recent problems of Norwalk virus outbreaks on ocean cruise liners and *E. coli* from fast food vendors have certainly kept this in the public mind. Countless times epidemiologic methods have been used to help reduce the outbreak of a disease.

Unfortunately, infectious disease epidemiologists do not focus much on digestive diseases that do not seem to have an infectious basis. This can limit opportunities. The great case in point is the story of *Helicobacter pylori* (HP) [3,4]. A later chapter in this book will review this topic in more detail, but a brief summary is in order. For decades, peptic ulcer disease was thought to be a disease of gastric acid production. Gastric cancer was thought to be caused by diet. The incidence of gastric cancer started to decline and no one understood why. Later, peptic ulcers became less of a problem and this was ascribed to the development of acid-blocking medication. Then two people, a pathologist and a gastroenterology fellow, postulated that an unknown organism seen on silver staining of gastric biopsy material was associated with peptic ulcers. The organism was quite difficult to culture and many had assumed it was just a commensal. The conventional wisdom could not accept that ulcers were an infectious disease. Barry Marshall first cultured the bacteria and in a later experiment then ingested the organism, developed gastritis and then eradicated the organism to partially fulfill Koch's postulates. Eradication of *H. pylori* healed and helped prevent ulcers. In 2005, Barry Marshall and Robin Warren received the Nobel Price in Medicine and Physiology for their work discovering HP. One can argue that this Nobel Prize was awarded for work in GI epidemiology.

Before 1900, HP was endemic around the world. Over the past 100 years, the prevalence of HP has declined in developed countries and with that decline came the decline in gastric cancer and peptic ulcers. Epidemiologists have contributed greatly to our understanding of HP and have helped to prevent further digestive disease. One question to ask, however, is why did it take so long? Why wasn't HP discovered in 1930? The answer was there, right before our eyes. Perhaps the wrong eyes were looking at the problem. Traditional epidemiologists did not study ulcers. Gastroenterologists were not looking to epidemiologists for help as they thought they understood the problem well. Might the answer have come sooner if GI epidemiology was a more mature discipline? One can only wonder.

Epidemiologists have been interested in cancer for a long time. The epidemiology of colon and pancreatic cancer has been well studied. Still, numerous opportunities exist for an epidemiologist to contribute to the understanding of digestive disease. Unfortunately, gastroenterology is increasingly becoming a divided field. First hepatology established itself as distinct discipline. Subsequently the endoscopists, pancreatologists, esophagologists, neurogastroenterologists and experts in inflammatory bowel disease (IBD) followed suit. Each of these groups has focused its efforts on additional years of training, separate meetings and separate societies, and even certification. While this has greatly enhanced these fields, it has also made it harder to think of GI epidemiology as a single discipline. People consider themselves as IBD or *H. pylori* experts rather than GI epidemiologists even if they are doing population research. This helps explain the challenge of searching the literature as highlighted at the start of this chapter. People don't think of GI epidemiology like cardiovascular epidemiology; they think about the epidemiology of the individual diseases.

Yet diseases happen to an individual, not just an organ. Exposures can affect the entire GI tract. Diet and ingested organisms may impact the gut based on location, but the entire GI tract is exposed to cigarette smoking, alcohol ingestion and bloodstream infections. Why should one person study the impact of cigarettes on the pancreas and another assess the impact on the stomach? Epidemiologists are needed to think in a horizontal fashion and link digestive diseases together. Such people can understand all the nuances of measuring exposures and translate these skills from one disease to another.

The opportunities for an epidemiologist interested in gastroenterology are further enhanced by the availability of data. As medical science has progressed and data systems developed (e.g., death certificates, mandatory reporting of specific infections) the possible uses of epidemiologic techniques have grown. However, the key development has been the introduction of computers and subsequent improvements in speed and memory. With modern computers, the epidemiologist can conduct and analyze studies with many thousands of participants and even millions of data points.

With such studies has come the development of enormous databases. For example the United States Public Health Service has organized several large studies and made the data available for public use. The National Health Interview Study (NHIS), which began in 1957, has over 100 000 subjects. The National Health and Nutrition Examination Surveys (NHANES) have been in continuation since 1971. Similarly, the National Ambulatory Medical Care Survey (NAMCS) and the Surveillance, Epidemiology and End Results (SEER) program have existed for decades. Because these studies have included hundreds of thousands of patients they provide the statistical power that epidemiologists need. These studies have not specifically focused on digestive diseases but yet have included data on symptoms, diagnoses, incidence rates and even measures of liver function and ultrasound assessments for gallstones. What have been missing have been individuals with an understanding of these data sets who are interested in GI topics.

Similarly, several large cohort studies such as the Nurses' Health Study have collected data on digestive problems. The primary aim of these studies has not been in digestive disease but they serve as a great resource for individuals interested in GI and epidemiology.

What about the more modern epidemics? Epidemiologists have long been interested in nutrition, and recently their attention has focused on obesity. The growing waistlines of Americans represent perhaps the most important epidemic of our time. Traditionally, obesity has been viewed as a risk factor for digestive diseases such as gastroesophageal reflux and non-alcoholic liver disease, but now obesity is viewed as a disease itself. Digestion certainly plays a role in obesity and may offer clues for how to stop this epidemic. GI epidemiologists have the opportunity to make a major impact in this field.

So why is GI epidemiology important to an epidemiologist? The reasons are clear. There has been a long history of outstanding work that has earned the highest awards that medicine has to offer. The opportunities for study are almost endless as the available data sources have been underutilized for the multiple digestive diseases that exist. The sky is the limit for a young person interested in this field.

Why is GI epidemiology important to a gastroenterologist?

Although GI epidemiology has been in existence for over 100 years it has not been an area of focus. Years ago, gastroenterologists were mostly physiologists. More recently the field has shifted toward endoscopy. In the 1990s considerable attention was given to outcomes research. This field was defined by the American Gastroenterological Association as being a combination of epidemiology, health services research, clinical investigation and clinical trials. Now the focus is on quality. In the past, quality improvement has not been considered research. Organizations have kept this work confidential under the cover of peer review. However, in the modern environment quality metrics are being collected by insurers and placed on the internet. Although quality improvement has a skill set that was largely developed in industry; the skills of an epidemiologist can be very helpful in advancing this field. Gastroenterologists in both private practice and in academic medical centers need to understand the tools of epidemiology and out-

comes research to improve the performance of their practice and the lives of their patients.

Gastroenterologists may not appreciate the story of the Broad Street pump [2], but they certainly appreciate the story of HP [3,4]. Although this topic was covered earlier from the perspective of the epidemiologist, the perspective of the gastroenterologist is slightly different. People in training today may find it hard to appreciate the impact that HP has had on our field. In 1930, gastric cancer was the most common cancer in America. The pathway of gastric carcinogenesis was well described. People were concerned about diet, especially the absence of fruits and vegetables and the presence of smoked or grilled meat and salted fish. However, then the incidence of gastric cancer started to decline and no one understood why. However, along came the "discovery" of HP and our understanding all changed. The cohort effect of birth year is now evidence-based and well understood (people born today are much less likely to acquire the infection than 50 years ago) and in retrospect, this all makes sense [5].

On a similar note, in the early 1980s gastroenterologists thought they knew a lot about peptic ulcers. Acid production was one of the best-studied elements of GI physiology. "No acid no ulcer" was the rule of the day. Again along came HP and everything changed. Now it is hard to imagine a world where people routinely need vagotomies or antrectomies. The Nobel Prize winners, Drs Barry Marshall and Robin Warren, were not themselves epidemiologists but used epidemiologic techniques to establish the importance of HP.

The importance of epidemiology to the gastroenterologist is not limited to HP. Perhaps the second greatest discovery of the past 20 years in GI was that of the viral agent hepatitis C [6,7]. Here again, epidemiology played a key role. People recognized the entity of non-A non-B hepatitis, but what was the cause? The lettering system even left room for this elusive agent. Although the agent was discovered using molecular techniques, the discovery was driven by what was known about the epidemiology of hepatitis.

These examples from the past just illustrate the importance of epidemiology to the gastroenterologist. What about future challenges and opportunities? Where can epidemiology help? We are making progress against colon cancer based on our understanding that adenomatous polyps are the precursors for this condition. In the 21st century we have to hope that the incidence of colon cancer declines just like gastric cancer in the last century. We recognize the importance of Barrett's esophagus in the development of esophageal cancer. The incidence of adenocarcinomas of the esophagus is increasing at an alarming rate. When will this modern epidemic peak? We need some type of screening test of Barrett's. Will it be a capsule? Will it be a blood test? But would such screening reduce mortality? Only time and research will tell.

Why is GI epidemiology important to the gastroenterologist? For many, the issue is simply furthering their understanding of the specific condition that interests them. Experts in any disease need to know the prevalence, incidence, impact, cost and prognosis of every important condition. New diseases will almost certainly be discovered (like HP) and knowledge of their epidemiology will be crucial to understanding how to maximize health.

We also have to be very careful not to let conventional wisdom "blind" us to solutions to today's challenges. Could colon polyps be due to an infection? Might esophageal cancer be the result of the decreasing prevalence of HP? What are the environmental causes of obesity or irritable bowel syndrome? Gastroenterologists with an interest in epidemiology are needed to keep asking these types of questions even when it seems the "answers" are known.

Challenges in GI epidemiology

Surely opportunities abound in GI epidemiology. We now have the ability to visualize the GI tract in its entirety. We have blood tests for viruses, HP and celiac disease. We have enormous databases and powerful computers. What is there to stop us?

Of course the first answer is we need people. In order for us to make progress in GI epidemiology we need people interested in the field. At present GI epidemiology is practiced in two ways. People with expertise in a specific disease include epidemiology as a component of what they do, or epidemiologists who have developed or have access to large databases ask questions related to GI diseases. Just a few people are truly GI epidemiologists. Fortunately or unfortunately, GI embraces many diseases and thus the field is spread thinly. We hope that by reading this book you have or may develop an interest in this field, and that this book will help nourish that interest so you decide to commit yourself to this field. Without a cadre of skilled investigators, the field will go nowhere and public health will not be best served.

The next issue is money. Fortunately the National Institutes of Health (NIH) and similar agencies around the globe have been very supportive of GI epidemiology. Training opportunities and initial grant support are plentiful. Of course the challenge is doing good work and obtaining long-term funding. These challenges and opportunities are discussed in detail in later chapters.

Perhaps the harder step is developing new techniques. Population-based research needs simple tests. We need a blood test for Barrett's esophagus; and we need simple blood or stool tests for inflammatory bowel disease, irritable bowel syndrome and colon cancer.

None of these challenges is insurmountable. The opportunities far outweigh the challenges in this field.

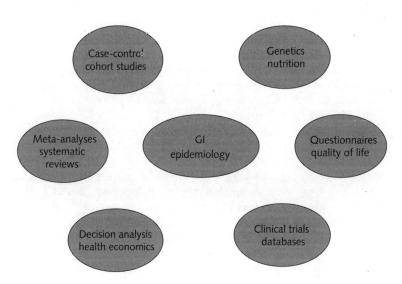

Fig. 1.1 The GI epidemiologist toolkit.

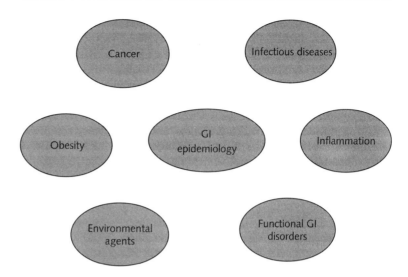

Fig. 1.2 The world of GI epidemiology.

Conclusions

This book embraces a broad definition of GI epidemiology. First the stage is set with a review of the burden of GI diseases. Then the tool box of the modern GI epidemiologist (Fig. 1.1) is reviewed in a series of chapters on traditional epidemiologic methods, patient-reported outcomes, meta-analyses, systematic reviews, decision analysis, health economics and even clinical trials. The specific areas of genetic, nutritional and infectious disease epidemiology are highlighted. The resources available to get a person started are discussed. The disease-specific chapters cover the world of the GI epidemiologist (Fig. 1.2). The diseases of the entire alimentary tract are reviewed from esophagus to anal canal as well as the liver and pancreas. Taken together this book represents an attempt at defining our field – GI epidemiology.

So why is GI epidemiology important? GI conditions are common and sometimes lethal. Many significantly impact on quality of life. GI conditions are expensive. The study of GI epidemiology is needed to understand how common, how deadly, how significant, and how expensive. But perhaps more importantly, GI epidemiology has

the potential to change significantly the way we understand disease and practice medicine. Changing the way we practice to benefit the people we see…what could be more important than that?

References

1. Jorgensen T *et al.* Epidemiology in gastroenterology. *Scand J Gastroenterol* 1996;**216**(Suppl.):199.
2. Johnson S. *The Ghost Map. The Story of London's Most Terrifying Epidemic and How it Changed Science, Cities, and the Modern World.* London: Riverhead Books, 2006.
3. Marshall BJ. The Lasker Awards: celebrating scientific discovery. *JAMA* 2005;**294**:1420.
4. Talley NJ, Richter J. Nobel Prize in Medicine awarded to a gastroenterologist in 2005. *Am J Gastroenterol* 2006;**101**:211.
5. Sonnenberg A. Causes underlying the birth-cohort phenomenon of peptic ulcer: analysis of mortality data 1911–2000, England and Wales. *Int J Epidemiol* 2006;**35**:1090.
6. Sherlock S. Landmark perspective: landmarks in viral hepatitis. *JAMA* 1984;**252**:402.
7. Purcell RH. The discovery of the hepatitis viruses. *Gastroenterology* 1993;**104**:955.

2   The Burden of Gastrointestinal and Liver Diseases

Nicholas J. Shaheen

Key points
- Gastrointestinal and liver diseases are among the most common conditions encountered and treated in primary care physicians' offices.
- The toll of these diseases in morbidity, mortality and healthcare costs is substantial.

- Several important trends in disease incidence, prevalence and mortality show that the impact of these diseases is dynamic.
- Given the changing epidemiology of gastrointestinal diseases, knowledge of disease trends is essential if policymakers and healthcare organizations are effectively to meet the needs of afflicted patients.

Introduction

Digestive and liver diseases impose a substantial burden. Over two million individuals were hospitalized in the USA with gastrointestinal (GI) and liver diseases in 2002. Gastrointestinal malignancies are among the most common cancers suffered by Americans, and colorectal cancer is the number three cancer killer of men and women in the USA [1]. Over 40 billion dollars of healthcare expenditure is used for gastrointestinal diseases annually [2].

Despite these sobering statistics, the USA lags behind several other nations in its ability to quantify and assess the toll of these diseases on society. This is in part due to the lack of nationalized healthcare, the presence of which in other nations allows centralized tracking of disease trends and utilization. Additionally, given that Americans frequently switch healthcare insurers, long-term, population-based longitudinal data on outcomes for a given disease state are difficult to obtain.

However, several privately and publicly held databases do allow us to make some assessment of disease trends and utilization in the USA. The purpose of this chapter is to use recent data from these databases to give a "snapshot" of the burden of gastrointestinal and liver diseases, with a focus on the US population. Although the primary focus of the chapter will be the morbidity and mortality of these diseases, the financial implications of gastrointestinal illness will also be considered.

Sources

Data presented below were garnered from several sources. The federal government maintains multiple databases with which to track disease incidence, prevalence and mortality. Private entities also track epidemiology and healthcare utilization, either as part of a billing scheme, or to improve allocation of resources. For each section below, the source of the data will be cited, and manipulations of the data after extraction from the source document will be explained. Next the limitations of the data will be presented and caveats for its interpretation will be discussed. Finally, the implications of the burden of gastrointestinal and liver diseases on policymakers and healthcare organizations will be considered.

What GI complaints and diseases bring patients to doctors?

A variety of symptoms and diseases cause patients to seek care in the primary care setting. One estimate of the conditions that bring patients to medical care can be derived from the National Ambulatory Medical Care Survey (NAMCS), a yearly national survey sponsored by the US Centers for Disease Control and Prevention (CDC) to provide information about the use of ambulatory services in the USA. These data are available on the National Center for Health Statistics website (www.cdc.gov/nchs/about/major/ahcd/ahcd1.htm). We used the NAMCS to determine the leading symptoms prompting an outpatient visit, and leading physician diagnoses. Excluded in NAMCS are federally funded providers, hospital-based clinics and emergency department visits.

The survey sampling unit for NAMCS is the provider–patient encounter in office-based practices. The 2002 NAMCS used a multistage probability design utilizing patient visits within physician practices sampled from 1900 geographically defined primary sampling units. Each provider was randomly assigned 1 week from the reporting year. The study design incorporates a patient visit weight (inflation factor) to derive national estimates from the survey. The principal, or first listed, reason for appointment was used in the analysis.

About two-thirds of physicians participating in NAMCS are primary care providers (family practice, internal medicine, gynecology, pediatrics). One quarter are from the following specialties: surgery, orthopedics, cardiovascular (CV) disease, dermatology, urology, neurology, ophthalmology, otolaryngology and psychiatry. The remaining specialties, including gastroenterology, are grouped under "other specialties." Less than 1% of the surveyed practices are gastroenterology specialty practices.

Table 2.1 demonstrates the symptoms for which Americans are most likely to seek healthcare referable to the gas-

trointestinal tract. "Upper abdominal pain" was included in the dyspepsia categorization. "Heartburn and indigestion" was used to estimate gastroesophageal reflux disease, but may have included patients with isolated dyspepsia. Symptoms of abdominal swelling, changes in girth, mass and fullness were grouped together under "abdominal distension." Anorectal symptoms were also grouped, with the exception of rectal bleeding. Gastroenteritis included both infectious and noninfectious forms. Diverticular disease included both diverticulosis and diverticulitis.

Abdominal pain, diarrhea, nausea and vomiting top this list. These top four complaints were unchanged when the dataset was restricted to only those providers who identified themselves as primary care physicians. Table 2.2 demonstrates the physician-derived GI diagnoses that were reported from the cohort. GERD has surpassed abdominal pain as the principal gastroenterology-related-provider diagnosis. Abdominal pain, gastroenteritis, constipation, dyspepsia and anorectal disorders (rectal bleeding, anorectal symptoms) follow. A significant increase in hepatitis C infection was noted, probably due to increased national awareness among patients and providers alike (1 237 708 vs 756 774 in 2000). Again, in subgroup analysis of family practice, internal medicine, gynecology and pediatrics, there was no change in the rankings of the top six diagnoses.

What GI diseases cause patients to be hospitalized?

The most common inpatient gastroenterology and hepatology discharge diagnoses may be compiled using the Nationwide Inpatient Sample (NIS). The NIS is one of the databases in the Healthcare Cost and Utilization Project (HCUP) (http://hcup.ahrq.gov/HCUPnet.asp). NIS is the only national hospital database with charge information on all patients, regardless of payer. The most recent version, NIS 2002, contains all discharge data from 995 hospitals located in 35 states, representing a 20% stratified sample of community hospitals in the USA.

The NIS database was queried using the following criteria: rank order of the disease, specific diagnosis according to the *International Classification of Disease, Ninth Revision, Clinical Modification* (ICD-9-CM), principal diagnosis, presence in the top 100 most common disease entities, and total number of patient discharges, for all patients in all hospitals. From this top 100 list, 14 gastroenterology and hepatology diagnoses were identified and tabulated. Two similar diagnoses were combined

Table 2.1 Leading gastrointestinal symptoms prompting an outpatient clinic visit, 2002. (Adapted from Shaheen NJ *et al.* The burden of gastrointestinal and liver diseases, 2006. *Am J Gastroenterol* 2006;**101**:2128, with permission from Blackwell Publishing.)

Rank	Symptom	Estimated visits
1	Abdominal pain	11 876 657
2	Diarrhea	3 766 261
3	Vomiting	2 653 944
4	Nausea	2 198 454
5	Constipation	1 830 406
6	Rectal bleeding	1 529 450
7	Heartburn	1 473 436
8	Dyspepsia, upper abdominal pain	918 935
9	Other GI symptoms, unspecified	897 052
10	Anorectal symptoms	873 119
11	Melena	811 019
12	Abdominal distension	786 901
13	Dysphagia	766 241
14	Lower abdominal pain[a]	751 521
15	Appetite decrease[a]	547 817

Source: NAMCS, 2002.
[a]Estimates based upon less than 30 encounters, which may be unreliable.

Rank	Diagnosis	Estimated visits	ICD-9 codes
1	GERD	5 512 159	530.11, 530.81
2	Abdominal pain	4 169 406	789.00, 789.09
3	Gastroenteritis	3 324 158	558.90, 008.xx, 009.xx
4	Constipation	2 562 166	564.0
5	Dyspepsia, gastritis	2 285 676	535.xx, 536.80, 536.90
6	Irritable bowel syndrome	2 063 539	564.1
7	Hemorrhoids	1 537 746	455.xx
8	Diverticular disease	1 493 865	562.1x
9	Hepatitis C infection	1 237 708	070.51, 070.54
10	Hernia, noninguinal	1 232 170	553.00, 553.10, 553.20, 553.90
11	Colorectal cancer	1 208 752	153.xx, 154.0, 154.1, 154.8, V10.05
12	Gallstone disease	1 109 408	574.xx, 575.0, 575.1, 575.2
13	Rectal bleeding	1 083 662	569.30
14	Hernia, inguinal	969 788	550.xx
15	Colon, benign neoplasm	853 037	211.30, 211.40
16	IBD[a]	834 856	555.xx, 556.xx
17	GI bleed, melena	753 680	578.xx

Table 2.2 Leading physician diagnoses for gastrointestinal disorders in outpatient clinic visits in the USA, 2002. (Adapted from Shaheen NJ *et al.* The burden of gastrointestinal and liver diseases, 2006. *Am J Gastroenterol* 2006;**101**:2128, with permission from Blackwell Publishing.)

Source: NAMCS, 2002.
GERD, gastroesophageal reflux disease; IBD.
[a]Estimates based upon less than 30 encounters, which may be unreliable.

into one entry: ICD-9 codes 574.10 (cholelithiasis with cholecystitis Nec) and 574.00 (cholelithiasis with acute cholecystitis).

Table 2.3 demonstrates the most common GI and liver causes of hospitalization, ordered by number of reports at discharge. The diagnosis "chest pain NOS" was included because this represents non-acute-myocardial-infarction chest pain, and a substantial number of these admissions were likely due to a gastrointestinal cause. This was the leading GI-related diagnosis. Gallstone disease and pancreatitis were each also responsible for over 200 000 hospitalizations. Aspiration pneumonitis and acute appendicitis rounded out the top five causes of hospitalization, and each of these entities was also in the overall top 30 causes of hospitalization for any disease entity.

What GI diseases cause mortality in the USA?

Gastrointestinal causes of death are available from the Division of Vital Statistics, National Center for Health Statistics (http://www.cdc.gov/nchs/data/statab/mortfinal2001_workI.pdf). Causes of death are classified using the *International Classification of Diseases, Tenth Revision*

(ICD-10). The causes of death are determined from hospital death certificates, which are entered into local and state databases. Data are transferred to the US Division of Vital Statistics after data entry into a standardized form.

In order to collate the data into clinically applicable diagnoses, multiple ICD-10 codes have been grouped by anatomic site to create a single disease entity. For instance, colorectal/anal cancer includes subjects with a cause of death reported as appendiceal cancer (C18.1), ascending colon cancer (C18.2), hepatic flexure cancer (C18.3), etc. Cancer diagnoses in the National Center for Health Statistics database are not subdivided by histologic type.

Table 2.4 reports the most common causes of death referable to the gastrointestinal tract. Colorectal cancer continues to be the most common GI-related cause of death. However, deaths from this condition have trended downward, and the 56 887 attributed deaths in 2002 represent a slight decrease from 2000, when 57 477 deaths were attributed to colorectal cancer. Also notable is an increase in the number of deaths from fibrosis/cirrhosis of the liver, from 14 003 in 2000 to 18 283 in 2002. Additionally, the number of deaths from esophageal cancer of all histologic types has now surpassed the number of deaths from gastric cancer, making esophageal cancer the number five etiology of gastrointestinal deaths.

Table 2.3 Most common gastrointestinal discharge diagnoses from inpatient admissions, 2002. (Adapted from Shaheen NJ *et al.* The burden of gastrointestinal and liver diseases, 2006. *Am J Gastroenterol* 2006;**101**:2128, with permission from Blackwell Publishing.)

Rank among GI DX	Rank among all DX	Diagnosis (ICD-9)	Total no. of discharges	Median LOS (days)	Median charges ($)	In-hospital deaths
1	16	Chest pain NOS (786.50)	324 618	1.0	7164	342
2	43 (574.1)	Cholelithiasis with cholecystitis NEC (574.1)	262 972	2.0	13 392	705
	46 (574.00)	Cholelithiasis with acute cholecystitis (574.00)		3.0	15 460	876
3	21	Acute pancreatitis (577.0)	243 332	4.0	11 402	3896
4	28	Food/vomit pneumonitis	188 555	6.0	16 274	34 562
5	30	Acute appendicitis NOS (540.9)	185 550	2.0	10 759	—[a]
6	31	Diverticuli of the colon w/o hemorrhage(562.11)	179 462	4.0	11 729	1821
7	36	Noninfectious gastroenteritis Nec (558.9)	157 364	2.0	5414	399
8	51	Gastrointestinal hemorrhage NOS (578.9)	116 724	3.0	9514	5957
9	57	Intestinal obstruction NOS (560.9)	102 111	4.0	8204	2948
10	61	Esophageal reflux (530.81)	94 919	2.0	8060	—[a]
11	80	Diverticula of the colon with hemorrhage (562.12)	74 717	3.0	9742	1003
12	82	Morbid obesity (278.01)	74 179	3.0	23 122	236
13	87	Intestinal adhesions with obstruction (560.81)	70 437	8.0	21 871	2365

[a]Too few cases to calculate a stable estimate.
ICD-9, *International Classification of Diseases*, 9th edition; LOS, length of stay; NEC, NOS.

What are the most common infections of the GI tract?

Multiple infections of the gastrointestinal tract are subject to reporting to the Centers for Disease Control (CDC) via the National Notifiable Diseases Surveillance System (NNDSS), a computerized system monitored jointly by the CDC and the Council of State and Territorial Epidemiologists. Once yearly, summary whole-year statistics are presented in the CDC's *Morbidity and Mortality Weekly Report* (MMWR). The most recent summary statistics available are from 2003, and were published online in the MMWR on 22 April 2005. This report is available on the MMWR website (http://www.cdc.gov/mmwr/preview/mmwrhtml/mm5254a1.htm).

Figure 2.1 demonstrates the relative proportions of incident infection for the top six most common etiologies for reportable GI infectious disease. *Salmonella* was far and away the most common of these conditions, with *Shigella* and *Giardia* second and third. The hepatotropic viruses, A and C, each had approximately 7500 reported cases. Certainly, because the acute phase of hepatitis C usually goes unrecognized, the incidence of the latter is underestimated. Of note is the continuing downward incidence of reported *E. coli* O157:H7. Only 2671 cases were reported in 2003, from a peak of 4744 cases in the late 1990s. Improved processing methods that decrease the potential for contamination of beef are credited for this decrease. Hepatitis A rates are also in decline since routine childhood immunization was recommended in 1996.

What are the current trends in causes of death from liver and biliary disease?

Data regarding the causes of liver-related mortality are available from the US Department of Health and Human Services, the Centers for Disease Control and Prevention,

Table 2.4 Leading 20 gastrointestinal causes of death in the USA, 2001. (Adapted from Shaheen NJ *et al*. The burden of gastrointestinal and liver diseases, 2006. *Am J Gastroenterol* 2006;**101**:2128, with permission from Blackwell Publishing.)

Rank	Cause of death	Number of deaths[a]	ICD-10 codes[b]
1	Colorectal/anal cancer	56 887	C18.0–C18.9, C19, C20, C21.0–C21.2, C21.8
2	Pancreatic cancer	29 803	C25.0–C25.4, C25.7, C25.9
3	Fibrosis/cirrhosis of liver and hepatic failure NOS	18 283	K72.0–K72.1, K72.9, K74.0–K74.1, K74.3–K74.6
4	Malignant neoplasms of the liver and intrahepatic ducts	13 351	C22.0–C22.4, C22.7, C22.9
5	Esophageal cancer	12 530	C15.0–C15.9
6	Stomach cancer	12 319	C16.0–C16.9
7	Alcoholic liver disease	12 207	K70.0–K70.4, K70.9
8	Vascular disorders of the intestine	9109	K55.0–K55.2, K55.8–K55.9
9	GI hemorrhage, unspecified	7804	K92.2
10	Paralytic ileus and intestinal obstruction	5248	K56.0–K56.7
11	Ulcers (gastric/duodenal/peptic)	4491	K25.0–K25.7, K25.9, K26.0–K26.7, K26.9, K27.0, K27.3–K27.7, K27.9, K28.4–K28.6, K28.9
12	Acute hepatitis C	4104	B17.1
13	Diverticular disease	3438	K57.0–K57.3, K57.8–K57.9
14	Acute pancreatitis	3075	K85
15	Malignant neoplasms of the gallbladder	1971	C23
16	Biliary tract cancer	1630	C24.0–C24.1, C24.8–C24.9
17	Perforation of intestine (nontraumatic)	1600	K63.1
18	Peritonitis	1562	K65.0, K65.8–K65.9
19	Cholecystitis	1475	K81.0–K81.1, K81.8–K81.9
20	*Clostridium difficile* enterocolitis	1332	A04.7

Source: National Center for Health Statistics Website – Mortality Tables (http://www.cdc.gov/nchs/data/statab/mortfinal2001_workI.pdf).
[a]Of a total of 2 416 425 deaths in 2001.
[b]*International Classification of Diseases*, 10th edition.

the National Center for Health Statistics, and the Office of Analysis and Epidemiology compressed mortality file (http://wonder.cdc.gov/mortICD10J.html). The compressed mortality file is a country-level national mortality and population database that is derived from US death certificates since 1979. A death rate based on fewer than

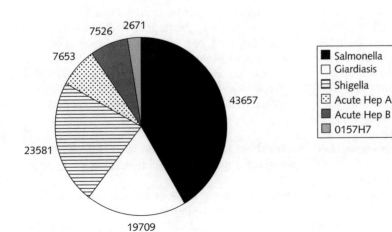

Salmonella
Giardiasis
Shigella
Acute Hep A
Acute Hep B
0157H7

Fig. 2.1 Reported cases of infectious gastrointestinal diseases in the USA, 2003. (Adapted from Summary of notifiable diseases – United States, 2003. *MMWR* 2005;**52**:1.)

Table 2.5 Causes of death from selected liver diseases in the USA, 2002. (Adapted from Shaheen NJ *et al.* The burden of gastrointestinal and liver diseases, 2006. *Am J Gastroenterol* 2006;**101**:2128, with permission from Blackwell Publishing.)

Cause of death	Rate per 100 000	No. of deaths	ICD-10 code
Liver cell carcinoma	4.9	14 047	C22
Alcoholic liver disease	4.2	12 121	K70.0–K70.4, K70.9
Acute hepatitis C	1.5	4 321	B17.1
Bile duct carcinoma	1.0	2 999	C22.1
Acute hepatitis B	0.2	659	B16, B16.0, B16.1, B16.2, B17.0
Chronic hepatitis C	0.2	518	B18.2
Primary biliary cirrhosis	0.1	418	K74.3
Acute hepatitis A	—[a]	76	B15, B15.0, B15.9
Chronic hepatitis B	—[a]	103	B18, B18.1

Source: US Department of Health and Human Services (US DHHS), Centers for Disease Control and Prevention (CDC), National Center for Health Statistics (NCHS), Office of Analysis and Epidemiology (OAE), Compressed Mortality File (CMF), computer tape, CDC WONDER Online Database.
[a]Too few cases to calculate a stable estimate.

20 deaths is considered statistically unreliable. Data are reported for deaths due to hepatobiliary disease for 2002, the most recent year for which these data are available.

Table 2.5 displays the leading causes of mortality from hepatobiliary disease. Compared with 1999, there has been an increase in the number of deaths from liver cell carcinoma, alcoholic liver disease and acute hepatitis C as well as acute hepatitis A. The greatest absolute increase in number of deaths occurred in hepatocellular cancer [3,4]. The number of deaths from acute hepatitis A almost doubled. This increase was due in part to a large, virulent outbreak in Pennsylvania that was caused by green onions contaminated during harvesting.

What are the most common gastrointestinal malignancies?

The Surveillance, Epidemiology and End Results (SEER) program (http://seer.cancer.gov) of the National Cancer Institute (http://www.cancer.gov) publishes annual estimates of cancer incidence in the USA. The SEER program is a population-based yearly epidemiologic survey of cancer incidence and survival. It provides data regarding cancer prevalence, incidence and mortality rates from nine population-based cancer registries including San Francisco-Oakland SMSA, Connecticut, Detroit (metropolitan), Hawaii, Iowa, New Mexico, Seattle (Puget sound), Utah and Atlanta (metropolitan). SEER uses a "first malignant primary only" method, meaning data reported include only the first malignant tumor in a specific anatomic site (breast, colon and rectum, stomach, etc.). The reported

prevalence rates for gastrointestinal cancers include all living cases that were diagnosed with gastrointestinal cancer. Once a case is counted, it will always be included as a prevalent case for as long as the individual is alive even if the individual has been treated and cured (e.g., undergoes surgery to excise the cancer).

Table 2.6 displays gastrointestinal cancer incidence and prevalence rates. Colorectal cancer continues to have the highest prevalence and incidence rates, eclipsing all other gastrointestinal malignancies by a factor of 10. Gastric, pancreatic and esophageal cancers form the next group of cancers. These malignancies are impressive for their high mortality [5,6] – despite the fact that colon cancer is 20 times more common than pancreatic cancer, the mortality rate of pancreatic cancer per 100 000 persons is more than half that of colon cancer. Consistent with previous trends [7], both the incidence and mortality trends for stomach cancer continued to decline.

What do Americans spend on GI illness?

Although a complete reckoning of the monetary toll of gastrointestinal illness is beyond the scope of this chapter, data sources are available with which to estimate the financial toll of these diseases.

The American Gastroenterological Association recently commissioned a study of the financial costs of gastrointestinal illness [2]. Using a variety of databases to estimate costs and utilization, they were able to estimate costs for 17 common gastrointestinal illnesses. Total cost estimates included direct costs (costs directly associated with pro-

Table 2.6 Prevalence and incidence of gastrointestinal cancers in the USA. (Adapted from Shaheen NJ *et al.* The burden of gastrointestinal and liver diseases, 2006. *Am J Gastroenterol* 2006;**101**:2128, with permission from Blackwell Publishing.)

Rank among GI cancers	Rank among all sites	Cancer site	Prevalence[a]	Incidence[b]	Incidence trend[d]	Mortality[c]	Mortality trend[d]
1	3	Colon and rectum	468 964	53.7	−0.8*	20.8	−1.8*
2	21	Stomach	34 105	8.9	−1.6*	4.7	−2.9*
3	22	Pancreas	21 534	11.0	−0.5	10.5	−0.1
4	23	Esophagus	21 156	4.5	0.3	4.4	0.6*
5	25	Liver and intrahepatic ducts	12 593	6.0	3.4*	4.6	1.9*

[a]Prevalence based on the SEER registry and 1 January 2001 US population estimates. These prevalences are for all ages, races/ethnicity and genders, and for diseases diagnosed between 1996 and 2000, from nine SEER registries.
[b]Age-adjusted incidence per 100 000 for all ages, races/ethnicity and genders, and for diseases diagnosed between 1997 and 2001.
[c]Death rates per 100 000, based on data provided by the National Center for Health Statistics (NCHS) public use data file (http://www.cdc.gov/nchs). The data are for the whole US population between 1997 and 2001 and are age adjusted to the 2001 US standard population.
[d]Annual percent change (APC) over the time interval (1992–2001 for both incidence and mortality trends) and for all ages, races/ethnicity and genders.
*The annual percent change is significantly different from zero ($P < 0.05$).

curing the goods and services associated with treatment, including expenses such as physician visits, medications and surgical costs), as well as indirect costs (costs not directly associated with care, but attributable to disease, such as decreased productivity due to impaired function, and opportunity costs associated with the time necessary to treat the disease). Indirect costs are most difficult to estimate [8]. In the AGA report, indirect costs were almost certainly underestimated, as the analysts estimated only one source of indirect costs, that being time away from work due to hospitalizations or physician visits.

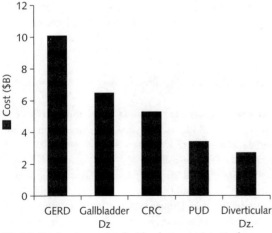

Fig. 2.2 Total costs associated with select gastrointestinal diseases in the USA, 2002. (Data from Sandler [2].)

Figure 2.2 demonstrates the five most expensive gastrointestinal conditions, in terms of total costs, both direct and indirect. Gastroesophageal reflux disease (GERD) was found to be the most costly, at over $10 billion in year 2000 estimates. Gallbladder disease, colorectal cancer, peptic ulcer disease and diverticular disease completed the top five conditions.

With respect to indirect costs, gastroenteritis and intestinal infections were the most costly, given the great toll of lost productivity and high number of patient visits associated with these diseases. The direct costs associated with GERD were more than 50% greater than the next highest disease, mostly owing to the high costs of chronic pharmacological therapy for the condition. Table 2.7 demonstrates the most common drugs prescribed in the USA for the year 2005, the most recent year for which these statistics are available, as estimated by a private marketing firm. As can be seen, 3 of the top 12 medications used in the USA were for GERD.

Some caveats – limitations of these data

Although the above data are the highest quality information available with which to assess the impact and trends of gastrointestinal diseases, several shortcomings must be recognized. Several of the data collection algorithms require recoding and/or interpretation by a third party of a source document. This interpretation introduces po-

Table 2.7 Top 12 selling branded prescription medications by retail dollars, 2005

Rank	Medication	Retail sales ($1000s)	Percent change from previous year
1	Lipitor	6 320 522	+6.0
2	Nexium[a]	3 436 794	+16.0
3	Prevacid[a]	3 327 919	+4.1
4	Zocor	3 106 628	−1.4
5	Adair Diskus	2 830 047	+21.8
6	Zoloft	2 561 069	−2.4
7	Plavix	2 480 042	+14.3
8	Effexor XR	2 219 469	−2.7
9	Singulair	2 089 348	+13.0
10	Norvasc	2 060 364	+9.4
11	Protonix[a]	1 957 950	+2.5
12	Ambien	1 932 940	+12.4

[a]Gastrointestinal medications.

Source: http://www.drugtopics.com/drugtopics/data/articlestandard/drugtopics/082006/309440/article.pdf.

tential error, especially if the third party is insufficiently skilled, or if the source data are ambiguous. These errors may be important in the categorization of causes of death listed on death certificates. Also, the presented data may inadequately express the complexity of these diseases, given that multiple diseases often coexist. Our NAMCS data, particularly, may underestimate the burden of GI disease, given that the primary or first-listed diagnosis was the one used for the calculations, as opposed to secondary diagnoses. Similarly, data derived from administrative databases, such as the NIS data, may suffer because the data are used primarily for billing purposes. Finally, the disease definitions of the datasets introduce limitations. For instance, the prevalence data from the SEER registry count any cancer survivor as a prevalent case. Therefore, a subject who underwent a Whipple procedure and had successful resection of a pancreatic cancer in 1980 would still be considered a prevalent case of pancreatic cancer today. While classification of such a patient as a prevalent case is somewhat imprecise, it does avoid the difficult question of when to consider a prevalent case of cancer "cured."

Implications

Gastrointestinal and liver diseases are among the costliest treated by American physicians, with respect to morbidity, mortality and financial burden. The above statistics attest to the toll of these diseases. Beyond merely describing the terrible impact of these diseases, these data should be used by gastroenterologists, epidemiologists and other inter-

ested parties to champion care of and research in these disease states. Additionally, frequent accounting of these diseases is necessary to spot trends in disease incidence and prevalence, both to serve as a "report card" for how we are doing in caring for these diseases, as well as to spot temporal trends in disease burden that might merit reallocation of resources to address the changes.

References

1. Jemal A *et al.* Cancer statistics, 2006. *CA Cancer J Clin* 2006;**56**:106.
2. Sandler RS, *et al.* The burden of selected digestive diseases in the United States. *Gastroenterology* 2002;**122**:1500.
3. El Serag HB *et al.* The continuing increase in the incidence of hepatocellular carcinoma in the United States: an update. *Ann Intern Med* 2003;**139**:817.
4. Davila JA *et al.* Hepatitis C infection and the increasing incidence of hepatocellular carcinoma: a population-based study. *Gastroenterology* 2004;**127**:1372.
5. Cleary SP *et al.* Prognostic factors in resected pancreatic adenocarcinoma: analysis of actual 5-year survivors. *J Am Coll Surg* 2004;**198**:722.
6. Polednak AP. Trends in survival for both histologic types of esophageal cancer in US surveillance, epidemiology and end results areas. *Int J Cancer* 2003;**105**:98.
7. Russo MW *et al.* Digestive and liver diseases statistics, 2004. *Gastroenterology* 2004;**126**:1448.
8. Koopmanschap MA, Rutten FF. A practical guide for calculating indirect costs of disease. *Pharmacoeconomics* 1996;**10**:460.

Part 2

Methodological Issues in GI Epidemiology

3

Overview of Epidemiologic Methodology

L. Joseph Melton III and Steven J. Jacobsen

Key points

- A "population" perspective complements the usual clinical view of disease based on the care of individual patients.
- Descriptive studies measure the impact of a disease on the population with respect to its frequency, morbidity and/or mortality. Methodological problems relate mainly to the identification of affected patients in the context of the population from which they arose.
- Analytic studies measure the association of various risk factors (exposures) with disease onset or progression. Methodologic

problems relate mainly to the identification of representative groups of cases and controls and accurate assessment of the exposures.

- Patient self-selection into exposed and unexposed groups (as opposed to random assignment in a controlled clinical trial) presents the main difficulty in interpreting the results of observational epidemiology studies.
- Epidemiologic studies represent the appropriate designs for addressing many important clinical questions.

In contrast to a clinical view of disease based on care of individual patients, epidemiology is concerned with the distribution and determinants of health and disease in populations. This community perspective more accurately reflects the impact of gastrointestinal (GI) diseases on society, which establishes priority for research support and control efforts. By determining the circumstances under which such disorders occur in the population, epidemiologic investigations can also identify subgroups at particularly high or low risk. This information can be used to design treatment or prevention programs, or to generate etiologic hypotheses for testing in subsequent research. In addition, epidemiologic studies among unselected community patients reflect the true spectrum of each disease and therefore provide the best information about prognosis. This may help optimize patient management. Finally, epidemiologic studies can evaluate the impact of new diagnostic tests and therapies, as well as environmental and behavioral factors, on disease trends over time. The interpretation of such information requires an appreciation for the epidemiologic methods used in its generation. These methods include descriptive studies of the frequency and impact of disease, as well as analytic studies of risk factors for disease onset or progression.

Descriptive epidemiologic methods

As the name implies, descriptive studies measure the impact of a disease on a population with respect to its frequency, morbidity and/or mortality, and they are often directed at "who, when and where" (person, place and time) questions. In qualifying the impact, most measures relate a number of affected persons (numerator) to population at risk (denominator). Thus, methodologic issues relate mainly to the accuracy of numerator and denominator data used to compute various disease rates. Specifically, the numerator depends on a precise definition of the disorder, as well as complete ascertainment of all affected individuals in the population of interest. Ascertainment, in turn, may depend on clinical, technical or systems capabilities. Of particular interest are technological advances that enable the detection of previously unrecognized cases. Generally, as diagnostic tests become more sensitive, the disease becomes more common (as milder cases are identified) and, simultaneously, appears less severe on average. Problems with the denominator relate to difficulty in defining the exact population from which the affected individuals actually arose. If a portion of the population is systematically missed, the condition may appear more common than it truly is.

Incidence (i.e., measure of risk of acquiring the disease)

$$\text{Incidence per 100,000 person-years} = \frac{\text{number of new disease cases during a specified time period}}{\text{person-years at risk during the same period}} \times 100,000$$

Prevalence (i.e., measure of risk of having the disease)

$$\text{Prevalence per 1000 population} = \frac{\text{number of persons with history of disease at a specified time}}{\text{population at that time}} \times 1,000$$

Fig. 3.1 Measures of disease frequency.

The most useful measure for assessing disease trends over time, identifying high-risk groups or measuring differences between populations is the **incidence rate** (Fig. 3.1). To determine the incidence of a particular disorder, all new cases that occur in some circumscribed population during a specified time period must be identified. In the typical clinical study, some new cases are identified but the population from which the cases originated cannot be precisely described. This precludes the ability to measure incidence. Strictly speaking, the incidence rate refers to the occurrence of disease among those actually at risk (e.g., genetic predisposition). Because this information is rarely available, however, incidence rates are typically calculated for an entire population, with the implication that everyone is at risk.

In other instances, the denominator (e.g., the population of a city or country for which census data exist, members of a health plan, etc.) may be known, but the exact number of new cases cannot be determined. This may result from an inability to canvass all local medical care providers or from inherent difficulty in finding new cases. Thus, discrepancies in reported incidence rates can result when one investigation defines new cases on the basis of symptoms among presenting patients and another employs physiological measurements on study volunteers (detection bias). Surveillance studies are often based on diagnostic codes from large administrative datasets where the actual grounds for making a given diagnosis may be unknown.

If the incidence of a particular GI disease cannot be determined, it may still be possible to determine its **prevalence**, that is, the proportion of persons in a population at some specific time who have the condition (Fig. 3.1). Prevalence is often estimated on a particular date (**point prevalence**) but can be assessed over a longer calendar period or as of some specific event such as birth or death. Prevalence and incidence are related (prevalence ≈ incidence × duration of disease), but prevalence is also influenced by survival, migration and other factors that do not reflect underlying disease risk in the population. Because these factors help to determine who has a condition at a certain point in time (as opposed to new onset), prevalence is less desirable than incidence for assessing the likelihood of disease occurrence (risk). Conversely, prevalence data are preferred for evaluating the burden of disease in the community because the number of affected people can be substantial when survival is good, as it is in many GI disorders, even when incidence rates are low.

Generally, the true spectrum of any given GI disease is best reflected by the incidence cases, who represent all occurrences in the population under study. The prevalence cases represent survivors (or immigrants), who may have very different characteristics. The apparent clinical spectrum found in patient series described from a medical center may be even more distorted because the cases can present a mixture of old and new and because referral patterns can impose intense patient selection (referral bias) even if medical center investigators report "unselected" cases.

Additional problems may be encountered when populations (e.g., different countries/environments, different personal/social settings) are compared to obtain insights about possible etiologic factors. If, for example, there are systematic differences in the age and sex distributions of the populations, the overall ("crude") incidence might appear to be unequal even when rates for each specific sex- and age-group within the two populations were identical. For a fair comparison, these systematic differences must be taken into account by weighting sex- and age-specific rates equally between the two groups. This is usually accomplished (direct adjustment) by multiplying the incidence rates for each age and gender subgroup by the number of comparable persons from some standard population (e.g., US population in 2000); the estimated number of cases that result from this step are then summed and divided by the total standard population to arrive at a new, "adjusted" incidence rate. By removing systematic differences between the populations, a comparison of adjusted rates answers the question "Would the overall rates differ if the age and sex distributions of the populations were the same?"

Analytic epidemiologic methods

Enumerating those with a given GI disorder is not usually

an end in itself. Instead, the emphasis more often is on discovering causative agents or factors associated with disease development, progression or complications. To do so, an investigator generally compares the relative proportions with disease between exposed and nonexposed groups, or proportions with the exposure between diseased and nondiseased groups. The underlying assumption is that if there is no association between exposure and disease, these proportions should be the same. It is relatively easy to determine the characteristics of a group of patients with a specific GI disease but much harder to decide whether or not those characteristics (risk factors) differ from expected. Consequently, appropriate referent (control) subjects from the population are needed for comparison. Hospital or referral center patients are rarely representative of the underlying general population in this regard, and using them as controls routinely leads to overestimation or underestimation (bias) of the association of specific risk factors with disease risk. Merely describing differences in the proportions of cases and referent subjects who have each putative risk factor (exposure) is not sufficient either. To assess the degree of risk associated with any particular etiologic or protective factor in a cross-sectional or case-control study, it is necessary to calculate an **odds ratio** (Fig. 3.2). The odds ratio is an estimate of the **relative risk**, or risk ratio/rate ratio (also shown in Fig. 3.2), which can be obtained directly from a cohort study.

Cross-sectional studies assess an entire population (or sample thereof) simultaneously for cases of a particular disease, and the presence of one or more risk factors (Fig. 3.3). With this information, one can calculate an odds ratio and also estimate the prevalence of that condition, as well as the prevalence of specific risk factors. This is inefficient if the disease and/or exposures are uncommon because effort is mostly expended on collecting data from subjects who have neither the disease nor the exposure of interest. Besides inefficiency, this approach is hampered by use of subjects with prevalent disease and prevalent exposures, thereby precluding the opportunity to assess temporal order. There are instances, however, where such diverse diseases and risk factors are being evaluated that the cross-sectional design is appropriate. The best example is the National Health and Nutrition Examination Survey (NHANES), which periodically samples the US population.

For studies of specific diseases, it is usually much easier (faster and cheaper) to conduct a comparable case-control study. In fact, case-control studies are generally required to investigate the etiology of uncommon GI disorders, and they are especially valuable for evaluating multiple risk factors simultaneously in order to generate pathophysiological hypotheses. In such a study, one begins with individuals who already have the disease in question (cases) and a comparable referent group, perhaps matched on extraneous factors (e.g., age, sex), without the disease (controls). Because the number of controls usually equals the number of cases (or some multiple, i.e., 2:1 or 3:1), this is much more efficient than evaluating the entire population, in which nondiseased individuals often greatly outnumber cases (100:1 or more). As illustrated in Fig. 3.4, the case and control groups are then compared for the prior presence or absence of factors (exposures) thought to be related to disease occurrence. The odds ratio calculated from these data is a good estimator of relative risk, which is the quantity actually desired, if three conditions are met:

1 the cases studied are representative of all cases in the underlying population in terms of the exposure of interest;

2 the controls are representative of all unaffected individuals in the population in terms of the exposure; and

3 the disease is rare.

The latter condition is easily fulfilled in practice because most diseases are rare enough (e.g., prevalence <5%). If either cases or controls are unrepresentative of their respective groups, however, the odds ratio will not accurately reflect the true relative risk. In addition, it is important that exposures be assessed consistently in both cases and controls; this is particularly important when knowledge of the disease outcome can influence assessment of the risk factor (measurement bias). Discrepancies often observed between case-control studies can usually be attributed to failure to satisfy one or more of these conditions.

Odds ratio (i.e., odds of disease
if exposed versus odds if unexposed)

$$\frac{\text{number of disease cases}}{\text{number of disease cases}} \times \frac{\text{number of controls}}{\text{number of controls}}$$

$$\frac{\text{number of disease cases with the risk factor}}{\text{number of disease cases without the risk factor}} \times \frac{\text{number of controls without the factor}}{\text{number of controls with the risk factor}}$$

Relative risk (i.e., risk of disease
if exposed versus risk if unexposed)

$$\frac{\text{incidence of disease among those exposed to the risk factor}}{\text{incidence of disease among those unexposed to the risk factor}}$$

Fig. 3.2 Measures of disease association.

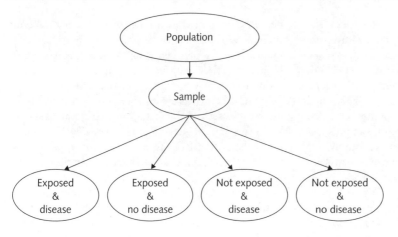

Fig. 3.3 Schematic of a cross-sectional study.

As a result of such problems, some prefer a cohort design. In a cohort study (Fig. 3.5), individuals with a characteristic thought to be related to disease etiology (exposed) and a comparable group without that characteristic (unexposed) are observed over time for the development of some disease outcome. Alternatively, it is sometimes possible to dispense with the unexposed group by estimating the number of disease outcomes that would have been expected in the cohort on the basis of the incidence of those outcomes in the general population (implicitly assuming that almost everyone in the population is unexposed). In order to establish a positive association between exposure and the outcome, it is necessary to show that the rate of developing disease is higher in the exposed than in the nonexposed group (relative risk). However, it is important to keep in mind that the "intervention" in a cohort study is not randomly assigned as it is in a clinical trial. Instead, patients self-select into the exposed and unexposed categories. This raises the possibility that any

observed increase in disease risk is not really due to the risk factor in question but rather to some unmeasured characteristic that, in turn, is associated with exposure status (confounding).

Cohort studies are usually expensive and time-consuming because of the large number of subjects needed and the lengthy follow-up often required to observe a sufficient number of outcome events. Indeed, the disease outcome must be relatively frequent for such studies to be feasible at all. Therefore, cohort studies are generally restricted to fairly common disorders, although they can be employed in smaller groups of people at high risk of disease. Cohort studies are also needed if it is important to assess several different clinical outcomes resulting from a single risk factor. While cohort studies are often carried out prospectively (concurrent cohort study) with baseline exposure assessed now and patients followed into the future, they can also be done retrospectively (historical cohort study) where the exposure is assessed at some earlier time point and disease outcomes are determined now. The latter approach is especially valuable for evaluating late outcomes when a cohort can be identified whose past exposure status can be reliably assessed.

Strengths and weaknesses of epidemiologic methods

The study designs described above are all "observational" in that the investigator neither allocates nor randomly assigns the exposure of interest as is done in a controlled clinical trial. This is an important distinction because randomization neutralizes, on average, the effects of any unmeasured or unknown determinants of the outcome in

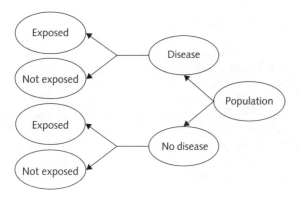

Fig. 3.4 Schematic of a case-control study.

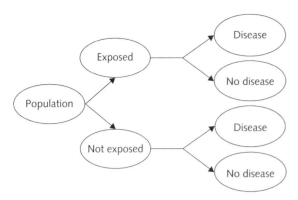

Fig. 3.5 Schematic of a cohort study.

the treated and untreated groups. Observational studies (natural experiments) do not enjoy this advantage and, because of the resulting potential for bias, are often given less credence than true experimental study designs. However, observational designs may be the only ones possible for addressing critical clinical questions. Thus, some important disease determinants clearly cannot be subjected to experimentation. It would obviously be unethical to randomize subjects to excessive weight gain, although trials may be possible where interventions are directed at

reducing weight. In addition, it is generally not feasible to extend controlled trials for a sufficient length of time to determine the effects of an intervention on long-term outcomes decades later, and the intermediate (surrogate) endpoints employed to reduce costs may not reflect clinically relevant endpoints. Moreover, the fact that efficacy is demonstrated under the idealized conditions of a trial does not necessarily mean that a given treatment is equally effective among the broader range of patients seen in routine clinical practice. Finally, many questions arise in medicine that experiments were never designed to answer: What set of clinical characteristics best defines a disease entity? What is the magnitude of the disease burden on society? What factors are associated with the risk of developing a disease? And which ones influence prognosis? These issues can be addressed in observational studies, including descriptive, cross-sectional, case-control and cohort studies. All of these applications of epidemiology are relevant to gastroenterology and are exploited in the following chapters that describe current knowledge concerning the frequency, etiology and impact of GI diseases.

The Mayo Foundation retains copyright on all original artwork.

4 Patient-Reported Outcomes

Ingela Wiklund

Key points
- Many gastrointestinal diseases are symptom-driven, so the patient's perspective is particularly important in this area.
- Patient-reported outcomes (PROs) provide essential information that objective measures and clinician assessment may fail to capture.
- PROs can be measured in a scientific, reliable and valid manner.
- Generic, disease-specific and treatment-specific PRO instruments exist.
- PRO instruments are valuable for use in clinical trials, to measure treatment outcomes, and also in clinical practice, to describe the burden of illness and to facilitate diagnosis and patient management.

Introduction

The medical community has traditionally preferred to use objective measures to confirm the presence of disease or to monitor treatment response. For example, these could be a positive test for a disease-causing microorganism, such as *Helicobacter pylori*, or the results of an endoscopy showing reflux esophagitis. However, many gastrointestinal (GI) diseases have a high symptom burden but little objective evidence for disease or poor correlation with tests for abnormality. Furthermore, because endoscopic and colonoscopic examinations are not generally performed in primary care, the GI tract is largely inaccessible to fur-

ther investigation in this setting. Primary care physicians are therefore required to rely on the patient's subjective report. Symptoms that are only felt by the patient, such as heartburn or abdominal pain, represent the most common self-reported outcome. The classification of medical outcomes into biological, clinician-reported, caregiver-reported and patient-reported is shown in Fig. 4.1.

Despite their common use, objective measures do have limitations. The interpretation of objective markers of disease activity, such as endoscopic findings, may differ between clinicians (often referred to as poor inter-rater reliability) [1]. Also, improvements in clinical measures may not correspond to improvements in how a patient

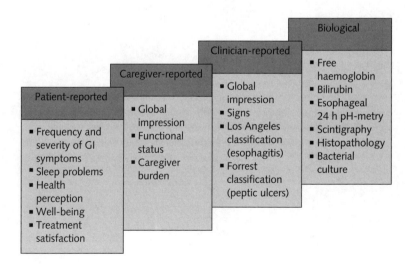

Fig. 4.1 Classification of medical outcomes, with examples from gastroenterology.

feels or is able to function. Some aspects of disease, such as pain intensity and relief, are known only to the patient. In the absence of objective measures, a physician relies on information from the patient in order to make a diagnosis or to assess whether a treatment is successful.

There is therefore a real need to help patients describe their own symptoms in a consistent, standardized way. One way to do this is to use patient-reported outcome (PRO) measures. The US Food and Drug Administration has recently put together draft guidance on the use of PRO measures in clinical trials to support labeling claims (summarized in Fig. 4.2), reflecting the growing recognition of the value of these tools [2]. In general, patients' well-being is increasingly being regarded by the medical community as an important factor in assessing treatment response. For example, assessment of PROs and health-related quality of life is now considered to be a standard part of care for patients with gastroesophageal reflux disease (GERD) [3]. The aim of this chapter is to describe some of the PRO instruments available for GI diseases and to review their value both in clinical trials and everyday practice.

What are PRO measures?

A PRO measure is a standardized instrument that assesses any aspect of health status or the benefit of therapy directly from the patient's perspective. PRO measures include a defined list of items to which patients respond using standardized response options and with respect to a defined recall period. They can be broadly grouped into generic, disease-specific and treatment-specific instruments (Fig. 4.3).

Generic PROs report overall health and its effect on aspects of everyday life, and can be used in various patient populations. Examples of generic instruments are the Short-Form 36 general health questionnaire (SF-36) [4] and the Psychological General Well-Being index (PGWB) [5]. These measures allow comparisons to be made be-

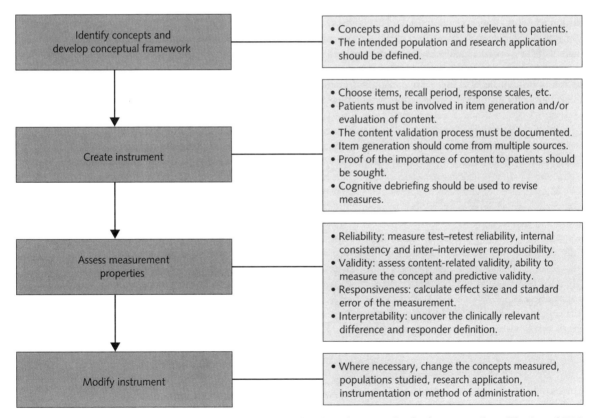

Fig. 4.2 Summary of the US Food and Drug Administration (FDA) guidance on the development and modification of PRO instruments.

Generic	Disease-specific		Treatment-specific
• Short Form-36 general health questionnaire (SF-36) • Psychological General Well-Being index (PGWB)	**Symptoms** • Reflux Disease Questionnaire (RDQ) • Gastrointestinal Symptom Rating Scale (GSRS)	**Quality of life** • Quality Of Life in Reflux and Dyspepsia questionnaire (QOLRAD)	• Functional Assessment of Cancer Therapy – Biologic Response Modifier (FACT–BRM)

Fig. 4.3 Classification of PRO instruments.

tween diseases but tend to be less sensitive than the more specific instruments to differences within groups of patients with the same condition [6]. In contrast, disease-specific PRO instruments are highly focused on the problems associated with a specific disease and so minimize the amount of "noise" that could be introduced by irrelevant items. These instruments allow patients to describe their symptoms (symptom scales) or the effect that their symptoms have on their lives. Disease-specific measures include the Reflux Disease Questionnaire (RDQ) [7] and the Gastrointestinal Symptom Rating Scale (GSRS) [8]. They also include disease-specific quality of life instruments, which measure how much a particular disease affects activities such as working, sleeping and eating; examples include the Quality Of Life in Reflux And Dyspepsia (QOLRAD)

questionnaire [9] and the Inflammatory Bowel Disease Questionnaire (IBDQ) [10]. Lastly, PROs can be treatment-specific. For example, a PRO could measure specific effects of a certain class of drug or type of therapy, such as the Functional Assessment of Cancer Therapy – Biologic Response Modifier (FACT-BRM) [11].

The value of PROs (Fig. 4.4)

Increasing understanding and recognition of diseases

Many individuals with GI diseases do not visit their physician about their symptoms. For example, population-based studies have shown that the majority of individuals

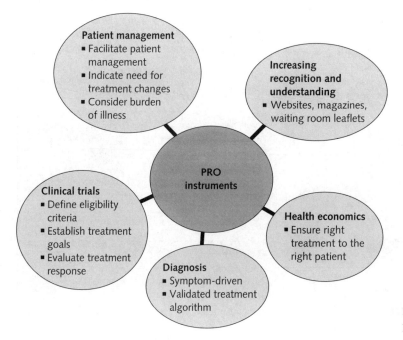

Fig. 4.4 The value of PROs in clinical practice and clinical trials.

with gastroesophageal reflux symptoms do not visit their primary care physician about them [12,13]. This may be because GI symptoms are generally not perceived as serious. Individuals with GI symptoms also often delay visiting their physician until they have another reason to go [14]. Websites, magazines or waiting-room leaflets that include questionnaires about symptoms can alert patients to recognize their true symptom load and its consequences, thereby encouraging individuals to talk to a physician about GI problems. Leaflets encouraging patients to raise their concerns with a physician have been associated with increased patient satisfaction [15].

PROs can also improve a physician's understanding of the burden that their patients have. There is increasing evidence of a communication gap between patients and physicians in the reporting of symptoms, which has the potential to lead to underestimation of patients' symptom burden [16–20]. For GI diseases specifically, data from clinical trials have shown that clinicians tend to underestimate symptom presence and severity and overestimate the benefits of treatment [21,22]. An improved understanding of the effect that GI symptoms can have on quality of life can also help physicians to highlight possible consequences.

PROs in clinical trials

Increasingly, the importance of taking into account the patient's perspective during drug development is being recognized [23]. In clinical trials, PRO tools can be used to establish the eligibility criteria that should be used, and also the results that can be expected after treatment. PRO tools should be used before other investigations, to uncover baseline levels, and then later, to assess treatment response. Because some treatment effects are known only to the patient, such as relief of pain, PROs can be essential for assessing the effectiveness of treatments in clinical trials.

Tools for diagnosis

PROs facilitate symptom-driven diagnosis. Symptoms are a good starting point for diagnosis because the presence and severity of symptoms drive individuals to consult [12,24]. For many GI diseases, a spectrum of symptoms exists. In the absence of objective evidence, PROs can help to establish a standardized cut-off point at which the severity and frequency of symptoms are considered to indicate disease. For example, heartburn is one of the primary symptoms of GERD, yet over 50% of the general population experience heartburn at least once a year. Clearly not all of these individuals are suffering from GERD. A PRO tool that assesses the frequency and severity of symptoms would assist physicians in diagnosing GERD in a standardized way. PROs that are not yet validated may also contribute to more accurate diagnosis. For example, the Reflux Disease Questionnaire (RDQ) assesses GERD-related symptoms and gives information on the presence and severity of patient-reported symptoms. This questionnaire has been preliminarily validated for this purpose [25].

Facilitating patient management

PROs can be used after diagnosis, to assist with the long-term management of patients. If physicians are made more aware of the burden of illness that their patients experience, including the effect that symptoms have on patients' everyday lives, they can more readily assess whether a patient will benefit from treatment. PROs can help a physician to understand the effect that GI symptoms have on health-related quality of life in a standardized way, and so identify where there is a need to treat. For example, the GERD Impact Scale (GIS) is a short, patient-completed questionnaire for patients who have been diagnosed with GERD. It can be used for patients with a new diagnosis, to determine the appropriate level of treatment, and also to help physicians identify currently treated patients who would benefit from changes to their treatment [26].

PROs can help physicians make sure that the most effective treatments are offered to the patients who will benefit most from them. In particular, PROs that evaluate health-related quality of life enable physicians to factor in the patient's burden of illness when considering how best to manage their symptoms.

PROs may also help to predict response to treatment. For example, a recent study has shown that a high level of anxiety or a low total well-being score at baseline predicts against a positive response to acid suppression therapy [27]. PROs can also predict mortality over and above traditional measures available to physicians, such as history and risk factors [28].

Health economic evaluation

Incorporating PROs into health economic analyses ensures that the benefit of a therapy as felt by the patient is quantified and included in economic decisions. PROs can therefore help make sure that, from a health economic perspective, each individual receives the most appropriate treatment. Standardized ratios such as cost per Quality Adjusted Life Year (QALY) allow the cost-effectiveness of different treatments to be compared. QALYs can also be used to compare treatment outcomes for different diseases, while the derived utility values are useful for comparing the burden of illness of various chronic conditions. PROs can help quantify the savings in cost associated with a treatment. For example, self-rated measurement of increased productivity at work can contribute to assessing the indirect costs saved.

Construction and validation of PRO instruments

The value of a PRO instrument is dependent on the quality of its development, and it is important that patients are involved during this process. Using patient and physician focus groups reduces the risk of measuring irrelevant symptoms. The reliability and validity of each instrument need to be confirmed [29]. In addition, their ability to detect change and interpretability also need to be tested if they are to be used in clinical trials [6].

Limitations of PROs

There are some limitations to the usefulness of PROs. Individuals may not answer honestly, especially if diagnosis of a particular disease via a PRO instrument offers access to treatment. As well as the possibility that they may not remember their experiences and so answer incorrectly, they may seek to fulfill a role as a "good patient." For example, they may report that their symptoms have improved as they feel that this is an appropriate response after having received treatment or because they feel grateful for the effort that a physician has shown.

Conclusions

Physicians can often underestimate the presence and severity of symptoms, and so there is a clinical need for standardized patient-reported symptom assessment. PROs capture the patient's perspective directly, and can be measured in a scientific, reliable and valid manner. PROs are useful both in clinical trials and for symptom-driven diagnosis in clinical practice. They are particularly valuable in diagnosing and assessing GI diseases because many of these diseases have a high symptom burden with little or inaccessible objective evidence for disease. PROs have the potential to increase and improve the understanding of the extent of patient suffering as a consequence of GI diseases. Because the wide-ranging effects of GI disorders are not always recognized and well understood by the medical community, PROs have particular importance in this area.

In the future, more research is needed on issues such as measuring the cost-effectiveness of GI treatment. Incorporating PROs into cost analysis will help to ensure that when the costs of various treatments are compared, the benefits that patients themselves experience can be taken into account.

References

1. Rath HC *et al.* Comparison of interobserver agreement for different scoring systems for reflux esophagitis: Impact of level of experience. *Gastrointest Endosc* 2004;**60**:44.
2. Food and Drug Administraton. Patient-reported outcome measures: Use in medical product development to support labeling claims. Rockville, MD: US Department of Health and Human Services, 2006 (http://www.fda.gov/cder/guidance/5460dft.htm).
3. Dent J *et al.* on behalf of the Genval Workshop Group. An evidence-based appraisal of reflux disease management – the Genval Workshop Report. *Gut* 1999;**44**(Suppl. 2):S1.
4. Ware JE. *SF-36 Health Survey: Manual and Interpretation Guide.* Boston: New England Medical Centre, 1993.
5. Dupuy HJ. The Psychological General Well-being (PGWB) Index. In: Wenger NK *et al.* (eds), *Assessment of Quality of Life in Clinical Trials of Cardiovascular Therapies.* Le Jacq Publishing Inc, 1984:170.
6. Talley NJ, Wiklund I. Patient reported outcomes in reflux disease: an overview of available measures. *Qual Life Res* 2005;**14**:21.
7. Veldhuyzen van Zanten S *et al.* Validation of the reflux disease questionnaire (RDQ), a new symptom scale for use in patients with upper gastrointestinal symptoms. *Gastroenterology* 2004;**126**(Suppl. 2):T1166.
8. Svedlund J *et al.* GSRS – a clinical rating scale for gastrointestinal symptoms in patients with irritable bowel syndrome and peptic ulcer disease. *Dig Dis Sci* 1988;**33**:129.
9. Wiklund IK *et al.* Quality of life in reflux and dyspepsia patients. Psychometric documentation of a new disease-specific questionnaire (QOLRAD). *Eur J Surg Suppl* 1998;**583**:41.
10. Guyatt G *et al.* A new measure of health status for clinical trials in inflammatory bowel disease. *Gastroenterology* 1989;**96**:804.
11. Bacik J *et al.* The functional assessment of cancer therapy-BRM (FACT-BRM): a new tool for the assessment of quality of life in patients treated with biologic response modifiers. *Qual Life Res* 2004;**13**:137.
12. Rey E *et al.* Medical consultation for gastro-oesophageal

reflux symptoms: reasons and associated factors. *Digestion* 2004;**70**:173.

13. Wong WM *et al.* Prevalence, clinical spectrum and health care utilization of gastro-oesophageal reflux disease in a Chinese population: a population-based study. *Aliment Pharmacol Ther* 2003;**18**:595.

14. Niemcryk SJ *et al.* Outpatient experience of patients with GERD in the United States: analysis of the 1998–2001 National Ambulatory Medical Care Survey. *Dig Dis Sci* 2005;**50**:1904.

15. Little P *et al.* Randomised controlled trial of effect of leaflets to empower patients in consultations in primary care. *Br Med J* 2004;**328**:441.

16. Corley DA *et al.* Accuracy of endoscopic databases for assessing patient symptoms: comparison with self-reported questionnaires in patients infected with the human immunodeficiency virus. *Gastrointest Endosc* 2000;**51**:129.

17. Fontaine A *et al.* Physicians' recognition of the symptoms experienced by HIV patients: how reliable? *J Pain Symptom Manage* 1999;**18**:263.

18. Justice AC *et al.* Clinical importance of provider-reported HIV symptoms compared with patient-report. *Med Care* 2001;**39**:397.

19. Suarez-Almazor ME *et al.* Lack of congruence in the ratings of patients' health status by patients and their physicians. *Med Decis Making* 2001;**21**:113.

20. Nekolaichuk CL *et al.* A comparison of patient and proxy symptom assessments in advanced cancer patients. *Palliat Med* 1999;**13**:311.

21. Fallone CA *et al.* Do physicians correctly assess patient symptom severity in gastro-oesophageal reflux disease? *Aliment Pharmacol Ther* 2004;**20**:1161.

22. McColl E *et al.* Assessing symptoms in gastroesophageal reflux disease: how well do clinicians' assessments agree with those of their patients? *Am J Gastroenterol* 2005;**100**:11.

23. Acquadro C *et al.* Incorporating the patient's perspective into drug development and communication: an ad hoc task force report of the Patient-Reported Outcomes (PRO) Harmonization Group meeting at the Food and Drug Administration, February 16, 2001. *Value Health* 2003;**6**:522.

24. Kennedy T, Jones R. The prevalence of gastro-oesophageal reflux symptoms in a UK population and the consultation behaviour of patients with these symptoms. *Aliment Pharmacol Ther* 2000;**14**:1589.

25. Shaw MJ *et al.* Initial validation of a diagnostic questionnaire for gastroesophageal reflux disease. *Am J Gastroenterol* 2001;**96**:52.

26. Jones R *et al.* Validation of the Gastroesophageal Reflux Disease Impact Scale – a patient management tool for primary care. *Gastroenterol* 2006;**130**(4 Suppl 2):M1974.

27. Wiklund I *et al.* Psychological factors as a predictor of treatment response in patients with heartburn: A pooled analysis of clinical trials. *Scand J Gastroenterol* 2006;**41**:288.

28. Heistaro S *et al.* Self rated health and mortality: a long term prospective study in eastern Finland. *J Epidemiol Community Health* 2001;**55**:227.

29. Guyatt GH *et al.* Methods to explain the clinical significance of health status measures. *Mayo Clin Proc* 2002;**77**:371.

5 GI Questionnaires

G. Richard Locke III

Key points
- Questionnaires should be evaluated prior to use just like any other diagnostic test.
- Questionnaires should be assessed for reliability and validity.
- Reliability is like precision; the answer is the same on repeated measures.
- Validity is like accuracy; the answer represents the truth.

Introduction

As discussed in the preceding chapter, patient-reported outcomes are of importance every day in GI epidemiology. Often physicians and researchers ask: "How are you doing?" The patient or study subject gives an answer, but sometimes it is hard to know how poorly they are doing and whether they are better or worse than before. How does one compare one answer with another from the same patient or study subject? How does one compare one patient with another? Fortunately, techniques have been developed to measure patient responses in a way that is accurate and precise. This chapter reviews the development of GI questionnaires. The goal is not to create a catalog of the existing instruments but rather to highlight what to look for when choosing an instrument for research or practice or assessing an article in the medical literature.

Before creating a questionnaire, one should first try to identify whether an appropriate measure already exists. Developing and testing a questionnaire requires specific knowledge, can take months to years to perform and can be quite expensive. It is more efficient to use something already developed even if it is not absolutely "perfect" for the study at hand. Ideally, the questionnaire has been constructed in a thoughtful manner and tested for reliability and validity. No one would accept a brand new diagnostic test without some evaluation of its accuracy or precision, and the same is true for patient-reported measures. Although many simply create a study questionnaire out of convenience, a questionnaire should not be just "made up." Like any test, thoughtful development and evaluation are needed. This chapter will explain the steps needed for appropriate questionnaire development (Box 5.1).

Drafting a questionnaire

If a new questionnaire is deemed necessary for a particular study, the first issue in design is scope. What needs to be measured? What are the appropriate topics? Often a questionnaire will ask several questions about related issues that can then be combined into some type of scale. These content areas are called domains. Scope can be determined by focus groups or interviews with experts.

The next decision is the mode of administration. Questionnaires can be administered face-to-face, by telephone or sent in the mail. They can be administered by people or by computerized voice response systems. Personal interactions are good for asking open-ended questions and following up with additional questions based on specific responses. However, this flexibility must be weighed against the issues related to socially desirable answers and expense. When human beings interact they usually want to be seen in a positive light. People are less likely to give socially unacceptable answers (even if those answers represent the truth) during a personal interview. Sensitive topics are best addressed in a less personal fashion. In addition, interviews are expensive. The interviewers have to be trained to administer the questionnaires in a systematic manner and, of course, be paid for their effort. The alternatives are written surveys that can be sent by mail or telephone, or web-based surveys that are conducted via a computer on-line. Such surveys are much less expensive and thus useful for large sample sizes. The trade-off is the ability to clarify answers with the respondent.

The next step is to write the questions. Each question should only address one item at a time. Combination questions can confuse the reader. If one asks a patient if

Box 5.1 Questionnaire development and validation

I. Questionnaire development
A. Mode of administration
   1. Face-to-face
   2. Phone interview
   3. Written, self-report
B. Response options
   1. Yes/no
   2. Likert scale
   3. Visual analog scale
   4. Open-ended questions
C. Item generation
   1. Focus groups
   2. Literature review

II. Questionnaire testing
A. Feasibility
   1. Time to completion
   2. Missed questions/blanks
   3. Misunderstood questions
   4. Ability to follow directions
B. Reliability
   1. Test–retest
   2. Internal consistency
C. Validity
   1. Face validity
   2. Content validity
   3. Concurrent validity
   4. Criterion validity
   5. Discriminant validity
   6. Responsiveness

they have heartburn or acid regurgitation, one has to be very clear whether the response should be an "either-or" or a "both." The other downside is that the answer does not identify which of the problems the person has. This fact might be important in a later analysis. Similarly, if one asks whether something bothers someone without asking if it is present one does not know if a negative answer means "present and not bothersome" or "absent."

The response options are important. Some questions are yes/no type issues but most have some shades of gray. Often people use categorical scales with a natural order (Likert scales); others will use a visual analog scale (VAS). The questions should not be leading in any specific direction. The language needs to be as neutral as possible.

Visual analog scales allow a very precise quantification of the response. Typically the respondent reads the question and then is offered a 10 centimeter horizontal line with an anchoring statement at each end:

"worst possible"_____"best possible"

The respondent then places a mark on the line to reflect their response. The downside of such scales is the expense of data entry. Study personnel must measure with a ruler how many millimeters the mark is from the start of the line. This is fine for a survey of 20 people but much more expensive for 2000.

The reading level of the survey is important. Software can be used to assess reading level. A fourth grade reading level is often recommended. Physicians and scientists are often poor judges of reading level, so it is best to get expert help. Many people cannot read, whether due to age, education, culture or visual acuity. Pediatric surveys often use pictures. For example, pain can be measured using a series of facial expressions. Verbal administration of the questionnaire may be necessary for some populations.

Language is important. Ideally questionnaires are available in multiple languages. They must be available in the languages spoken by the population of interest for the study and should be validated in each language. During development or prior to use, the questionnaire should be translated from one language to another and then a different person "back translates" the questionnaire from the new language back to the original. This allows a comparison of the two versions of the questionnaire. The "back translation" version of the questionnaire should mirror the original.

Typically the initial version of a questionnaire has more questions than planned for the final questionnaire. During the course of testing the questionnaire, questions that do not perform well or are redundant should be eliminated. This selection should be data-driven, not just expert opinion. Such item reduction is a common aspect of questionnaire development.

Testing a questionnaire

Feasibility

Once a questionnaire is developed, the next step is to test feasibility. The questionnaire should be administered to a small group to be sure they can actually complete it without confusion. The time to completion is measured in order to assess responder burden as this will affect response rates. The questionnaire should be reviewed to assess for missed questions or blank answers. The person can be interviewed to assess for misunderstood questions. Often questionnaires have "go to" directions that allow people to skip questions. The issue is whether those instructions are easily understood.

The goal is to make questionnaires measure patient-reported outcomes with the accuracy and precision that are expected of any other measure in medicine. In psychometrics, the terms validity and reliability are used in place of accuracy and precision. A questionnaire is reliable if it provides the same result on repeated measurement under stable conditions (precision) and valid if it measures what it intends to measure (accuracy).

Reliability

Reliability can be measured by administering the questionnaire on two separate occasions close together. The goal is to make the interval long enough so the respondents cannot remember their answers but short enough so that no change in their condition will have occurred. These two answers can then be compared. However, one must remember that high levels of agreement can occur by random chance. If a question measures an issue for which just 5% of people say "yes" then 95% will say "no." This is like flipping a coin that has only a 5% chance of heads. If flipped a second time, the coin will give the same answer 90% of the time $[(0.05 \times 0.05) + (0.95 \times 0.95)]$. A high level of agreement has occurred just by random chance. Certainly a different standard is needed to decide if this question is reliable.

The kappa statistic is a chance-corrected measure of agreement that is used to assess such dichotomous (e.g., yes–no) type answers. A weighted kappa statistic can be calculated for multilevel responses. This statistic is calculated as:

(Observed – Expected Agreement)/(1 – Expected Agreement)

A value of 0.4 is needed but 0.7 is better. Kappa statistics will be low for rare answers; questions that have closer to 50–50 responses will have better results.

An alternative approach to assessing reliability is to ask nearly identical questions on the same questionnaire. This approach is most useful in longer questionnaires; otherwise the respondents will clearly notice that they are being asked the same thing twice. The correlation between the answers to these similar questions can then be assessed.

Validity

Validity has several forms and is best thought of as a continuum – that is, a measure is not simply valid or invalid,

but rather has a degree of validation. One should not ask whether the questionnaire is valid, but rather, how valid is it? Face validity, content validity, criterion validity, discriminant validity, construct validity and responsiveness are all features that an instrument can have, and these issues need to be addressed as the instrument is developed and tested.

Face validity is a simple concept: does the questionnaire look valid to an expert? Often this is the only level of validity that a questionnaire has; people just make up questions to suit the purposes of the study. The next level is **content validity**: does the questionnaire measure the appropriate issues? Does a reflux questionnaire measure heartburn and acid regurgitation? Does it measure chest pain, dysphagia, dyspepsia and respiratory symptoms? Does a bowel questionnaire measure all the elements of diarrhea and constipation? Content validity is also typically determined by panels of experts.

The next level is **concurrent validity**: how well does a new questionnaire compare with the gold standard? For many symptom surveys, the gold standard is a face-to-face physician interview. In some situations the gold standard may be a long survey from which a newer shorter version has been derived. For example, the sickness impact profile (SIP) has over 100 questions and was later modified to create the Short Form-36 (SF-36), which in turn was further modified to give the Short Form-12 (SF-12). Gold standards can also be called criterion standards and thus comparing a new questionnaire to a gold standard can be called **criterion validity**. However, often no gold standard exists. The new questionnaire is designed to be better than existing instruments. This makes assessing concurrent validity much more difficult. What is the truth? In this case multiple measures can be used to develop a consensus definition of the truth and then the new questionnaire can be compared to that standard.

Perhaps the most difficult concept to understand is **construct validity**. In this case the designer develops a construct of how the questionnaire should perform. Based on this construct some patients should have worse scores than others; and then the survey is administered to see if this holds true. The survey needs to perform in a predictable fashion.

Discriminant validity refers to the concept that a questionnaire should be able to identify distinct groups. Can the survey responses distinguish one group from another? **Responsiveness** is yet another attribute a questionnaire should have; especially one that will be used in a clinical trial. Is the questionnaire sensitive to change? The challenge to testing responsiveness is that there must be an intervention or something that leads to a change in the person's condition. Typically responsiveness is assessed in the setting of a clinical trial. Most responsive questionnaires must be developed in one clinical trial before they can be used to assess the effects in another.

Not all questionnaires need to be tested and shown to fulfill all these forms of validity. In some situations a discriminant questionnaire is needed; for others the questionnaire needs to be responsive. The questions needed to address these two tasks might be quite different. At a minimum, questionnaires must have face and content validity. However, an assessment of concurrent validity is preferred.

Conclusions

Many physicians and researchers conducting clinical studies do not need to know all these details of questionnaire development. The important message of this chapter is that researchers need to be sure that the instrument they are using was developed with rigor. This is similar to the laboratory assays that are used every day for patient care and research. The user may not know how they were tested but does know that they were tested before being used. Ideally, the questionnaire development and assessment of validity has been published in a peer-reviewed journal. When reading a journal article, one should be sure to look for a reference of the validation. Authors should not just "make up" the questions they use.

Fortunately, well-validated measures exist to measure most GI symptoms and diseases. Additional measures exist to measure quality of life, physical functioning, work productivity and other outcomes. A catalog of these is beyond the scope of this chapter but such instruments can easily be found. Sometimes the actual questionnaires are published as appendices to a journal article. This places them in the public domain and available for use. Most often the authors need to be contacted for permission. Some questionnaires are proprietary and can only be used for a fee.

The goal of this chapter was to familiarize the reader with the steps required rigorously to develop and test a GI questionnaire. Alternatively, one can and should search the literature for existing measures and write the authors to obtain permission for their use. By using well-tested measures the physician and researcher can assure that we know what is being measured when we ask people "How are you doing?"

Further reading

Eisen GM *et al.* Health-related quality of life: A primer for gastroenterologists. *Am J Gastroenterol* 1999;**94**:2017.

Eypasch E *et al.* Gastrointestinal Quality of Life Index: development, validation and application of a new instrument. *Br J Surg* 1995;**82**:216.

Guyatt G *et al.* A new measure of health status for clinical trials in inflammatory bowel disease. *Gastroenterology* 1989;**96**:804.

Guyatt GH *et al.* Measuring health-related quality of life. *Ann Intern Med* 1993;**118**:622.

Hahn BA *et al.* Evaluation of a new quality of life questionnaire for patients with irritable bowel syndrome. *Aliment Pharmacol Ther* 1997;**11**:547.

Patrick DL *et al.* Quality of life in persons with irritable bowel syndrome: development and validation of a new measure. *Dig Dis Sci* 1998;**43**:400.

Provenzale D *et al.* Health-related quality of life after ileoanal pull-through evaluation and assessment of new health status measures. *Gastroenterology* 1997;**113**:7.

Spilker B (ed.) *Quality of Life and Pharmacoeconomics in Clinical Trials*. Philadelphia: Lippincott-Raven, 1996.

Svedlund J *et al.* GSRS – a rating scale for gastrointestinal symptoms in patients with irritable bowel syndrome and peptic ulcer disease. *Dig Dis Sci* 1988;**33**:129.

Testa MA, Simonson DC. Assessment of quality-of-life outcomes. *N Engl J Med* 1996;**334**:835.

Ware JE. The status of health assessment 1994. *Annu Rev Public Health* 1995;**16**:327.

Yacavone RF *et al.* Quality of life measurement in gastroenterology: what is available? *Am J Gastroenterol* 2001;**96**:285.

Clinical Trials

William J. Sandborn

Key points
- Clinical trials evaluating drug efficacy in gastrointestinal disease have evolved considerably over the last several years.
- Crucial features of the study must be carefully considered during the study design planning phase.
- Study designs used in inflammatory bowel disease trials can be used as a model for other gastrointestinal disease trials.

Introduction

The design and conduct of clinical trials in gastroenterology requires that a variety of issues be addressed including: (i) defining the study population; (ii) defining the instruments that will be used to measure disease activity; (iii) defining the treatment indications; (iv) defining the efficacy outcome measures; (v) defining the study design; (vi) defining the control group and the expected rate of response for the control group; and (vii) selecting the dose(s) of drug to be used in the study.

This chapter will use the design and conduct of clinical trials in patients with inflammatory bowel disease as an illustrative example for diseases in gastroenterology generally.

Defining the study population

A variety of inclusion and exclusion criteria are used to define the study population in patients with inflammatory bowel disease.

1 Diagnosis. The diagnoses of Crohn's disease (CD) or ulcerative colitis (UC) are based on standard clinical, endoscopic, radiographic and pathologic criteria.

2 Disease extent. Colonoscopy and small bowel radiography can be used to classify patients with CD and UC according to the macroscopic extent of disease. Patients with CD typically have ileitis, ileocolitis or isolated colitis [1]. Patients with UC typically have disease limited to the rectum (ulcerative proctitis), to the rectosigmoid colon (ulcerative proctosigmoiditis) or the left colon (left-sided

UC), or disease extending proximal to the splenic flexure or involving the entire colon (extensive UC or substantial UC and pancolonic or universal UC) [2]. These anatomic classifications are useful for selecting appropriate patients for treatment with targeted delivery systems (e.g., budesonide for ileal CD; suppositories for UC of the rectum).

3 Disease behavior. Most patients with CD will eventually develop complications of disease including fibrostenosis with intestinal obstruction, fistulization and/or abscess formation. Classification systems for CD, such as the Rome Classification, Vienna Classification and Montreal Modification of the Vienna Classification [3–5] incorporate both disease location and disease behavior. In general, patients with abscesses or fibrostenotic and obstructive symptoms are typically excluded. Some trials permit the enrollment of patients with draining fistulas as long as there is active inflammatory disease as well or fistula closure is the primary treatment indication for the study.

4 Disease activity. Patients with CD are generally classified as being in remission, or as having mildly, moderately or severely active CD according to the CD activity index (CDAI) (see below) [6,7]. Similarly, patients with UC are generally classified as being in clinical remission, or having mildly, moderately or severely active disease. No one index (instrument) dominates for classification of disease severity in patients with UC. For outpatients in remission or with mildly or moderately active disease, the Mayo Score is frequently used [8,9]; for inpatients with severely active disease, the Truelove and Witts Index is frequently used [10]. In most instances, hospitalized patients with severe CD or UC are excluded from clinical trials. In patients with UC, clinical (symptomatic) remission must have endoscopic confirmation of remission; conversely, patients with mildly, moderately or severely active disease must have endoscopic confirmation of disease activity.

5 Concomitant medications. In patients with CD or UC, concomitant medications are permitted at stable doses during clinical trials including the oral 5-aminosalicylate medications, antibiotics (CD only), systemic corticosteroids, budesonide (CD only), azathioprine, 6-mercaptopurine and methotrexate. In general, patients receiving rectal mesalamine (mesalazine), rectal corticosteroids, tacrolimus, cyclosporine (ciclosporin) and infliximab are excluded. Patients who are unable to discontinue corticosteroids without experiencing a symptomatic relapse are considered to be steroid-dependent [11].

6 Other clinical circumstances. Patients with surgical resection of more than 100 cm of small bowel are usually excluded from clinical trials in order to avoid enrolling patients with short bowel syndrome. Patients with ostomies are also excluded – the CDAI has not been validated in CD patients with ostomies, and an ostomy implies that the colon is either diverted or surgically resected in patients with UC. Patients with a diagnosis of low-grade or high-grade dysplasia of the colon within 5 years are excluded from clinical trials because they have a high rate of progression to cancer [12].

Defining the instruments that will be used to measure disease activity

A variety of instruments have been developed to measure disease activity (Table 6.1). Many of the instruments are those used to define baseline disease activity described in the previous section.

In CD, the predominant instrument is the validated CDAI [6,7]. In summary, scores range from 0 to approximately 600, with scores below 150 defining remission, scores of 150–219 defining mildly active disease, scores of 220–450 defining moderately active disease, and scores above 450 points defining very severe disease. The calculation of the CDAI score is based in part on a symptom diary maintained by the patient for 7 days prior to evaluation.

In UC, the Mayo score has achieved widespread use in recent years in patients with UC in remission or mildly or moderately active UC [8,9]. Scores range from 0 to 12 points based on symptom presence, endoscopic findings and physician's global assessment. A patient's functional assessment is included in the measure of general well-being when determining the Physician's Global As-

sessment score. The Sutherland Index, Clinical Activity Index, and Baron score are alternatives to the Mayo score [9,13–15]. In patients with severely active UC, the Lichtiger score (modified Truelove and Witts Index) and the Mayo score can be utilized [8,9]. There is no dominant index for measuring histologic disease activity. The Geboes Index has been validated and tested for reproducibility [16]; scores range from 0 to 5.4, with higher scores indicating more severe histologic inflammation. An alternative to the Geboes Index is the Riley Index [17].

Defining the treatment indications

The treatment indications for clinical trials in CD and UC have been extensively reviewed elsewhere in systematic reviews [7,9]. In addition, the Food and Drug Administration (FDA) has developed draft guidelines for the clinical evaluation of drugs for CD and UC, and the European Agency for the Evaluation of Medicinal Products (EMA) has developed Points to Consider on Clinical Investigation of Medicinal Products for the Management of CD that address treatment indications [18,19].

In CD, treatment indications include: induction of response and remission; maintenance of response and remission; steroid-sparing and steroid-free remission; mucosal healing; induction and maintenance of fistula improvement and fistula remission. The defined treatment indication has direct impact on study duration. For example, induction of response and remission trials, which enroll patients with active inflammatory CD, are 4–16 weeks in duration. Maintenance of response and remission has been assessed with several different study designs including a randomized induction trial with late (6-month) endpoints [20], a randomized induction trial followed by re-randomization of responding patients in a maintenance trial [21], and an open label induction trial followed by a randomized maintenance trial in responding patients [22,23]. The minimum duration of a maintenance study should be 6 months, and 1 year is preferred. Steroid sparing has been assessed with several different study designs including maintenance of a steroid-induced remission [24], steroid withdrawal in steroid-dependent patients [25,26], and steroid withdrawal in patients with moderately to severely active CD despite corticosteroid therapy [21,22,27]. The indication of mucosal healing in CD is still evolving. To date, this indication has only been evaluated in controlled trials as a substudy in relatively small groups of patients [28,29]. There is only very limited experience with randomized trials for the indications of

Table 6.1 Commonly used disease activity indices. (Reproduced from Baumgart DC, Sandborn WJ. Inflammatory bowel disease: clinical aspects and established and evolving therapies. *Lancet* 2007;**369**: in press, with permission from Elsevier.)

Ulcerative colitis

Index types and names	Variables taken into account								Reference(s)
Clinical indices	Stool frequency	Bleeding	Temperature	Pain	General well-being	EIM	Labs	Endoscopy	
Truelove–Witt Severity Index	x	x	x	x	x		x		10
Powel–Tuck Index (St Mark's Index)	x	x	x	x	x	x		x	55
Clinical Activity Index (CAI) (Rachmilewitz Index)	x	x	x	x	x	x	x		14
Physician's Global Assessment (PGA)				x	x				37
Lichtiger Index (aka modified Truelove–Witt Severity Index (MTWSI))	x	x		x	x				56
Investigator Global Assessment (IGA)					x				57
Simple Clinical Colitis Activity Index (SCCAI)	x	x	x		x	x			58
Ulcerative Colitis Clinical Score (UCCS)	x	x			x				47
Mayo Score (aka Mayo Clinic Score, Disease Activity Index (DAI))	x	x			x			x	8
Sutherland Index (Disease Activity Index (DAI) or UCDAI)	x	x			x			x	13
Endoscopic indices	Mucosal appearance	Mucosal vulnerability	Ulcers						
Baron Score	x	x							15
Modified Baron Score	x	x	x						47
Mayo Endoscopy Subscore	x	x	x						8
Endoscopic Index (Rachmilewitz Endoscopic Activity Index (EAI))	x	x							14

Crohn's Disease

Index types and names	Variables taken into account										
Clinical indices	Stool frequency	Perianal lesions	Temperature	Pain	General well-being	EIM	Labs	Endoscopy	Weight	Abdominal mass	Reference(s)
Crohn's Disease Activity Index (aka Best Index or CDAI)	x	x	x	x	x	x	x				6
Simple Index (Harvey Bradshaw Index)											59
Organization Mondiale de Gastroenterologie Index (OMGE)	x	x	x	x	x	x	x		x	x	60
Cape Town Index	x	x	x	x	x	x	x		x	x	61
Fistula indices	Discharge	Induration	Number of fistulas	Impaired sexual activity							
Perianal Crohn's Disease Activity Index (PDAI)	x	x	x	x							62
Fistula Drainage Assessment	x	x	x	x							30
Endoscopic indices	Quality of ulcers	Surface involved	Disease extent	Strictures							
Crohn's Disease Endoscopic Activity Index of Severity (CDEIS)	x	x	x								63
Endoscopic Crohn's Disease Index (SES-CD)	x	x		x							64
Rutgeerts Score	x	x	x	x							65

induction and maintenance of fistula improvement and fistula remission [30–32].

In UC, treatment indications include: treatment of signs and symptoms, induction of clinical response and clinical remission; induction of remission, mucosal healing, maintenance of remission; and steroid-sparing and steroid-free remission. Induction trials for the first group of indications are typically 4–8 weeks in duration for patients with mildly to moderately active disease, and 1–2 weeks in duration in patients with severely active disease [8,33–36]. Induction trials for mucosal healing, which enroll patients with mucosal inflammation seen at endoscopy, are typically 4–8 weeks in duration [35,37,38] (package insert with prescribing information for Pentasa (mesalamine), 2005).

Maintenance of response and remission has been assessed with several different study designs including a randomized induction trial in patients with active UC with late endpoints at 6 and 12 months [35] and a randomized maintenance trial in patients in endoscopic remission [39]. The minimum duration of a maintenance study should be 6 months, and 1 year is preferred. Steroid-sparing has been assessed with the study design of steroid withdrawal in patients with moderately to severely active UC despite corticosteroid therapy [35].

Defining the efficacy outcome measures

Representative efficacy outcome measures for clinical trials in CD and UC for the treatment indications discussed above are shown in Table 6.2. These have been extensively reviewed elsewhere [7,9], and again, there are FDA draft guidelines for the clinical evaluation of drugs for CD and UC and EMA points for the management of CD that address efficacy outcome measures [18,19]. The selection of efficacy outcome measures requires that a number of considerations be taken into account, including: whether or not validated disease activity instruments and outcome measures exist; what outcome measures have led to regulatory approval of drugs for a given treatment indication; whether the outcome measure is sensitive and/or specific for a treatment effect; and whether or not a given outcome measure is clinically relevant. A specific efficacy outcome measure must be selected for the primary endpoint of the study. The primary endpoint should measure a dichotomous clinically relevant endpoint that can be determined at a specific point in time – for instance, induction of remission at week 8. Endpoints based on continuous measures of disease activity, such as median CDAI scores or the

median time to loss of response, are not appropriate as the primary endpoint for a clinical trial because they are of uncertain clinical relevance.

The power calculations to determine the sample size for the trial should be based on the primary endpoint. If two primary endpoints are desired, then a statistical penalty must be paid such that the alpha level is set at 0.025 rather than 0.05, or alternatively a contingent sequential analysis design with co-primary endpoints can be employed such that primary endpoint is assessed, and if statistical significance at the 0.05 level is achieved, then the co-primary endpoint is assessed for statistical significance at the 0.05 level [21,22]. Other secondary endpoints should be prespecified. Any secondary endpoints that are not prespecified will need to be designated as *post hoc* endpoints at the time of the statistical analysis when the trial is completed.

Defining the study design

Randomized controlled trials can be designed as superiority trials or non-inferiority trials. Superiority trials test the hypothesis that treatment A is superior to treatment B, with a two-sided alpha set at 0.05. Superiority trials for efficacy can either be placebo-controlled or have an active comparator. In situations where a safe and effective therapy for a given treatment indication in a given disease exists, and where there is the potential for harm from withholding treatment, it may not be ethical to perform a placebo-controlled trial. In this instance, in order to evaluate a new therapy as a potential alternative to an effective existing therapy when the new therapy may not be more effective than the existing therapy, a non-inferiority (equivalence) study design is required [40,41]. Non-inferiority trials test the hypothesis that treatment B is non-inferior (equivalent) to treatment A. Most superiority clinical trials in patients with CD and UC are powered to detect differences ("superiority margin") in response and remission rates of 15–20%. Differences of this magnitude have generally been considered clinically important. The "non-inferiority margin" for an equivalence trial should be approximately 50% of a superiority margin that would be considered clinically important. Thus, the non-inferiority margin in clinical trials in patients with CD and UC is approximately 7.5–10%. An alternative approach is to use a value for the non-inferiority margin that is lower than the lower bound of the 95% two-sided confidence interval for the pooled data for the comparator therapy in this indication [46].

Table 6.2 Treatment indications and efficacy outcome measures

Treatment indication	Criteria	Efficacy outcome measure	Definition
Crohn's disease			
Induction of response 70	CDAI[a] of 220–450	Response 70	Decrease from baseline CDAI score ≥70 points
Induction of response 100	CDAI of 220–450	Response 100	Decrease from baseline CDAI score ≥100 points
Induction of remission	CDAI of 220–450	Remission	CDAI score <150 points
Maintenance of response 70	CDAI <220 and decrease from baseline CDAI score ≥70 points	Relapse	CDAI ≥220 points and an increase from baseline ≥70 points
Maintenance of remission	CDAI <150	Relapse	CDAI ≥150 points and an increase from baseline ≥70 points
Steroid sparing	Steroid therapy at baseline	Steroid discontinuation	Complete steroid discontinuation
Steroid-free remission	Steroid therapy at baseline	Steroid discontinuation and remission	Complete steroid discontinuation and CDAI <150 points
Induction of mucosal healing	Mucosal ulcerations in the colon and terminal ileum by video colonoscopy	Mucosal healing	Complete absence of mucosal ulcerations in the colon and terminal ileum in patients in whom these lesions were present at the start of the study
Induction of fistula improvement	Draining fistulas at baseline	Fistula improvement	Closure of individual fistulas defined as no fistula drainage despite gentle finger compression. Improvement defined as a decrease from baseline in the number of open draining fistulas of ≥50% for at least two consecutive visits (i.e., at least 4 weeks)
Induction of fistula remission	Draining fistulas at baseline	Fistula remission	Remission defined as closure of all fistulas that were draining at baseline for at least two consecutive visits (i.e., at least 4 weeks)
Ulcerative colitis			
Treatment of signs and symptoms	Physician's Global Assessment of 1 or 2 points	Treatment success	Improvement (a minimum 1 point decrease from baseline) in the Physician's Global Assessment score AND improvement in at least one other clinical assessment (stool frequency, rectal bleeding, patient's functional assessment, endoscopy findings) AND no worsening in any other clinical assessment
Induction of clinical response	Mayo score 6–12, endoscopy subscore ≥2	Clinical response	Decrease from baseline in the total Mayo score ≥3 points and ≥30% and a decrease in the rectal bleeding subscore ≥1 point or an absolute rectal bleeding subscore of 0 or 1
Induction of clinical remission	Mayo score 6–12, endoscopy subscore ≥2	Clinical remission	Mayo score of ≤2 points with no individual subscore >1 point
Induction of remission	Mayo score of 0	Remission	Mayo score of 0
Induction of mucosal healing	Mayo endoscopy subscore ≥2	Mucosal healing	Absolute Mayo endoscopy subscore of 0 or 1

(*Continued.*)

Table 6.2 *(Continued.)*

Treatment indication	Criteria	Efficacy outcome measure	Definition
Maintenance of remission	Clinical remission (no clinical symptoms) and endoscopic remission	Relapse (increase in stool frequency ≥1–2 stools above normal for the patient and recurrence of rectal bleeding) confirmed by endoscopy	Absence of clinical relapse confirmed by endoscopy
Steroid sparing	Steroid therapy at baseline	Steroid discontinuation	Complete steroid discontinuation
Steroid-free remission	Steroid therapy at baseline	Steroid discontinuation and remission	Complete steroid discontinuation and Mayo score of ≤2 points with no individual subscore >1 point

[a]CDAI, Crohn's Disease Activity Index.

Defining the control group and the expected rate of response for the control group

As described earlier, the control group for clinical trials can either consist of a placebo or an active comparator. In general, placebo-controlled trials are the most efficient trials and permit smaller sample sizes, which is desirable from the perspective of limiting patient exposure to an agent of unknown efficacy and safety. However, because mesalamine is safe and effective for the induction and maintenance of response and remission in patients with UC, true placebo-controlled trials for UC may not be possible. Several options for conducting controlled trials in this patient population exist. One option is to perform a placebo-controlled superiority trial in which patients are randomized to standard therapy (mesalamine) plus placebo versus standard therapy plus the investigational agent. Patients entering such a trial could either be on no medical therapy, or could be currently receiving the standard therapy [47]. A second option is to perform an active comparator superiority trial in which patients not currently receiving treatment are randomized to standard therapy or the investigational agent [48]. A third option is to perform a non-inferiority trial in which patients not currently receiving treatment are randomized to standard therapy or the investigational agent.

When designing placebo-controlled trials and active comparator trials in patients with CD and UC, careful consideration must be given to the expected placebo-response or active comparator-response for the specific treatment indication and patient population, and taking into account the primary endpoint of the study and the instrument used to measure disease activity. A meta-analysis has been performed that quantified the placebo response and remission rates for induction trials in patients with active CD [49]. Similarly, three meta-analyses have been performed that quantify the placebo response and remission rates in patients with active UC [50–52]. These meta-analyses as well as the placebo response and remission rates outlined in systematic reviews of clinical trials in patients with CD and UC should be used to estimate the expected placebo or active comparator response and remission rates in order to perform power calculations when designing controlled trials [7,9].

Selecting the dose(s) of drug

A key factor in designing clinical trials is selecting doses of the active agent that demonstrate both efficacy and the optimum balance between efficacy and safety. Typically, a range of doses is established in phase I or has been established in phase II and/or III trials in other diseases. Phase II dose-ranging trials in inflammatory bowel disease typically will have a placebo-control group and 2–3 doses of the active agent. Each arm of the trial will typically contain 25–75 patients, leading to a study with a total of 75–300 patients [8,33,37–39,53,54]. A large phase III trial should not be undertaken until the optimum dose has been established.

Conclusions

During the last 10 years, the conduct of clinical trials in patients with CD and UC has become increasingly sophisticated and state-of-the-art. These trials evaluate defined populations for specific treatment indications using established instruments to measure disease activity and established efficacy outcome measures. Most trials are placebo-controlled superiority trials, but in some instances active comparator trials and non-inferiority trial designs are required. Knowledge regarding the expected placebo response has increased, as has experience in designing phase II studies to determine the optimum dose of the drug. These advances in the conduct of clinical trials have enhanced the development of new therapies for the treatment of these disorders. The lessons learned in this therapeutic area are generalizable to most gastrointestinal disorders.

References

1. Farmer RG *et al.* Clinical patterns in Crohn's disease: a statistical study of 615 cases. *Gastroenterology* 1975;**68**:627.
2. Langholz E *et al.* Incidence and prevalence of ulcerative colitis in Copenhagen county from 1962 to 1987. *Scand J Gastroenterol* 1991;**26**:1247.
3. Sachar D *et al.* Proposed classification of patient subgroups in Crohn's disease. *Gastroenterol Int* 1992;**5**:141.
4. Gasche C *et al.* A simple classification of Crohn's disease: report of the Working Party for the World Congresses of Gastroenterology, Vienna 1998. *Inflamm Bowel Dis* 2000;**6**:8.
5. Silverberg MS *et al.* Toward an integrated clinical, molecular and serological classification of inflammatory bowel disease: Report of a Working Party of the 2005 Montreal World Congress of Gastroenterology. *Can J Gastroenterol* 2005;**19**(Suppl. A):5.
6. Best WR *et al.* Development of a Crohn's disease activity index. National Cooperative Crohn's Disease Study. *Gastroenterology* 1976;**70**:439.
7. Sandborn WJ *et al.* A review of activity indices and efficacy endpoints for clinical trials of medical therapy in adults with Crohn's disease. *Gastroenterology* 2002;**122**:512.
8. Schroeder KW *et al.* Coated oral 5-aminosalicylic acid therapy for mildly to moderately active ulcerative colitis. A randomized study. *N Engl J Med* 1987;**317**:1625.
9. D'Haens G *et al.* A review of activity indices and efficacy endpoints for clinical trials of medical therapy in adults with ulcerative colitis. *Gastroenterology* 2007 (in press).
10. Truelove SC, Witts LJ. Cortisone in ulcerative colitis. Final report on a therapeutic trial. Br Med J 1955;**2**:1041.
11. Faubion WJ *et al.* The natural history of corticosteroid therapy for inflammatory bowel disease: a population-based study. *Gastroenterology* 2001;**121**:255.
12. Riddell RH *et al.* Dysplasia in inflammatory bowel disease: standardized classification with provisional clinical applications. *Hum Pathol* 1983;**14**:931.
13. Sutherland LR *et al.* A randomized, placebo-controlled, double-blind trial of mesalamine in the maintenance of remission of Crohn's disease. The Canadian Mesalamine for Remission of Crohn's Disease Study Group. *Gastroenterology* 1997;**112**:1069.
14. Rachmilewitz D. Coated mesalazine (5-aminosalicylic acid) versus sulphasalazine in the treatment of active ulcerative colitis: a randomised trial. Br Med J 1989;**298**:82.
15. Baron JH *et al.* Variation between observers in describing mucosal appearances in proctocolitis. Br Med J 1964;**1**:89.
16. Geboes K *et al.* A reproducible grading scale for histological assessment of inflammation in ulcerative colitis [see comment]. *Gut* 2000;**47**:404.
17. Riley SA *et al.* Microscopic activity in ulcerative colitis: what does it mean? *Gut* 1991;**32**:174.
18. Fredd S. Standards for approval of new drugs for IBD. *Inflamm Bowel Dis* 1995;**1**:284.
19. European Agency for the Evaluation of Medicinal Products. Points to consider on clinical investigation of medicinal products for the management of Crohn's disease, draft 5. EMEA, 2001 (http://www.emea.eu.int/pdfs/human/ewp/228499en.pdf).
20. Sandborn WJ *et al.* Certolizumab pegol administered subcutaneously is effective and well tolerated in patients with active Crohn's disease: results from a 26-week, placebo-controlled Phase III study (PRECiSE 1). *Gastroenterology* 2006;**130**:A-107 Abstract 743.
21. Sandborn WJ *et al.* Natalizumab induction and maintenance therapy for Crohn's disease. *N Engl J Med* 2005;**353**:1912.
22. Hanauer SB *et al.* Maintenance infliximab for Crohn's disease: the ACCENT I randomised trial. *Lancet* 2002;**359**:1541.
23. Schreiber S *et al.* Certolizumab pegol, a humanised anti-TNF pegylated FAb′ fragment, is safe and effective in the maintenance of response and remission following induction in active Crohn's disease: a phase III study (Precise). *Gut* 2005;**54**(Suppl. VII):A82.
24. Candy S *et al.* A controlled double blind study of azathioprine in the management of Crohn's disease. *Gut* 1995;**37**:674.
25. Feagan BG *et al.* Methotrexate for the treatment of Crohn's disease. The North American Crohn's Study Group Investigators. *N Engl J Med* 1995;**332**:292.
26. Feagan BG *et al.* CDP517, a humanized monoclonal antibody to tumor necrosis factor-α, for steroid-dependent Crohn's disease: a randomized, double-blind, placebo-controlled trial. *Aliment Pharmacol Ther* 2006;**23**:617.
27. Colombel JF *et al.* Adalimumab for maintenance of clinical response and remission in patients with Crohn's disease: the

CHARM trial. *Gastroenterology* 2007;**132**:52.

28. D'Haens G *et al.* Endoscopic and histological healing with infliximab anti-tumor necrosis factor antibodies in Crohn's disease: A European multicenter trial. *Gastroenterology* 1999;**116**:1029.

29. Rutgeerts P *et al.* Scheduled maintenance treatment with infliximab is superior to episodic treatment for the healing of mucosal ulceration associated with Crohn's disease [see comment]. *Gastrointest Endosc* 2006;**63**:433; quiz 464.

30. Present DH *et al.* Infliximab for the treatment of fistulas in patients with Crohn's disease. *N Engl J Med* 1999;**340**:1398.

31. Sandborn WJ *et al.* Tacrolimus for the treatment of fistulas in patients with Crohn's disease: a randomized, placebo-controlled trial. *Gastroenterology* 2003;**125**:380.

32. Sands BE *et al.* Infliximab maintenance therapy for fistulizing Crohn's disease. *N Engl J Med* 2004;**350**:876.

33. Sninsky CA *et al.* Oral mesalamine (Asacol) for mildly to moderately active ulcerative colitis. A multicenter study. *Ann Intern Med* 1991;**115**:350.

34. Hanauer SB *et al.* Delayed-release oral mesalamine at 4.8 g/day (800 mg tablet) for the treatment of moderately active ulcerative colitis: The ASCEND II trial. *Am J Gastroenterol* 2005;**100**:2478.

35. Rutgeerts P *et al.* Infliximab induction and maintenance therapy for ulcerative colitis. *N Engl J Med* 2005;**353**:2462.

36. Lichtiger S *et al.* Cyclosporine in severe ulcerative colitis refractory to steroid therapy. *N Engl J Med* 1994;**330**:1841.

37. Hanauer S *et al.* Mesalamine capsules for treatment of active ulcerative colitis: results of a controlled trial. Pentasa Study Group. *Am J Gastroenterol* 1993;**88**:1188.

38. Kamm MA *et al.* Once-daily high concentration MMX mesalamine in active ulcerative colitis: placebo and active comparator-controlled study. *Gastroenterology* 2007;**132**:66.

39. An oral preparation of mesalamine as long-term maintenance therapy for ulcerative colitis. A randomized, placebo-controlled trial. The Mesalamine Study Group. *Ann Intern Med* 1996;**124**:204.

40. Ware JH, Antman EM. Equivalence trials [see comment]. *N Engl J Med* 1997;**337**:1159.

41. Wiens BL. Choosing an equivalence limit for noninferiority or equivalence studies [see comment]. *Control Clin Trials* 2002;**23**:2. [Erratum appears in *Control Clin Trials* 2002;**23**:774.]

42. Kruis W *et al.* Maintaining remission of ulcerative colitis with the probiotic *Escherichia coli* Nissle 1917 is as effective as with standard mesalazine. *Gut* 2004;**53**:1617.

43. Sandborn WJ *et al.* Safety of celecoxib in patients with ulcerative colitis in remission: a randomized, placebo-controlled pilot study. *Clin Gastroenterol Hepatol* 2006;**4**:203.

44. Lemann M *et al.* A randomized, double-blind, controlled withdrawal trial in Crohn's disease patients in long-term remission on azathioprine. *Gastroenterology* 2005;**128**:1812.

45. Tinmouth JM *et al.* Are claims of equivalency in digestive diseases trials supported by the evidence? *Gastroenterology* 2004;**126**:1700.

46. Kaul S, Diamond GA. Good enough: a primer on the analysis and interpretation of noninferiority trials. *Ann Intern Med* 2006;**145**:62.

47. Feagan BG *et al.* Treatment of ulcerative colitis with a humanized antibody to the a4b7 integrin. *N Engl J Med* 2005;**352**:2499.

48. Thomsen OO *et al.* A comparison of budesonide and mesalamine for active Crohn's disease. International Budesonide-Mesalamine Study Group. *N Engl J Med* 1998;**339**:370.

49. Su C *et al.* A meta-analysis of the placebo rates of remission and response in clinical trials of active Crohn's disease. *Gastroenterology* 2004;**126**:1257.

50. Kornbluth AA *et al.* Meta-analysis of the effectiveness of current drug therapy of ulcerative colitis. *J Clin Gastroenterol* 1993;**16**:215.

51. Ilnyckyj A *et al.* Quantification of the placebo response in ulcerative colitis [see comment]. *Gastroenterology* 1997;**112**:1854.

52. Su CY *et al.* Factors that influence placebo remission rates in clinical trials of active ulcerative colitis: a meta-analysis. *Gastroenterology* 2005;**128**(Suppl. 2):A-326.

53. Targan SR *et al.* A short-term study of chimeric monoclonal antibody cA2 to tumor necrosis factor alpha for Crohn's disease. Crohn's Disease cA2 Study Group. *N Engl J Med* 1997;**337**:1029.

54. Hanauer SB *et al.* Human anti-tumor necrosis factor monoclonal antibody (adalimumab) in Crohn's disease: the CLASSIC I trial. *Gastroenterology* 2006;**130**:323.

55. Powell-Tuck J *et al.* Correlations between defined sigmoidoscopic appearances and other measures of disease activity in ulcerative colitis. *Dig Dis Sci* 1982;**27**:533.

56. Lichtiger S, Present DH. Preliminary report: cyclosporin in treatment of severe active ulcerative colitis [see comment]. *Lancet* 1990;**336**:16.

57. Hanauer SB *et al.* Budesonide enema for the treatment of active, distal ulcerative colitis and proctitis: a dose-ranging study. U.S. Budesonide enema study group. *Gastroenterology* 1998;**115**:525.

58. Walmsley RS *et al.* A simple clinical colitis activity index. *Gut* 1998;**43**:29.

59. Harvey RF, Bradshaw JM. A simple index of Crohn's disease activity. *Lancet* 1980;**i**:514.

60. Myren J *et al.* The O.M.G.E. Multinational Inflammatory Bowel Disease Survey 1976-1982. A further report on 2,657 cases. *Scand J Gastroenterol* (Suppl.) 1984;**95**:1.

61. Wright JP *et al.* A simple clinical index of Crohn's disease activity – the Cape Town index. *S Afr Med J* 1985;**68**:502.

62. Irvine EJ. Usual therapy improves perianal Crohn's disease as measured by a new disease activity index. McMaster IBD Study Group. *J Clin Gastroenterol* 1995;**20**:27.

63. Mary JY, Modigliani R. Development and validation of an

endoscopic index of the severity for Crohn's disease: a prospective multicentre study. Groupe d'Etudes Therapeutiques des Affections Inflammatoires du Tube Digestif (GETAID). *Gut* 1989;**30**:983.

64. Daperno M *et al.* Development and validation of a new, simplified endoscopic activity score for Crohn's disease: the SES-CD [see comment]. Gastrointest Endosc 2004;**60**:505-12.

65. Rutgeerts P *et al.* Predictability of the postoperative course of Crohn's disease. *Gastroenterology* 1990;**99**:956.

7 Decision Analysis

John M. Inadomi

Key points
- Decision analysis is used to compare competing strategies of management under conditions of uncertainty.
- Various methods may be employed to construct a decision model (decision tree, Markov model) and analyze the results (mean outcomes, Monte Carlo simulation, discrete event simulation).
- The results of decision analysis may assist policymakers to prioritize competing healthcare interventions, in addition to providing a framework to generate hypotheses for further research.

Background

Decision analysis is a research method designed to synthesize data in order to derive a summary conclusion [1]. The origins of decision analysis lie in game theory, historically associated with economics and business administration and subsequently extended to medical research [2,3]. In biomedical research, decision analysis is often used quantitatively to compare competing strategies of clinical management under conditions of uncertainty. The analysis generally consists of mathematical equations constructed to model idealized subjects or cohorts with various disease states, then superimposing different decision options. The results of these analyses may then be applied to individual patients or groups of patients to guide clinical decision-making and health policy [4–7].

This chapter will provide an overview of decision analysis and construct a framework by which one may intelligently critique studies that appear in published literature (Table 7.1). The intention is to allow the reader to become more familiar with the terminology, use and limitations inherent with this form of research.

Decision trees

The most basic form of decision analysis is a decision tree. As with all good research, a relevant question must be formulated that identifies the specific problem to be solved. A hypothesis should then be generated in a form that can be tested by the analysis. It is important to format the question in a manner that provides the opportunity to retrieve reliable data with which one may populate the variables of the model. If the question is too broad, insufficient data sources will be available and the model will suffer from inadequate information. However, a question that is too limited in scope may not be generalizable to relevant populations.

After the clinical problem and hypothesis are defined, a clinical scenario is developed at the point where a decision to pursue one of several strategies must be made. From this point, defined as the **decision node**, two or more arms of the tree are drawn, each depicting a different strategy In the example shown in Fig. 7.1, the clinical decision to be made is: "What is the best colorectal cancer screening test?" and four diagnostic testing strategies are presented. As it is likely that each strategy may result in numerous outcomes, this is depicted by the use of branching arms of each strategy. At each branch point, or **chance node**, the possibility of following an individual arm is set by the probability of achieving that outcome. Conventionally, the sequence is drawn from left to right, representing the progression of events in chronological order leading to the ultimate outcome of the analysis. Additionally, decision nodes are represented by squares, while chance nodes are designated by circles.

Outcomes of the tree are the terminal events of the model, and can be years of life, death and morbidity, but also any other state of health or disease. Because the goal of therapy may not necessarily be solely to increase life expectancy, but rather to improve quality of life, decision analysis has incorporated the concept of utilities, or pa-

Table 7.1 Description of various types of decision analysis methods

Method	Format	Description
Decision tree	Linear model	Model that initiates at a decision node then flows in a unidirectional fashion to chance nodes and terminal (outcome) nodes
Markov model	Recursive model	Model that involves transitions between various health states in a time-dependent fashion, allowing repetitive movement between nodes
Monte Carlo simulation	Static, stochastic	Form of analysis in which values for multiple variables are simultaneously varied. Inputs/outputs do not vary with time (static), but include random variation (stochastic)
Discrete event simulation (beyond scope of chapter discussion)	Dynamic, stochastic	Form of analysis in which variables are simultaneously varied. Inputs vary over time (dynamic), with accounting for random variation

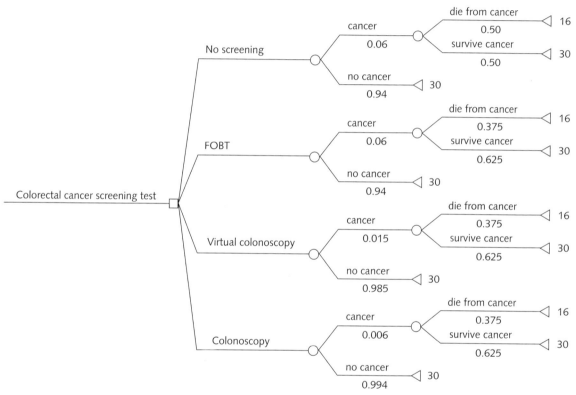

Fig. 7.1 Decision tree comparing strategies to reduce mortality from colorectal cancer: Examined strategies include: no screening, fecal occult blood testing (FOBT), colonoscopy and virtual colonoscopy (VC). The tree begins with a decision node (square) and branches to the four competing strategies after which the potential outcomes of each strategy, including cancer development, cancer cure or death from cancer are modeled. In this idealized model, mortality from competing causes is not considered, nor are complications from diagnostic or therapeutic interventions. Each strategy leads to chance nodes (circles) at which point the probability of achieving each outcome is based on the value of the variables emanating from the node. The example assumes that in the absence of screening there is a 6% lifetime risk of developing colorectal cancer, and 50% of cancer patients are assumed to die from their disease. FOBT is assumed to have an identical rate of cancer development but a 25% relative risk reduction in cancer mortality (50% − [50% × 25% = 12.5%] = 37.5% absolute mortality risk). Virtual (VC) and conventional colonoscopy (colonoscopy) are assumed to decrease cancer incidence by 75% and 90% respectively (1.5% and 0.6% cancer incidence), and have similar benefit on detected cancer mortality as FOBT. To simplify the example it is assumed that all patients who develop cancer do so at age 65 years, and either die within one year or achieve normal life expectancy if cured of cancer. In the absence of colorectal cancer mortality, patients are assumed to live to age 80 years (30 years of additional life expectancy).

tient preferences, to adjust benefit to reflect the fact that some health states are preferred over others [8–12]. For example, a year of life in perfect health may be valued more highly than a similar amount of time undergoing chemotherapy, or time spent after sustaining a complication of an intervention that sustains life. Quality-adjusted life years (QALYs) use utilities to adjust the absolute gain or loss in life in an effort to reflect morbidities associated with various diseases and interventions [12]. As decision trees are generally designed to compare competing strategies of management, the difference in strategies in terms of life years or QALYs saved or lost may be calculated. Outcomes may also include monetary gains or losses. In this manner, the difference in costs between strategies may be compared, either alone or simultaneously with comparison of benefit, thus providing the basis for cost-effectiveness analysis, which will be covered in another chapter. Outcomes are generally denoted by boxes or triangles in a decision tree.

After a clinical problem is identified and appropriately constructed in a model, such as a decision tree, information must be gathered to populate the variables in the tree. Specifically, values must be provided to indicate the probability of following each arm that emanates from a chance node in the model [13]. As it is desirable to use the best evidence to support the choice of value for each variable, a systematic review of the literature or meta-analysis should be performed for all variables [14]. Data retrieved through literature review should be examined for validity through evidence-based methods [14–21]. If multiple data sources are not available to provide sufficient information, "expert opinion" may be used although this method is less rigorous than the former. In all cases, the range of reasonable values for each variable must be entertained. A sensitivity analysis should be performed (see below) to determine whether variations in the initial assumptions of the model cause the conclusions of the analysis to change.

After constructing the decision tree, defining outcomes and specifying values for the variables in tree, the analysis may be performed. This is accomplished through "folding back" and "averaging" [1]. This process starts on the right side of the tree, with the "outcomes" boxes, and folds back to the left, finishing at the decision node. The value of each outcome is multiplied by the probability of achieving the outcome; these "weighted" values are then summed at the chance node that led to the outcomes. The process repeats from right to left, with each successive value at a chance node being multiplied by the probability of getting to that node, and again summed with the other weighted values at the next more "proximal" chance node in the tree. At the most proximal chance nodes, just before (to the right) of the decision node, there will be a single value representing each arm or strategy modeled in the tree (Fig. 7.2). The optimal strategy is identified by comparison of the values associated with each strategy. Thus, in the analysis shown in Fig. 7.2, the optimal colorectal cancer screening test is colonoscopy because this strategy yields the greatest number of life-years (29.97) compared with strategies using virtual colonoscopy (29.92), fecal occult blood testing (FOBT) (29.68) or no screening (29.58). This comparison represents the **base-case scenario** in which the initial assumptions of the model are utilized to calculate the outcome.

Although the base-case scenario is usually presented first in a study, the most important step in the analysis is performance of a sensitivity analysis. By varying the values of each variable in the model, one may test the stability of the conclusions of the analysis and determine which variables contribute most heavily to the results. Sensitivity analyses may be performed by varying one or more variables simultaneously, using the range of reasonable values for each variable that was determined from the literature, or from expert opinion. If small changes in a variable cause the conclusion of the analysis to change, the model is said to be sensitive to that variable. An important goal of decision analysis is hypothesis generation – if a model exhibits sensitivity to a particular variable, research should be pursued in an effort to define more precisely the value associated with that variable so as to establish more firmly the certainty of the conclusions of the analysis. If changing the values of other variables does not change the conclusions of the analysis, further research in these areas may be deemed less critical towards defining the optimal management.

Markov models

Note that in the example provided for decision trees, the age of cancer diagnosis was assumed to be constant because age was not included as a variable in the model. Although it is possible to construct a tree in which the age of cancer diagnosis varies, this requires addition of multiple additional branches to the tree increasing its complexity. In this situation, a more elegant solution is construction of a Markov model. This model may be used to answer research questions that examine transitions between various stages of health [22]. A Markov model is a recursive model, allowing movement back and forth between points in a model, unlike decision trees, which constrain

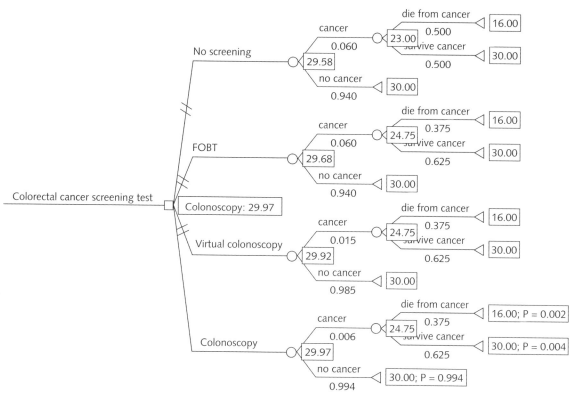

Fig. 7.2 The decision tree is analyzed by folding back and averaging. Starting from the right side of the tree, the value of each outcome is multiplied by the probability of achieving that outcome. This value is summed with the other weighted outcomes at the chance node leading to those outcomes. In turn, these values are weighted by the probability of following that branch of the tree and summed with other weighted outcomes at the next more proximal (to the left in the tree) chance node. At the most proximal branch of each strategy there will be a single value representing the weighted sum of outcomes associated with that strategy. This value may be compared to the competing strategies at the decision node in order to determine the optimal strategy. In this case screening colonoscopy is modeled to produce the greatest number of life years.

movement to occur in one direction. Markov models may be preferred to decision trees when it is important to incorporate the impact of time in the simulation, thus identifying when events occur. In addition, Markov models provide a means by which to introduce more complex interactions between health states.

Construction of a Markov model begins with identification of the health states that define a clinical scenario [1]. These include "healthy," "dead" and various states of disease. Second, allowable transitions from one state to another are drawn as arrows (Fig. 7.3). Some arrows may be bidirectional to illustrate the ability to move from one state to another and back again. Other arrows are unidirectional such as those leading to **sink states**, states that cannot be left once entered (i.e., death). Arrows may also indicate the ability to remain within a state. Third, a cycle

length must be chosen to represent the amount of time that elapses during transitions between states. The cycle should be chosen to reflect the clinical scenario modeled and is generally equal to the minimum amount of time required when moving from one state of health to another. Fourth, the values for variables representing the transitions are derived, usually from existing literature, as was described for the development of decision trees. Fifth, outcomes are defined for the analysis such as costs, life-years or QALYs. Unlike decision trees where outcomes are calculated only at the conclusion of the analysis, outcomes for a Markov model may be accumulated over the duration of the model by assignment of incremental "rewards" to each health state. As a result, several advantages are acquired including the ability to allow clinical events to occur multiple times during the simulation, and applica-

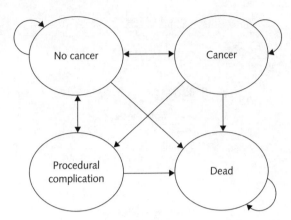

Fig. 7.3 Markov model. The ovals represent the modeled health states, the arrows illustrate the possible transitions between health states that occur during each cycle of the model. In this example, patients who do not have cancer may develop cancer, may sustain a complication from an intervention to decrease cancer mortality (e.g., a perforation during a screening colonoscopy) or die from non-cancer causes. Similarly, patients in whom cancer has developed may be cured of cancer, sustain complications related to cancer treatment or die of cancer. The looped arrows indicate the possibility that patients may remain in a particular health state during subsequent cycles.

tion of discounting, which is used to reflect patients' time preferences for receiving various outcomes.

Markov models can be analyzed in several different ways. The standard method in medical research involves calculation of the mean outcomes of a hypothetical cohort of patients. Alternative methods include stochastic simulations such as Monte Carlo analysis, which will be briefly discussed, discrete event simulation, and matrix algebra, which is dealt with by more detailed papers on the subject [22,23]. Analysis of a hypothetical cohort is generally performed with assistance from computer programs, although the mathematical functions required are generally limited to multiplication and addition. The general scheme for analysis involves distribution of a hypothetical group of patients into the initial health states, according to the proportions appropriate for the question that is being asked. For every cycle, the hypothetical cohort is redistributed among various health states in a manner regulated by the transition rates specified in the model. Simply stated, a proportion of the cohort in a given state will exit that state and enter another state based on the rate established for that transition. Once all transitions into and out of each health state have been performed, outcomes for each cycle are reassigned. Outcomes may be costs, clinical events (gastrointestinal bleeds, can-

cers, surgeries, etc.) or life years proportioned to the cycle length, which may be further adjusted by utilities to derive QALYs. This process is repeated for each cycle specified by the investigator and the various outcomes are summed to calculate the results. For the base-case analysis, the results would be expressed as the mean or average expected outcomes such as the costs, number of cancers or life-years associated with each strategy. Additionally, comparison between strategies should be provided to estimate outcomes such as the mean number of cancers averted, life-years gained or difference in costs between competing strategies.

Markov models may also be analyzed using a specialized form of stochastic analysis known as a Monte Carlo simulation [24]. This is a multiple-way sensitivity analysis in which any or all of the variables in the model are varied simultaneously. Furthermore, the values for each variable may be randomly picked from a predefined distribution of possibilities that may be in the form of a normal, exponential, bimodal or other distribution (second-order simulation). The model is run multiple times, each run using a different set of values for each variable. The use of distributions allows certain values to be chosen more frequently than others to represent a particular variable. The results of a Monte Carlo simulation include expected values and the range of outcomes in the form of a density function (such as the mean and 95% confidence intervals in the case of normal distributions), and thus give a more complete picture of the range of probable results of the analysis. Monte Carlo simulation uses variable inputs that do not vary over time, thus it is generally considered a static analysis. Discrete event simulation, in contrast, allows the model inputs to vary over the duration of the simulation period, and thus it is considered a dynamic analysis.

Limitations of decision analysis

It is important to understand the inherent limitations of decision analytic studies. Greatest among these is the reliance of models on the assumptions upon which they are constructed. Although assumptions are generally limited to the values assigned to variables in the model, they should also pertain to the structure of the model or the manner in which the various elements interact with each other. To examine the impact of base-case assumptions, rigorous sensitivity analysis is performed to test whether the model conclusions are robust to changes in the parameter estimates (values of variables in the model) or changes in the model structure. If clinically plausible changes in the value assigned to a variable result in differing conclusions, the model is stated to be sensitive to that variable. Sensitive variables are logical targets for further research, because they are identified to be important parameters required to define optimal management. Variables that are not associated with changes in outcome in sensitivity analysis are either well defined through previous research, or are less important in defining disease management. In this manner decision analysis fulfills one of its primary functions, which is hypothesis generation, or the identification of relevant research questions. Structural assumptions are necessary in order to simplify complex medical events but are more difficult to identify and test. The challenge of model construction is to include key variables relevant to the clinical question being raised while excluding less important ones. Simplification of "real world" events is essential and requires input from investigators who are experts in the field in question. Full disclosure of the model including parameter and structural assumptions is essential for validation of its conclusions.

Despite its limitations, decision analysis remains an essential tool for health services and outcomes research. These techniques allow comparison of competing management strategies in a quantitative fashion, summarize existing literature into a single metric, and generate hypotheses based on the important factors governing clinical management.

Conclusions

Decision analysis is conducted to compare outcomes between competing strategies of management under conditions of uncertainty. A variety of tools, including decision trees and Markov models, have been adapted to biomedical research in order to calculate a quantitative summary of existing data concerning a research topic that may guide clinical decision-making and even health policy. Of potentially greater impact is the ability of these studies to generate hypotheses that inform future research efforts to optimize health benefits.

References

1. Petitti DB. *Meta-analysis, Decision analysis and Cost-effectiveness Analysis*. New York: Oxford University Press, 1994.
2. Von Neumann J, Morgenstern O. *Theory of Games and Economic Theory*. New York: Wiley, 1947.
3. Henschke UK, Flehinger BJ. Decision theory in cancer thera-py. *Cancer* 1967;**20**:1819.
4. Pauker SG, Kassirer JP. Decision analysis. *N Engl J Med* 1987;**316**:250.
5. Weinstein M, Fineberg H. *Clinical Decision Analysis*. Philadelphia: Saunders, 1980.
6. Sox HC *et al. Medical Decision Making*. Stoneham, MA: Butterworth, 1988.
7. Kassirer JP. The principles of clinical decision making: an introduction to decision analysis. *Yale J Biol Med* 1976;**49**:149.
8. Froberg DG, Kane RL. Methodology for measuring health-state preferences – II: Scaling methods. *J Clin Epidemiol* 1989;**42**:459.
9. Froberg DG, Kane RL. Methodology for measuring health-state preferences – I: Measurement strategies. *J Clin Epidemiol* 1989;**42**:345.
10. Froberg DG, Kane RL. Methodology for measuring health-state preferences – IV: Progress and a research agenda. *J Clin Epidemiol* 1989;**42**:675.
11. Froberg DG, Kane RL. Methodology for measuring health-state preferences – III: Population and context effects. *J Clin Epidemiol* 1989;**42**:585.
12. La Puma J, Lawlor EF. Quality-adjusted life-years. Ethical implications for physicians and policymakers. *JAMA* 1990;**263**:2917.
13. Richardson WS, Detsky AS. Users' guides to the medical literature. VII. How to use a clinical decision analysis. A. Are the results of the study valid? Evidence-Based Medicine Working Group. *JAMA* 1995;**273**:1292.
14. Oxman AD *et al.* Users' guides to the medical literature. VI. How to use an overview. Evidence-Based Medicine Working Group. *JAMA* 1994;**272**:1367.
15. Guyatt GH *et al.* Users' guides to the medical literature. II. How to use an article about therapy or prevention. B. What were the results and will they help me in caring for my patients? Evidence-Based Medicine Working Group. *JAMA* 1994;**271**:59.
16. Jaeschke R *et al.* Users' guides to the medical literature. III. How to use an article about a diagnostic test. B. What are the results and will they help me in caring for my patients? The Evidence-Based Medicine Working Group. *JAMA* 1994;**271**:703.
17. Jaeschke R *et al.* Users' guides to the medical literature. III. How to use an article about a diagnostic test. A. Are the results of the study valid? Evidence-Based Medicine Working Group. *JAMA* 1994;**271**:389.
18. Guyatt GH *et al.* Users' guides to the medical literature. II. How to use an article about therapy or prevention. A. Are the results of the study valid? Evidence-Based Medicine Working Group. *JAMA* 1993;**270**:2598.
19. Oxman AD *et al.* Users' guides to the medical literature. I. How to get started. The Evidence-Based Medicine Working Group. *JAMA* 1993;**270**:2093.
20. Laupacis A *et al.* Users' guides to the medical literature. V. How to use an article about prognosis. Evidence-Based Medi-

cine Working Group. *JAMA* 1994;**272**:234.

21. Levine M *et al*. Users' guides to the medical literature. IV. How to use an article about harm. Evidence-Based Medicine Working Group. *JAMA* 1994;**271**:1615.

22. Beck JR, Pauker SG. The Markov process in medical prognosis. *Med Decis Making* 1983;**3**:419.

23. Platell CF *et al*. Flexible sigmoidoscopy screening for colorectal neoplasia in average-risk people: evaluation of a five-year rescreening interval. *Med J Aust* 2002;**176**:371.

24. Doubilet P *et al*. Probabilistic sensitivity analysis using Monte Carlo simulation. A practical approach. *Med Decis Making* 1985;**5**:157.

8 Health Economics

Dawn Provenzale and Joseph Lipscomb

Key points
- An understanding of economic analysis in gastroenterology is helpful in shared decision-making by physician and patient.
- The essential components of economic analysis are outlined and the reader is provided with the necessary definitions to read these analyses critically and determine if the results can be applied to their practice.
- Understanding the costs of gastroenterology practices, how they are calculated, and how they compare with the costs of other medical practices provides the gastroenterologist with important information for interacting with patients, other providers and payers.
- It is important to understand the distinctions between the different types of economic analyses and when each should be applied. Information on the different types of economic analyses and the settings in which they are used is given.
- Published criteria for performing economic analyses are outlined; these can be used to evaluate the quality of published economic analyses and their validity.

Introduction

In an era of rising national healthcare expenditures, gastroenterology has faced increased scrutiny of its practices and costs. Economic considerations permeate our day-to-day practice styles, and economic analyses are increasingly common in the gastrointestinal literature. In order to evaluate these economic analyses and determine their value for guiding clinical practice, the reader must have an understanding of certain economic concepts and principles and how they are used (and sometimes misused) in the medical literature. In addition, the criteria for performing an economic analysis must be clearly understood so that the reader may critically evaluate these economic analyses and determine which can be applied to their practice [1].

This chapter is divided into three parts, which focus in turn on: (i) the concept of economic cost; (ii) different types of economic analyses; and (iii) the criteria for performing an economic analysis, including applications of these criteria to screening of patients with gastroesophageal reflux disease (GERD) and to surveillance of patients with Barrett's esophagus.

Defining "cost" for health economic analyses

The concept of cost

In economic terms, cost is defined in terms of foregone opportunities. Specifically, the cost of any good or service is measured in principle as the value of the resources required to produce that item, with each resource valued ("costed out") in terms of what it could earn in its next best use – called its "opportunity cost." Thus, the concept of economic cost recognizes that the personnel, equipment, supplies and other inputs employed to produce a particular medical service **could** have been used to produce other goods or services of value. Moreover, it is generally assumed that each of these inputs is paid roughly according to the value it contributes to producing goods and services; for example, if the prevailing wage rate for a medical technician is $20/hour, that is the technician's opportunity cost because he or she is able to earn this (and no more than this) in some other productive employment opportunity. Hence, the economic (opportunity) cost of the medical service is defined as the sum of the opportunity costs of the resources required to produce it. That is, cost is the monetary value of the resources used for the services [2].

Domains of cost

As defined and frequently used in health economic studies, economic costs span a number of domains [2], which may be classified as follows [3]:

Direct costs

These are defined as the value of the goods, services and other resources consumed in the provision of a healthcare intervention or in responding to the current and possibly future side effects of the intervention. Thus, direct costs are incurred in the process of treating, detecting or attempting to prevent a disease or illness. They include **direct healthcare costs** (e.g., medical personnel, supplies, drugs, facilities) for resources traditionally employed within the healthcare system proper; **direct non-healthcare costs** (e.g., transportation to care, child care while the parent is being screened or treated, special dietary products) for resources absorbed in the care delivery process (other than patient time) that lie outside the healthcare system; and **patient time cost** for the foregone productive opportunities associated with the individual's participation in his or her own healthcare process (and often measured in terms of market wages foregone in principle).

It is particularly important to distinguish between the direct cost of a healthcare service – from an economic opportunity cost perspective – and the posted price (charge) for that service. In fee-for-service healthcare in the USA, rarely will charges be a reflection of true opportunity cost [4]. Historically, and still frequently, the posted price of a service is often set strategically by the provider so as to maximize total net revenue for the services being billed [5]. For example, the charge for a frequently performed and well-insured procedure may be set at a level so that revenue flows from all payers can effectively subsidize a less frequently performed, high-cost procedure – allowing its posted price to remain "reasonable." In general, higher prices for services that are less price sensitive can open the way for lower prices for services that are more price sensitive. Consequently, neither posted nor actually billed charges will necessarily reflect economic opportunity cost. By the same token, the amount that third-party payers reimburse for a service will not reflect opportunity costs either, unless the insurer bases payments on its own (successful) efforts to estimate the opportunity cost. In fact, the Medicare program's diagnosis-related group (DRG) system for reimbursing hospitals and other facilities, as well as its fee schedule system for reimbursing physicians and other outpatient services, are intended to

result in payment amounts that roughly approximate (on average) the opportunity cost of the services rendered [3]. (Whether those aims have been achieved remains a prime topic for discussion in the healthcare community.)

Productivity (indirect) costs

These are defined in terms of the value of the lost economic output as a result of an individual's illness or death. Specifically, **morbidity costs** are measured by the lost earnings due to illness or treatment for illness, while **mortality costs** are measured by the lost earnings due to premature death.

Two practical points should be noted. First, in an economic analysis that includes both patient time costs and morbidity costs, it is important not to double-count by incorporating the former also in the latter; instead, the sum of the costs from the two categories should reflect a mutually exclusive and exhaustive accounting of the total productivity burden of the disease and treatment regarding the individual. Second, it has become common to acknowledge that in an economy with less than full employment of labor resources, firms will adjust to employees' lost time due to illness or death by hiring and training replacement workers. Thus, using the (lifetime) morbidity or mortality cost estimate for a worker lost because of (transient) illness or death may significantly overstate the true productivity cost to the firm, and to the economy. Nonetheless, the firm (and economy) will bear some short-term costs in searching for, hiring, training and fully integrating the replacement labor; the economic value of the resources absorbed in this process is known as the **frictional cost** associated with the lost worker's illness or death [6].

There are two other basic issues that arise in almost all cost calculations used in health economics evaluations: analytical perspective and effects of time and place.

Perspective (or point of view) of the analysis

The cost burden imposed by a given health condition or healthcare intervention depends on the perspective from which it is calculated. For example, for a 58-year-old employed individual undergoing colon cancer surgery, the economic costs of undergoing the procedure include whatever direct healthcare and direct nonhealth costs are incurred beyond what insurance covers, plus patient time costs and any additional morbidity costs (all as defined above). From the standpoint of the hospital and surgeons involved in the surgery, the (net) economic cost is the amount of reimbursements received from all sources, minus the provider's estimated opportunity cost of performing the procedure. For the patient's health insurer, the cost is the dollar volume of the claims paid. For the individual's employer, the cost is the dollar value of the firm's output that is lost and/or the frictional cost associated with replacing the worker's productivity during his absence. From the perspective of the individual's family, the economic cost of the surgery is the value of the time diverted to assisting and caring for the individual (which may include foregone marketplace earnings).

The absolute dollar cost estimate for the surgery will probably vary significantly depending on which of these perspectives is selected. And there is one additional viewpoint from which the costs of the surgery can be computed, and it is in fact the one most common in health economics evaluations: the **societal perspective**. From this vantage point, the cost of the surgery is the sum of all opportunity cost components, regardless of how they are distributed across and borne by individuals and institutions.

Computing and comparing costs across time and place

Whatever the perspective assumed, the cost associated with a disease or of a specific intervention may vary depending on when and where it occurs and how long the effects are felt over time. Economic evaluations generally should acknowledge and adjust for these considerations, as discussed briefly now.

EVALUATING COST FLOWS OVER TIME FROM A PRESENT-VALUE PERSPECTIVE: THE PROCESS OF DISCOUNTING
In economic evaluations in which the costs of different interventions are being compared (and this is typically the case), it is important that the time flows of costs associated with each intervention be stated in a way that allows for valid comparisons [2]. For example, in comparing a preventive intervention with a treatment intervention, the former may involve very substantial upfront costs and may (if successful) generate significant cost savings downstream, whereas the latter may involve little cost in the early going but large cost once disease develops, is detected and requires treatment. The challenge is calculating the overall cost impact of each intervention in a way that reflects the differential timing of these cost flows, so that they can be appropriately evaluated from a present-time perspective (i.e., in the here-and-now). The process for achieving this is called discounting [7].

To illustrate, consider the simple case in which $1000 is invested for 1 year at a real (i.e., inflation-adjusted) rate of return of 3%. One year from now, the total of principal plus interest is $1000(1+0.03) = $1030. It follows that the **present value** of $1030 received 1 year from now is $1000 – and, similarly, that the present value of $1030 of costs that might be incurred in 1 year is $1030/(1+0.03) = $1000. Put differently, to cover $1030 in costs expected to be incurred a year from now, we need to set aside only $1000 today. In general terms, the present value of X of costs incurred in year n is $\$X_n/(1 + i)^n$, where i is the selected annual discount rate (assumed to be 0.03 in the example here). For an intervention associated with a stream of economic costs over N years from its initiation, the present value of that cost stream can be denoted as $C_{PV} = \Sigma X_n/(1 + i)^n$, where the sum is from $n = 1$ to N.

ADJUSTING FOR INPUT PRICE INFLATION AND GEOGRAPHIC VARIATIONS IN INPUT COSTS
The costs of the inputs used in the production of healthcare goods and services tend to increase over time simply due to general price inflation; in addition, input costs may vary geographically at any point in time (e.g., between urban and rural facilities or across regions of the country) because of cross-sectional cost-of-production differences. Consequently, in economic evaluations that use data drawn from multiple years, from multiple geographic sites, or both, it is important to first adjust for those input price differences attributable to inflation and/or geographic variation before combining them to arrive at representative (and clearly interpretable) estimates of the economic cost of a disease or of an intervention. Standard formulas for doing this are discussed in Brown et al. [2]. To illustrate what is at issue, suppose one is estimating the total direct cost impact of a program to increase the rate of screening colonoscopy in the 50+ age population, and that the available cost data come from 10 geographically spread, population-based study sites and across the five-year time span from 2000 to 2005. The standard formulas cited in Brown et al. [2] would then allow one to derive (for example) a "nationally representative" cost estimate stated (for example) in "2005 dollars."

Finally, note that the rationales for discounting costs to present value and for adjusting cost estimates for inflationary effects are separate and distinct. It is a common perception that one discounts simply to adjust for inflation effects. In fact, one discounts to reflect the underlying time-value of money, and would do so even if there were no price inflation. In the economic analyses defined in the next section, the standard approach is first to purge opportunity cost estimates of inflation (and geographic variation) effects, and only then to discount to present value using some selected, real (i.e., inflation-adjusted) rate of interest.

So far our discussion has been about "costs" – yet it is intuitively evident that the economic evaluation of healthcare interventions inevitably requires measuring and comparing both costs **and** benefits. As we turn now to define and compare the alternative types of health economic analyses, it will become clear in each case how "benefits" are conceptualized and how costs and benefits are then analyzed jointly to arrive at conclusions about the economic merits of alternative interventions.

Types of economic analyses

We now briefly discuss the major types of economic analyses used to evaluate healthcare interventions, with particular attention to the one type (cost-effectiveness analysis) carried out most often in the gastroenterology literature.

Cost identification analysis

In some instances, decision-makers may be principally concerned with the economic cost burden associated with one or more healthcare interventions or policies [2]. Depending on the issue being examined, the scope of such a cost analysis may include direct (healthcare plus non-healthcare) costs and productivity costs, or only direct costs, or only direct healthcare costs. To be sure, each intervention may have implications for individual and population health outcomes; but the decision focus in these instances is the net cost impact of the intervention. For example, there has been great interest in recent years about whether patients participating in cancer clinical trials generate significantly greater direct healthcare costs than otherwise [8]; studies exploring this issue have essentially been cost identification analyses [2]. While these studies calculate costs of care or interventions, they do not consider costs in relation to health effects or outcomes.

Cost-effectiveness analysis

When the decision-maker is interested in both the health effects and the costs of an intervention – and, specifically, with whether the intervention generates a sufficient improvement in health outcomes to merit the associated increase in cost – the methodology of choice in recent years is cost-effectiveness analysis (CEA).

More formally, cost-effectiveness analysis designates the current (status quo, or comparator) intervention for addressing a given health problem as x, and some alternative intervention under consideration as i. To evaluate the 'cost-effectiveness' of intervention i (relative to x), we perform a cost-effectiveness analysis and calculate the incremental cost-effectiveness ratio, CER = $(C_i - C_x)/(E_i - E_x)$, where C_i and C_x are the costs associated with interventions i and x, and E_i and E_x are the health outcome effectiveness measures associated with i and x. In classic CEA, the effectiveness measure is a unidimensional outcome. By far the most frequently employed effectiveness measure in the literature is some variant of survival or life expectancy, for example life-years gained [2]. In that case, CER can be interpreted as the increment in cost per life-year gained from adopting intervention i rather than the status quo intervention x. In other words, it is the additional cost incurred for the additional gain in life expectancy from adopting intervention i rather than the status quo (intervention x). For cost-effectiveness analysis (and its variants, to be discussed shortly), cost is typically assumed to encompass direct healthcare and direct non-healthcare costs, plus frictional costs – but not productivity (indirect) costs [2]. The rationale for excluding the latter is that such morbidity and mortality cost effects are reflected, albeit very imperfectly, in effectiveness measures such as life-years (and in survival measures adjusted for quality-of-life effects, as found in the cost-utility analyses defined below). Consequently, to avoid double-counting certain costs and benefits in both the denominator and numerator of CER, the conservative approach is to exclude the productivity cost consequences associated with increments in life expectancy (or quality-adjusted life expectancy). Also, in multi-year cost-effectiveness analyses, both the cost estimates **and** the effectiveness estimates in the CER are discounted to present value, with cost estimates further purged of inflation or geographic variation effects, as described previously. The US Panel on Cost-Effectiveness in Health and Medicine has recommended that both costs and effectiveness be discounted at the same, inflation-adjusted, interest rate – specifically, at an annual rate of 3% in the base-case analysis, with the rate being allowed to vary between 0% (no discounting) and 7% in sensitivity analyses [7].

Cost-utility analysis

When effectiveness is to be regarded as a multidimensional construct, reflecting both length of life **and** quality of life, it is common to express E_i and E_x in terms of "quality-adjusted life-years" (QALYs) [9]. This necessarily involves computing the effectiveness of an intervention as a type of weighted-average, which combines the decision-maker's perceived value (utility) associated with projected life expectancy with the perceived value of the quality of life during those years. In such a cost-utility analysis (CUA), the CER is phrased in terms of cost per QALY.

Drawing inferences from CEA and CUA ratios

In the vernacular, a cost-effective action is sometimes described as one yielding a big "bang for the buck." As operationalized in health economics, CEA compares options (instead) in terms of "bucks required per unit of bang achieved." When intervention i is both more effective and more costly than x – the situation most commonly encountered in analyses of new healthcare technologies – the smaller the computed value of CER, the better. But how small is "small enough" to indicate that i should be adopted instead of x? One approach to address this question systematically is to compare the CER of interest to a broad spectrum of ratios emerging from other cost-effectiveness analyses, as published in what has become known as "league tables" [2]. An example is given in Table 8.1, which is adapted from a comprehensive league table of cost-utility ratios for oncology interventions, as constructed by Earle *et al.* [10].

To illustrate, if a newly developed screening procedure for colorectal cancer had a cost-utility ratio of, say, less than $10 000 per QALY gained, it would be in the upper tier of this league table and, arguably, a candidate for adoption. However, there is no hard-and-fast rule for where to draw the line in such a table, nor an obvious socially constructed basis yet proposed for deriving such a consensus. Nonetheless, interventions with CEA and CUA ratios greater than $100 000 are often regarded as not cost-effective, while those with ratios below $20 000 are generally seen as cost-effective and those with ratios below $50 000 often regarded as cost-effective [2]. In addition, league tables can also assist the decision-maker who has an explicitly defined budget for competing healthcare interventions. The decision-maker would use the league table to choose interventions that both maximize effectiveness (e.g., increase life expectancy) and are within the explicitly stated budget (e.g., $50 000/LY gained).

When it is **not** the case that intervention i is both more effective and more costly than intervention x, other decision outcomes arise. If i is both more effective and less costly than x, then i is said to "dominate" x and is clearly the cost-effective choice. Similarly, if i is both less effective and more costly than x, then i is clearly not cost-effective (relative to x). Another possibility is that intervention i is

both less effective and less costly than x; in this case, one would choose i over x if the savings in healthcare dollars were sufficiently large to justify the associated decrement in health effectiveness (thus, the larger the CER, the better). However, given the long-held medical ethics credo to "first, do no harm," this is a somewhat troubling scenario, and in fact is rarely encountered in the published health economics literature.

One final possibility, often mentioned in the CEA literature though not often found in practice, should be noted: if the available options (here, interventions i and x) happen to be equally effective, for example, if the outcomes of the alternative strategies are equal in terms of life-years gained or quality-adjusted life-years gained, one simply selects the least costly option. To do so is to engage in **cost-minimization analysis (CMA)** [2].

When the cost and health consequences of competing interventions are systematically displayed and summarized, but no summary CEA or CUA ratios are computed, the resulting evaluation is often termed a **cost-consequence analysis** [2]. For example, if the analyst wished to examine the economic impact of alternative therapies for achalasia – e.g., pneumatic dilatation, botulinum toxin injection or surgery – he or she would calculate the costs for each of these alternative strategies, and also the outcomes or health consequences in terms of dysphagia-free days or symptom relief. The analyst would then simply report the costs and the benefits of each of these strategies. Once the information on costs and outcomes is explicitly stated, it would be up to the decision-maker to determine which strategy to choose based on the information provided. This type of information could be very useful in the clinical setting in which the provider and patient are considering alternative management strategies. Joint decision-making is facilitated when all of the costs and potential risks and benefits of the alternative strategies are explicitly stated.

Cost-benefit analysis

A distinguishing feature of cost-benefit analysis (CBA) is that both the costs and health effects associated with an intervention are expressed in monetary units. Costs are computed just as in CEA or CUA, but now the added life-years or quality-adjusted life-years generated by the intervention must be valued in dollar terms. More formally, in CBA one estimates the net benefit (NB) = $E^s_i - C_i$ for intervention i. The intervention passes the cost-benefit test if, and only if, NB > 0. Note there is no requirement now to compare i with the status quo or any other inter-

Table 8.1 League table of cost/QALY in 1998 $US

Description of interventions, their alternatives and the target population	Cost utility
Biopsy versus no biopsy for 50-year-old men with elevated PSA levels	<$0
Second-line paclitaxel vs vinorelbine for metastatic breast cancer	<$0
Second-line docetaxel versus paclitaxel for metastatic breast cancer	<$0
One-time Pap smear screening program vs no screening program for a low-income 70-year-old black woman seeking medical care from a municipal hospital outpatient clinic	<$0
Endorectal surface coil for MR imaging vs conventional MR imaging for otherwise healthy men with biopsy-proven prostate cancer	$1300
Current treatment vs no treatment for patients with Hodgkin's disease at a university hospital in Norway	$2000
Immediate biopsy vs 6-month observation for a 50-year-old woman with abnormal findings on mammography	$2500
Second-line treatment with docetaxel vs paclitaxel for patients with recurrent widely disseminated metastatic breast cancer who are failing on standard treatments	$4100
Triennial breast cancer screening in 50–65-year age group vs no screening program for the population of Dutch women	$4200
Universal screening program for breast, cervical and colorectal cancers vs no screening program for Nordic population	$4700
Alternating CAV and VP-P chemotherapy vs standard CAV chemotherapy for patients with extensive SCLC	$5400
Adjuvant tamoxifen vs no treatment for a 45 year-old premenopausal woman with node-positive, ER-positive breast cancer	$5700
Adjuvant chemotherapy vs tamoxifen for a 45-year-old premenopausal woman with node-positive, ER-negative breast cancer	$6400
Adjuvant chemotherapy vs tamoxifen for a 45-year-old premenopausal woman with node-negative, ER-negative breast cancer	$6500
Adjuvant chemotherapy, assuming lifelong benefit, vs no adjuvant chemotherapy for women aged 45 with stage I or IIa node-negative, ER-negative breast cancer	$6700
Biennial breast cancer screening in 50–70-year age group versus triennial breast cancer screening in 50–65-year age group for the population of Dutch women	$6900
Adjuvant chemotherapy after surgery, assuming a 15% gain in life expectancy, vs surgery alone for Dukes' B or C colorectal cancer patients	$8100
Paclitaxel, cisplatin and tamoxifen vs cyclophosphamide and cisplatin for women with stage III/IV ovarian cancer	$8800
Adjuvant chemotherapy, assuming lifelong benefit, vs no adjuvant chemotherapy for women aged 60 with stage I or IIa node-negative, ER-negative breast cancer	$9700
Bone marrow transplantation vs no BMT for patients with a variety of hematologic malignancies	$9900
Adjuvant chemotherapy after surgery, assuming a 10% gain in life expectancy, vs surgery alone for Duke's B or C colorectal cancer patients	$11 000
Paclitaxel, cisplatin, and hexamethylmelamine vs cyclophosphamide and cisplatin for women with stage III/IV ovarian cancer	$11 000
Adjuvant chemotherapy vs tamoxifen for a 45-year-old premenopausal woman with node-positive, ER-positive breast cancer	$12 000
High-specificity vs normal-specificity endorectal surface coil for MR imaging for otherwise healthy men with biopsy-proved prostate cancer	$12 000
Adjuvant tamoxifen vs no adjuvant treatment for a 45-year-old premenopausal woman with node-negative, ER-positive breast cancer	$15 000
Adjuvant chemotherapy vs tamoxifen for a 45-year-old premenopausal woman with node-negative, ER-positive breast cancer	$15 000
First-line 5-FU-based chemotherapy vs supportive care alone for patients with surgically noncurable colorectal cancer	$15 000
Biopsy vs no biopsy for 60-year-old men with elevated PSA levels	$15 000
Adjuvant high-dose interferon alfa-2b therapy vs no interferon treatment for newly diagnosed resectable primary cutaneous melanoma patients	$16 000
Surgery plus adjuvant chemotherapy vs surgery alone for patients with Dukes' stage C colon cancer	$17 000

(Continued.)

Table 8.1 *(Continued.)*

Description of interventions, their alternatives and the target population	Cost utility
TP-ifosfamide versus CP for women with stage III/IV ovarian cancer	$18 000
Mammography screening vs no population-based screening for women aged 45 to 69	$18 000
Adjuvant combined chemohormonal therapy vs chemotherapy alone for a 45-year-old premenopausal woman with node-positive, ER-positive breast cancer	$19 000
Breast cancer screening every 2 years vs no breast cancer screening past age 69	$19 000
Interferon alfa-2b with melphalan and prednisone versus conventional treatment for patients with multiple myeloma	$19 000
Follow-up program, including carcinoembryonic antigen monitoring, vs no follow-up for Norwegian patients with resected colorectal cancer	$19 000
Breast cancer screening in 40–70-year age group every 1.3 years vs biennial breast cancer screening for the population of Dutch women	$20 000
Adjuvant chemotherapy, assuming 5 years of benefit, vs no adjuvant chemotherapy for women aged 45 with stage I or IIa node-negative, ER-negative breast cancer	$20 000
Adjuvant chemotherapy vs no adjuvant chemotherapy for 45-year-old premenopausal women who have undergone surgery for node-negative, ER-negative stage I or IIa breast cancer	$20 000
Sequential testing strategy using sputa, FNA and expectant management vs no testing for a 50-year-old man with a radiographically detected large (>3 cm) peripheral lung mass	$20 000
Flutamide plus orchiectomy versus orchiectomy alone for 70-year-old men with newly diagnosed, untreated, severe metastatic prostate carcinoma with good performance status	$21 000
Breast-conserving surgery vs modified radical mastectomy for women with stage I and II breast cancer	$21 000
Adjuvant chemotherapy, assuming 5 years of benefit, vs no adjuvant chemotherapy for women aged 60 with stage I or IIa node-negative, ER-negative breast cancer	$25 000
Chemotherapy vs no chemotherapy for 60-year-old premenopausal women who have undergone surgery for node-negative, ER-negative stage I or IIa breast cancer	$25 000
Adjuvant chemotherapy after surgery, assuming a 5% gain in life expectancy, vs surgery alone for Dukes' B or C colorectal cancer patients	$28 000
First-line 5-FU-based chemotherapy versus supportive care alone for patients with surgically noncurable gastric cancer with no previous chemotherapy	$30 000
Flutamide plus orchiectomy versus orchiectomy alone for 70-year-old men with newly diagnosed, untreated, minimal metastatic prostate carcinoma and good performance status	$30 000
First-line 5-FU-based chemotherapy vs supportive care alone for patients with surgically noncurable gastric, pancreatic/biliary, or colorectal cancer	$31 000
High-dose chemotherapy with ABMT vs standard chemotherapy for a 45-year-old woman with metastatic breast cancer	$34 000
Chemotherapy vs no chemotherapy for a 60-year-old woman with node-negative breast cancer	$37 000
Adjuvant chemotherapy versus no adjuvant chemotherapy for a 60-year-old woman with early-stage node-negative, ER-negative breast cancer	$37 000
Interferon alfa versus hydroxyurea for 50-year-old patients with chronic-phase, Ph-positive chronic myelogenous leukemia (CML)	$37 000
Chemotherapy vs no chemotherapy for a 65-year-old woman with node-negative breast cancer	$41 000
Sequential testing strategy using sputa, FNA and thoracoscopy vs sputa, FNA and expectant management for a 50-year-old man with a radiographically detected large (>3 cm) peripheral lung mass	$42 000
Combined chemohormonal therapy vs chemotherapy alone for a 45-year-old premenopausal woman with node-negative, ER-positive breast cancer	$44 000
Chemotherapy vs no chemotherapy for a 70-year-old woman with node-negative breast cancer	$48 000
Chemotherapy vs no chemotherapy for a 75-year-old woman with node-negative breast cancer	$58 000
Adjuvant chemotherapy versus no adjuvant chemotherapy for 75-year-old woman with early-stage node-negative, ER-negative breast cancer	$58 000
Adjuvant chemotherapy, assuming an increase in disease-free survival but no change in overall 10-year survival with treatment, versus no adjuvant chemotherapy for women aged 45 with node-negative breast cancer	$64 000

(Continued.)

Table 8.1 *(Continued.)*

Description of interventions, their alternatives and the target population	Cost utility
Biennial breast cancer screening in 40–70-year age group years vs biennial breast cancer screening in 50–70-year age group for the population of Dutch women	$70 000
Adjuvant chemotherapy, assuming an increase in disease-free survival but no change in overall 10-year survival with treatment, vs no adjuvant chemotherapy for women aged 60 with node-negative breast cancer	$75 000
Chemotherapy vs no chemotherapy for an 80-year-old woman with node-negative breast cancer	$75 000
Breast cancer screening every 2 years vs no breast cancer screening past age 75	$80 000
Routine preoperative brain CT vs no preoperative brain CT for patients with potentially resectable lung cancer and no clinical evidence of CNS involvement	$81 000
Interferon alfa vs conventional chemotherapy for 45–50-year-old patients diagnosed with chronic myelogenous leukemia in the early chronic phase	$96 000
Adjuvant combined chemohormonal therapy vs chemotherapy alone for a 45-year-old premenopausal woman with node-positive, ER-negative breast cancer	$110 000
High-dose chemotherapy with ABMT vs standard chemotherapy for a 45-year-old woman with metastatic breast cancer	$120 000
First-line 5-FU-based chemotherapy vs supportive care alone for patients with surgically noncurable pancreatic/biliary cancer	$120 000
Breast cancer screening in 40–70-year age group every 1.3 years vs biennial breast cancer screening in 50–70-year age group for the population of Dutch women	$140 000
Antiemetic therapy with ondansetron vs metoclopramide for a 40-kg patient receiving cisplatin chemotherapy (≥ 75 mg/m^2) who had not previously been exposed to antineoplastic agents	$190 000
CXR screen vs no testing to follow patients with resected intermediate-thickness, local cutaneous melanoma	$220 000
Adjuvant combined chemohormonal therapy vs chemotherapy alone for a 45-year-old premenopausal woman with node-negative, ER-negative breast cancer	$240 000
Adjuvant tamoxifen vs no treatment for a 45-year-old premenopausal woman with node-negative, ER-negative breast cancer	$280 000
Antiemetic therapy with ondansetron versus metoclopramide for a 70-kg patient receiving cisplatin chemotherapy (≥ 75 mg/m^2) who had not previously been exposed to antineoplastic agents	$460 000
IV immunoglobulin versus no IV immunoglobulin for chronic lymphocytic leukemia and hypogammaglobulinemia	$7 900 000
Prostate cancer screening with +/– PSA +/– DRE +/– TRUS vs no screening in a 50-year-old male	D
Biopsy vs no biopsy for an asymptomatic 70-year-old man with elevated PSA levels	D
Clinical monitoring + CEA vs clinical monitoring alone for patients undergoing follow-up after colon cancer resection	D
Follow-up of various intensities vs no follow-up for colorectal cancer patients previously treated by surgery	D
ABMT vs five additional courses of CHOP chemotherapy for patients between 15 and 60 years of age with intermediate- or high-grade NHL	D
Thoracoscopy vs sequential strategies including sputa, FNA and thoracoscopy for a 50-year-old man with a >3-cm peripheral lung mass on CXR	D

Note. <$0: cost-saving. D: dominated (more costly but not more effective).

Abbreviations: ABMT, autologous bone marrow transplant; BMT, bone marrow transplant; CAV, cyclophosphamide, doxorubicin and vincristine; CEA, carcinoembryonic antigen; CHOP, cyclophosphamide, doxorubicin, vincristine and prednisone; CLL, chronic lymphocytic leukemia; CML, chronic myelogenous leukemia; CP, cyclophosphamide and cisplatin; CT, computerized tomography; CXR, chest X-ray; DRE, digital rectal exam; ER, estrogen receptor; FNA, fine-needle aspiration; 5-FU, fluorouracil; IV, intravenous; MR, magnetic resonance; NHL, non-Hodgkin's lymphoma; NSCLC, non-small-cell lung cancer; PSA, prostate-specific antigen; SCLC, small-cell lung cancer; TP, paclitaxel and cisplatin; TRUS, transrectal ultrasound; VP-P, etoposide and cisplatin. (Reproduced from Earle CC *et al.* [10], with permission from the American Society of Clinical Oncology.)

vention to reach a judgment. Thus, a cost-benefit analysis provides an explicit decision about whether the cost of the practice is worth the benefit obtained from it. If two or more **mutually exclusive** programs have positive net benefits, one chooses the program with the greatest net benefit [1].

A variety of methods have been used to obtain monetary evaluations of "benefit" for CBA [2]. One frequently seen in the early health economics literature is termed the "human capital" approach, wherein benefit is essentially defined in terms of the mortality and morbidity productivity costs **averted** as a result of the intervention. The most commonly used tactic for estimating benefits in CBA currently is the willingness-to-pay (WTP), or contingent valuation, approach, wherein the analyst attempts to determine the individual's (or a population's) subjective valuation of the health consequences of the intervention by ascertaining the maximum dollar amount the decision maker(s) are willing to pay to attain the intervention's projected outcomes. The most frequently used approach is to interview individuals, typically by survey, to ascertain their WTP for explicitly defined outcomes linked to the interventions of interest. An alternative, "revealed preference" approach involves the statistical analysis of real-world decision-making (e.g., the extra wage payment a worker requires for a hazardous job, or the market price people are willing to pay for smoke detectors and other safety devices) to provide a basis for inferring WTP for the health intervention of interest.

In addition to being familiar with the different types of economic analyses, it is important to understand how they are performed and how the results can be applied to clini-

cal practice. The following steps are useful for determining the validity of an economic analysis (Box 8.1) [11]. The criteria have been reviewed and discussed elsewhere [1].

Criteria for performing and evaluating economic analyses

1 Was a well-defined question posed in answerable form?

The first step in the assessment of an economic analysis is to decide whether a well-defined question has been posed in an answerable form [11]. Alternative strategies for comparison should be stated, and the perspective of the analysis (e.g., that of the patient, an HMO or society) defined. As an example, the investigator who wishes to examine the cost-effectiveness of screening individuals with gastroesophageal reflux disease (GERD) for Barrett's esophagus might pose the following question: taking the perspective of an HMO, is screening for Barrett's esophagus in patients with longstanding GERD cost-effective compared with common medical practices such as breast and cervical cancer screening?

2 Was a comprehensive description of the competing alternatives given?

In the second step of a critical appraisal, the reader should assess the report for a complete description of the competing alternatives (the alternative practices, strategies, interventions, etc.). In the case of screening GERD patients the analysis should explicitly state the results that will trigger further analysis (e.g., columnar epithelium with goblet cells on biopsy), and what additional analysis will be performed (e.g., endoscopic surveillance). The reader should also seek some definition of the events that will result in evaluation of patients in the no screening strategy (worsening of GERD symptoms, dysphagia, etc.). Enough information should be provided to the reader so that he or she can judge the generalizability of the program to his or her own practice and to determine if the relevant costs or consequences have been included.

3 Was there evidence that the program's effectiveness had been established?

The third step in assessing an economic analysis is to determine that the effectiveness of the program under study has been established; that is, that a causative link of the program to the outcome exists. In the case of screening

---

Box 8.1 Criteria for evaluating an economic analysis [3]

1 Was a well-defined question posed in an answerable form?
2 Was a comprehensive description of the competing alternatives given?
3 Was there evidence that the program's effectiveness had been established?
4 Were all the important and relevant costs and consequences for each alternative identified?
5 Were costs and consequences measured accurately in appropriate physical units?
6 Were costs and consequences valued credibly?
7 Were costs and consequences adjusted for differential timing?
8 Was an incremental analysis of costs and consequences of alternatives performed?
9 Was a sensitivity analysis performed?
10 Did the presentation and discussion of study results include all issues of concern to users?

for GERD, the reader should be provided with some evidence that screening reduces mortality from esophageal cancer. We are interested in economic evaluations of cost-effective approaches to effective practices. Therefore, if the effectiveness of the practice under study has not been established, the reader should not waste his or her time on the remainder of the report. With respect to screening for GERD, there is no direct evidence (results of randomized trials) that this practice actually reduces mortality from esophageal cancer, but indirect evidence (case series) related to early diagnosis and surveillance of patients with Barrett's esophagus suggests that screening individuals with GERD may be beneficial [12–16].

4 Were all the important and relevant costs and consequences for each alternative identified?

The next step in the evaluation requires that all the important and relevant costs and consequences, or benefits, of the alternative strategies be identified. The different types of costs, and the distinctions between them, have been described earlier. Most economic analyses consider only the direct healthcare costs of providing a particular service. This would include the costs of equipment, supplies, facility costs, salaries for physicians and support personnel and other operating and organizational costs. Direct non-healthcare costs incurred by patients and their families, such as any out-of-pocket expenses not covered by insurance, may also be included in some analyses, although this is uncommon because direct non-healthcare costs are highly individualized and difficult to measure. Productivity or indirect costs created by time lost from work or the psychosocial costs reflected in pain or distress suffered by the patient are typically not included in economic analyses because of the difficulty in measuring them.

The costs of screening for GERD would include costs for endoscopy plus biopsies if taken, salaries of technical staff and physicians, endoscopists, pathologists, and also any out-of-pocket expenses to the patient. In addition to cost, a summary of the health consequences or effects (risks and benefits) of the program should be listed. These consequences may include changes in the physical, psychological or emotional functioning of the patient, and may be measured in terms of life-years gained, disability prevented or quality-adjusted life-years gained. Thus, a list of relevant consequences of a screening program for GERD patients would incorporate any increase in life expectancy from cancer prevention and some measure of disability or

work loss days prevented by this program. With regards to costs, direct healthcare cost consequences that should be considered would include changes in physician visits and hospitalizations and the ordering of follow-up tests such as endoscopy.

5 Were costs and consequences measured accurately in appropriate physical units?

In the next component of the critical appraisal, the reader must determine if the costs and consequences have been measured accurately and in the appropriate physical units. In this step, the reader should seek a list of the elements of the analysis described in section 4 and the units for their measurement. For example, in a screening program for GERD, endoscopy might be performed for $600 per test [17]. Other screening tests should be similarly listed, and physician visits and fees should be included. The consequences and the units for their measurement should be explicitly stated. In the screening example, the reader should search for evidence that benefits such as years of life gained from early diagnosis, disability days avoided, cancers prevented, etc. are valued and are measured in the appropriate units (days, years, visits, etc.).

6 Were costs and consequences valued credibly?

In the sixth step of a critical evaluation of an economic analysis, the reader must determine if the costs and consequences included in the analysis are comprehensive and plausible. The most appropriate concept of the cost of a service or procedure is the economic "opportunity cost" value of the components of the service, or the items used to produce the service. Costs may be estimated in a variety of ways, and a clear explanation of the data and the methods used to calculate them should be presented.

The newer information systems that measure resource consumption [18] have promoted the accurate assessment of costs for economic analysis. Hospital accounting departments may also provide information about costs. If estimates of costs (of resources consumed) are not available, charges that have been adjusted to reflect costs may be used as proxy for them. One approach to adjusting charges for acute inpatient care is to calculate cost-to-charge ratios (computable from the cost reports submitted by most hospitals to Medicare). These ratios can be used to convert billed charges to resource cost estimates. Third-party reimbursement levels, for example, the Medicare diagnosis related group (DRG) [19] payment, have also been used as a proxy for the opportunity cost. Thus, there are diverse methods for obtaining costs. The reader should seek an explanation of the method that was used to determine costs for each analysis [1].

An explanation of how benefits are calculated should also be provided. In a cost-effectiveness analysis, for example, health consequences are often measured in terms of life-years saved, or life-years gained. Therefore, assigning a value to benefits is straightforward – each life-year gained or lost (at a point in time) counts the same. Productivity or indirect costs, such as the cost of time lost from work or school, and benefits, as required for one form of cost-benefit analysis, may be more difficult to ascribe. For example, the productivity cost of lost work time may be difficult to calculate for certain groups such as housewives, the elderly, children and the unemployed. Because productivity benefits are even more difficult to measure, their incorporation into economic evaluations remains controversial [1].

In cost-utility analysis, a variant of cost-effectiveness analysis, benefits are often measured in terms of quality-adjusted life-years. The analysis examines both the number of years of life gained from a practice, and the quality of those years. In other words, a cost-utility analysis considers that certain practices may be associated with discomfort and disability. Outcomes are adjusted to account for these quality-of-life effects. The studies that incorporate quality-of-life measures, also known as patient preferences or utilities, attempt to quantify how much better the quality of life is in one health state compared with another, for example, without cancer than with cancer. The results are reported in quality-adjusted life units (e.g., days, months or years) gained from a particular strategy. For a GERD screening program, the quality of life of those in the screened and the unscreened strategies would be measured and compared. The quality-of-life measurements should evaluate the short-term inconvenience or disability associated with screening, and the long-term disability associated with potential outcomes including the diagnosis of Barrett's esophagus, the risk of adenocarcinoma, and the inconvenience associated with surveillance endoscopy. The results of a cost-utility analysis are reported as an incremental cost-utility ratio.

7 Were costs and consequences adjusted for differential timing?

The costs and health consequences for some interventions occur relatively close to the initiation of the program, for example, vaccination for influenza. For other interventions, particularly those involving screening, the timing of the expenditures and the timing of the health benefits of the program may differ significantly. In a cancer screening program, the costs will typically arise early on, while the benefits of screening (including increased life expectancy) will occur in the future. In order to adjust for these differences in the timing of outcomes, it is appropriate to apply standard discounting formulas, as discussed earlier, to calculate the present value of both costs and health consequences. That is, to determine their value as viewed by the decision-maker today [20]. An extensive discussion of discounting has been provided earlier, but briefly, discounting considers that a dollar today is worth more than a dollar in the future, and, because life-years are valued relative to dollars in economic analyses, they are also discounted. Most economic analyses use discount rates ranging from 3% to 7%, with 3% as the current recommended standard [9].

8 Was an incremental analysis of costs and consequences of alternatives performed?

In order to set priorities for resource allocation, it is necessary to consider the additional costs that one program incurs over another, compared with the additional benefits that are produced. The average costs (the total cost for the procedure or program) and average benefits obtained from the program are easily calculated, but do not provide the crucial information needed to determine health policy. It is the additional, or incremental, costs and benefits compared with an alternative practice or program that permits the policy-maker to maximize health benefits with a limited healthcare budget [1]. Costs and health consequences (benefits) should be listed and a cost-effectiveness ratio, the metric for evaluating trade-offs across treatment alternatives, should be calculated for each strategy being compared. As an example, Table 8.2 lists both the average and incremental cost-utility ratios for alternative strategies for surveillance of patients with Barrett's esophagus. Cost-utility ratios are similar to cost-effectiveness ratios except that the outcomes reflect not only quantity (e.g., life-years gained) but also the quality of those years and consider disability and discomfort associated with the health condition under analysis (QALYs). Costs, here, refer to the direct medical costs of the surveillance tests themselves, as well any "induced costs" due to complications of surveillance procedures, the treatment costs for cancers that might be detected through surveillance, and the costs for the evaluation and

Table 8.2 Average costs and incremental costs for surveillance of patients with Barrett's esophagus

Strategy	Total cost (average) ($)	Average remaining quality-adjusted life expectancy	Average cost per quality-adjusted life-year gained ($)	Incremental cost ($)	Additional gain in quality-adjusted life expectancy (years)	Incremental cost per quality-adjusted life-year gained ($/QALY gained)
No surveillance	4100	12.64	324.36	D	D	D
Surveillance every 5 years	13 900	12.74	1091.05	9800	0.10	98 000
Surveillance every 4 years	15 116	12.73	1187.43	1216	−0.01	D
Surveillance every 3 years	6779	12.72	1319.10	1663	−0.01	D
Surveillance every 2 years	19 207	12.71	1511.72	2428	−0.01	D
Yearly surveillance	23 199	12.68	1829.57	3992	−0.03	D

D: dominated – costs more yet yields a lower quality-adjusted life expectancy. (Reproduced from Drummond MF *et al.* [11], with permission from Oxford University Press.)

treatment of cancers detected in those who are not undergoing surveillance, but who develop symptoms that lead to evaluation for cancer.

First, we focus on the average cost-utility ratio. The average cost-utility ratio, or cost per QALY gained, is calculated by dividing the total costs of a particular strategy by the gain in life expectancy for that strategy. For the no surveillance strategy, which serves as the basis for comparison, the costs amount to $4100 (Table 8.2, column 2) and the remaining quality-adjusted life expectancy is 12.64 years (column 3). The average cost-utility ratio is $4100 ÷ 12.64, or $324.36 per QALY gained, as shown in column 4. Moving to the next strategy, surveillance every 5 years, column 2 shows that the cost is $13 900 and column 3 shows that the quality-adjusted life expectancy is 12.74 years. In column 4, the average cost per QALY gained is $13 900 ÷ 12.74, or $1091.05.

Next, we will focus on the calculation of the incremental cost-utility ratio. Column 5 shows that the additional cost for adding surveillance every 5 years compared with no surveillance is $13 900 − $4100 = $9800. The average remaining quality-adjusted life expectancy for the individual who does not undergo surveillance is 12.64 years, while the quality-adjusted life expectancy for those undergoing surveillance every 5 years is on average 12.74 years. The years of life gained when surveillance every 5 years is initiated is 12.74 − 12.64 = 0.10 years (37 days) (column 6). The additional 0.10 years is the incremental benefit obtained by performing surveillance every 5 years. The incremental cost per QALY gained, or the incremental

cost-utility ratio as shown in column 7, is the incremental cost divided by the additional QALYs gained: $9800 ÷ 0.10 = $98 000, as shown in Table 8.2.

The incremental cost-utility ratios for the more aggressive surveillance strategies (every 1–4 years) are not calculated, as these strategies are dominated by surveillance every 5 years. In other words they cost more than surveillance every 5 years and they yield a lower quality-adjusted life expectancy than surveillance every 5 years as shown in Table 8.2 (columns 2 and 3). It is only with these incremental cost-utility or cost-effectiveness ratios that the policy-maker can determine if the additional benefit is worth the additional cost of adding surveillance compared with a previous policy of no surveillance.

Using these ratios, policy-makers who have a fixed budget can allocate funding based on incremental gains and losses. These cost-utility or cost-effectiveness ratios alone, however, cannot identify "cost-effective" practices. They must be placed in a decision context that is expressed in one of two forms. In the first form, an explicit threshold or maximum amount that the policy-maker is willing to spend is stated. For example, the policy-maker may be willing to spend $100 000/QALY gained to increase the length of life of patients with Barrett's esophagus by one year. Given our current estimates of cancer risk, surveillance every 5 years would increase quality-adjusted life expectancy and would not exceed the threshold of $100 000/ QALY gained. In the second form of decision context, a league table, as described earlier, which is a list of medical practices and their associated cost-utility ratios, is used as a basis for comparison with surveillance of patients with Barrett's esophagus. Table 8.1 lists incremental cost-utility ratios of practices in oncology. Surveillance of patients with Barrett's esophagus every 5 years has an incremental cost-utility ratio of $98 000/QALY gained. Referring to Table 8.1, this would be considered cost-effective compared with breast cancer screening in the 40–70-year age group every 1.3 years versus biennial breast cancer screening in the 50–70-year age group for the population of Dutch women, because it has a lower incremental cost utility ratio ($98 000/QALY vs $140 000/QALY).

Calculating incremental cost-effectiveness or cost-utility ratios for the alternative strategies is essential but does not provide us with a decision rule upon which to base health policy. Crucial parameters for decision-making include the cost of one strategy compared with another and the resources available to provide surveillance. Those who make health policy must also consider the number of patients affected by Barrett's esophagus and who might benefit from surveillance, and the number who would benefit from other comparison practices. In addition, the incidence of cancer is paramount in the decision-making process for Barrett's esophagus patients. Thus, the policymaker must consider several factors simultaneously when making decisions about funding. These include the budget, or willingness to pay threshold, the number of patients who would benefit from surveillance and the benefits to be gained, and the comparison between the cost of surveillance and the cost of other accepted medical practices.

From the patient's perspective, the quality of life associated with surveillance, the short-term discomfort and time lost from daily activities associated with procedures, and the long-term disability associated with esophagectomy, are also important factors.

9 Was a sensitivity analysis performed?

Due to variations in the literature estimates (each of which is affected by sampling and other types of errors) and differences in the opinions of experts in the field, there will be uncertainty surrounding one or more parameters in any economic analysis. To examine the effects of such variation on the results of the analysis, a sensitivity analysis should be performed. In sensitivity analysis, the value of each parameter of interest is varied over a broad range to determine the "sensitivity" of the results to variations in the parameter. The sensitivity of the preferred strategy to change in the underlying assumptions of the model is a measure of the strength, or robustness, of the conclusions. If the preferred strategy is altered by sensitivity analysis,

then the analysis is said to be sensitive to the value of that parameter. The reader of an economic analysis should seek some evidence that a sensitivity analysis has been performed. In an evaluation of surveillance of patients with Barrett's esophagus, a critical sensitivity analysis would be to vary the expected incidence of cancer over a broad range to determine the impact of an increase or decrease in the expected number of cases on the preferred strategy.

10 Did the presentation and discussion of study results include all issues of concern to users?

Assumptions and methodologic judgments are an integral part of an economic analysis. The reader should be provided with a list of the assumptions and value judgments that were made to perform the analysis, in order to determine the validity of the study and the applicability of the results to his or her practice. For example, in surveillance of patients with Barrett's esophagus, esophageal adenocarcinoma is assumed to occur as a progression from no dysplasia to low-grade dysplasia to high-grade dysplasia and finally to cancer. In addition, it is assumed that endoscopy is not a perfect test. There may be false positives or false negatives for dysplasia or cancer due to sampling error by the endoscopist and misinterpretation by the pathologist. The reader must decide if these assumptions are credible and the results applicable to his or her practice. In sensitivity analyses, the authors should consider a broad range of parameter assumptions to increase the generalizability of their analysis to populations that differ from their own.

These 10 criteria for economic appraisal provide a framework for reading and evaluating economic analyses in the medical literature. A more detailed discussion of these criteria for economic appraisal can be found in Drummond *et al.* [11], which provides a comprehensive review of the principles of health program evaluation.

In summary, this chapter provides an overview of the considerations involved in performing economic analyses, identifying cost-effective practices among alternative interventions and distinguishing between the different types of economic analyses. We have outlined the distinctions between costs and charges, and provided definitions of key terms used in the health economics literature. The types of economic analyses are outlined, and, finally, the criteria for evaluating economic analyses are presented. Examples are provided to illustrate both the concepts of economic analysis and the process of critically evaluating economic analyses to determine their applicability to clinical practice.

Acknowledgments

The work of the authors is supported in part by the NIDDK (Grant #5 K24 DK002926–07).

References

1. Provenzale D *et al.* A reader's guide to economic analysis in the GI literature. *Am J Gastroenterol* 1996;**91**:2461.
2. Brown ML *et al.* Economic analysis and clinical research. In: Gallin JI (ed.) *Principles and Practice of Clinical Research*. San Diego: Academic Press, 2002:275.
3. Luce BR *et al.* Estimating costs in cost-effectiveness analysis. In: Gold M *et al.* (eds) *Cost-Effectiveness in Health and Medicine*. New York: Oxford University Press, 1996:176.
4. Finkler SA. The distinction between cost and charges. *Ann Intern Med* 1982;**96**:102.
5. Fryback DG *et al.* Measuring economic outcomes in cancer. *J Natl Cancer Inst Monogr* 2004;**33**:134.
6. Weinstein MC *et al.* Productivity costs, time costs and health-related quality of life: a response to the Erasmus Group. *Health Economics* 1997;**6**:505.
7. Lipscomb J *et al.* Time preference. In: Gold M *et al.* (eds) *Cost-Effectiveness in Health and Medicine*. New York: Oxford University Press, 1996:214.
8. Brown ML. Cancer patient care in clinical trials sponsored by the National Cancer Institute: What does it cost? *J Natl Cancer Inst* 1999;819.
9. Gold MR *et al. Cost-Effectiveness in Health and Medicine*. New York: Oxford University Press, 1996.
10. Earle CC *et al.* Systematic overview of cost-utility assessments in oncology. *J Clin Oncol* 2000;**18**:3302.
11. Drummond MF *et al. Methods for the Economic Evaluation of Health Care Programs*. Oxford: Oxford University Press, 1987.
12. Cederqvist C *et al.* Cancer of the esophagus. II. Therapy and outcome. *Acta Chir Scand* 1978;**144**:233.
13. Skinner DB. En bloc resection for neoplasms of the esophagus and cardia. *J Thorac Cardiovasc Surg* 1983;**85**:59.
14. Ellis FH Jr *et al.* Esophagectomy. A safe, widely applicable, and expeditious form of palliation for patients with carcinoma of the esophagus and cardia. *Ann Surg* 1983;**198**:531.
15. Galandiuk S *et al.* Cancer of the esophagus. The Cleveland Clinic experience. *Ann Surg* 1986;**203**:101.
16. DeMeester TR *et al.* Selective therapeutic approach to cancer of the lower esophagus and cardia. *J Thorac Cardiovasc Surg* 1988;**95**:42.
17. Duke University Clinical Cost Manager. Transition Systems I, Boston, MA.
18 Transition System I: Clinical Cost Manager. Boston, MA: Transition Systems Inc.
19. *St. Anthony's DRG Working Guidebook*. Reston, Virginia: St. Anthony Publishing Inc., 1996.
20. Detsky AS *et al.* A clinician's guide to cost-effectiveness analysis. *Ann Intern Med* 1990;**113**:147.

Systematic Reviews

Philip Schoenfeld

Key points
- In order to deal with the exponential growth in digestive disease research, scientific data should be synthesized periodically in review articles.
- Systematic reviews utilize a standard methodology to search the literature, select appropriate articles for review, and for data extraction from these articles. Therefore, systematic reviews should be less biased than the standard narrative reviews, where the authors may ignore data that do not fit their conclusions.

- Systematic reviews are beneficial because they summarize the current knowledge about the treatment, diagnosis or natural history of a specific disorder. These reviews also provide insight about the methodologic weaknesses of current data and facilitate evaluation of specific subgroups of patients.
- Through this analysis, systematic reviews may be hypothesis-generating. Specific subgroups of patients that appear most likely to respond to a therapy may be identified. Because methodologic weaknesses of previous studies are highlighted, future studies can be designed to overcome these obstacles.

Introduction

The volume of published medical research is expanding exponentially. No practitioner can keep up with the enormous volume of published research. This research becomes a simple accumulation of facts unless practitioners pause to synthesize these data and consider how to apply them to the management of their individual patients. Therefore, review articles provide an appropriate forum to assess the methods and the results of research studies about a particular topic. Narrative reviews used to represent the vast majority of published review articles. In these articles, an "expert" discusses published data about a specific topic in a nonstandardized fashion. This approach frequently leads to biased presentations of data. If an "expert" holds a specific point of view about the management of a disorder, then that "expert" may simply focus on research studies that support his or her

point of view while ignoring research studies that refute their position. Systematic reviews avoid this bias because they utilize a standard methodology to retrieve articles, select articles for inclusion in a systematic review, and for a detailed analysis of methodology and results from individual studies. Thus, systematic reviews are more likely to provide an unbiased and comprehensive analysis of data about a specific topic.

In this chapter, we will provide a more detailed discussion about the differences between narrative reviews and systematic reviews while listing the methodology of well-designed systematic reviews (Box 9.1). Specifically, we will review techniques for comprehensive literature searching, development of study selection criteria, techniques to assess the validity of individual studies, techniques for data extraction from individual studies, and qualitative techniques to present results from individual studies.

Narrative reviews versus systematic reviews

In a traditional review article or narrative review, an "expert" usually provides their opinions about the management of a very broad topic. For example, a typical review article might discuss new diagnostic tests and new

Box 9.1 Criteria for a well-designed systematic review
1 Develop a focused question.
2 Specify study selection criteria.
3 Perform a comprehensive literature search.
4 Assess the validity of individual studies in the systematic review.
5 Demonstrate reproducibility of data extraction from individual studies.

therapies for the management of Crohn's disease, which is certainly a very broad topic. The "expert" will cite research studies that support their conclusions. These conclusions may be based on appropriately designed research studies and/or the author's clinical judgment and experience. This exercise is not a reproducible exercise and the validity or "foundation of evidence" for the conclusions of narrative reviews may be quite variable [1]. Research about narrative review articles actually demonstrated this by asking leading "experts" in different fields to judge the quality of narrative reviews written by their colleagues [2]. When reviewing this research, Sackett and colleagues noted that "experts could not agree, even among themselves, about whether other experts who wrote review articles had conducted a competent search for relative studies, generated a bias-free list of citations, appropriately judged the scientific quality of the cited articles, or appropriately synthesized their conclusions. Indeed, when these experts' own review articles were subjected to the same simple scientific principles, there was an inverse relationship between adherence to these standards and self-professed expertise." [3]

Therefore, evidence-based medicine principles endorse the use of systematic reviews to produce an unbiased synthesis of the research about a specific topic [4,5]. Systematic reviews utilize the methodology that is absent from narrative reviews. There is a comprehensive search of the medical literature for relevant studies. A bias-free list of citations is developed, and citations that refute the author's views are not excluded. The scientific quality of a study's research design is judged (e.g., for trials about therapy, authors will determine if randomization or double-blinding were utilized). Finally, the conclusions in the review article can be directly correlated to the data generated from all relevant articles identified in the literature search. Thus, a bias-free review of the literature should be provided by the systematic review whereas the narrative review is subject to multiple different types of bias, which may limit the validity of the narrative reviews' conclusions [2].

Should you do a systematic review?

Colleagues and trainees frequently ask me questions about how to design a research trial on a specific topic. I usually encourage my colleagues to search the literature for a systematic review on this topic. Because medical research is continually expanding, many research questions have been addressed by published studies. However, many of these studies provide biased results due to flaws in study methodology, selection of patient populations,

or use of clinically unimportant endpoints. Well-designed systematic reviews should identify hypotheses that have not been answered by published research and discuss the ideal design for future research studies about their topic. **If a recent systematic review is not available, then I advise my colleagues and trainees to perform a systematic review on their topic before embarking on their original research study.** By performing a systematic review, a new hypothesis about a specific disorder may be generated. You may identify specific patient populations that should be evaluated with a new therapy, or you may identify a more appropriate endpoint to utilize in your own study, or you may identify other methodologic flaws (e.g., lack of appropriate blinding) that limited the validity of results from other published studies and insure that you don't make the same mistake in your own original research study.

This chapter will outline the steps that should be performed when conducting a systematic review. However, if you are thinking of performing a systematic review, then I recommend that you obtain assistance from two types of "experts." First, health services researchers who have been trained in the performance of systematic reviews and meta-analyses will facilitate the design and execution of your systematic review. Health services researchers with this experience are present at most academic research centers. Also, you should collaborate with a "content expert" on your topic. A "content expert" is an experienced clinician who is considered a leading practitioner in this field and who has published research studies about your topic. With this background, your "content expert" should be very familiar with the published data about your topic. This "expert" should be able to identify areas of controversy in published research and methodologic flaws in the selection of patient populations or study endpoints. Therefore, your "content expert" can assist you with the development of focused questions while your systematic review is still in the planning stages. Overall, you should view the performance of a systematic review as a "team" effort that utilizes the skills of your methodology expert and your content expert.

Developing a focused question

A focused question consists of three parts: (i) patient population, (ii) intervention, and (iii) study endpoint. For example, a focused question might ask: *Among patients with ileocecal Crohn's disease* [patient population], *is 6-MP or placebo* [intervention] *more likely to maintain remission of Crohn's disease* [study endpoint]? Another example addresses this question for a diagnostic test study: *Among average-risk 50-year-old patients referred for colorectal cancer screening* [patient population], *how accurate is CT colonography compared to colonoscopy* [intervention] *for the diagnosis of large (≥1-cm) polyps* [study endpoint]? Focused questions may also be developed around epidemiologic issues: *In population-based studies* [patient population], *what is the prevalence of irritable bowel syndrome* [study endpoint] *based upon results of a questionnaire using ROME II criteria for the diagnosis of irritable bowel syndrome* [intervention]?

The development of your focused question is crucial because it guides the development of your study selection criteria. For example, if your systematic review will answer the question about efficacy of 6-MP for maintenance of remission of ileocecal Crohn's disease, then your systematic review will include all published research studies about patients with ileocecal Crohn's disease in remission who were treated with 6-MP or placebo with a study endpoint of duration of Crohn's disease remission.

Many investigators will add a fourth component to their focused question: study methodology. For example, focused questions about therapy might only utilize randomized controlled trials because these trials are less likely to produce biased results, or you might limit your systematic review to randomized, double-blind trials, which are least likely to produce biased results. If you utilize this criteria, then your focused question might become: *Based upon the results of randomized, double-blind trials* [study methodology] *in patients with ileocecal Crohn's disease* [patient population], *is 6-MP or placebo* [intervention] *more likely to maintain remission of Crohn's disease* [study endpoint]? Your "content expert" may be particularly valuable at this stage. He or she should be very familiar with the published research on this topic. If your "content expert" states that there are only 1–2 randomized, double-blind trials about this topic, then it would be futile to perform a systematic review. With this advice from your "content expert", you would probably revise your focused question.

Comprehensive literature search

It is only through the performance of a comprehensive literature search that the authors can ensure a bias-free list of citations. Therefore, authors of a systematic review should identify all studies that meet their inclusion criteria. Generally, this means that multiple bibliographic databases, including Medline, EMBASE (a European version of Medline), the Cochrane controlled trials database (which contains listing for more than 200 000 randomized controlled trials), and Current Contents (which lists recently published data) should be searched using search criteria that derive from your focused question. When the literature search has been completed, the authors should review the titles and abstracts of individual articles from the literature searches in order to identify articles that fit their study selection criteria. After obtaining relevant articles, the authors should also review the reference list or citations in these articles in order to identify additional relevant studies.

These electronic bibliographic searches should not be limited to articles published in the English language. Important articles may be published in Spanish, French, Japanese, etc. Don't despair about this process. The abstracts of these non-English language articles are usually available in English, and you can usually determine if an article meets your study selection criteria based upon the abstract. If a non-English language article does meet your study selection criteria, then you will need to obtain a copy and obtain a translation of the study.

Finally, authors of systematic reviews should beware "publication bias" [6–8]. This issue can be understood in the context of "positive studies" and "negative studies." The term "negative studies" is sometimes used to refer to studies that do not show a difference between a therapy and a placebo, or to studies that do not demonstrate a difference in diagnostic accuracy between a new diagnostic test and a standard or conventional diagnostic test. The term "positive studies" is sometimes used to refer to studies that do demonstrate statistically significant differences between a new therapy and placebo or between a new diagnostic test and a standard diagnostic test. Epidemiologic research demonstrates that "positive studies" are more likely to be accepted quickly for publication as a full manuscript compared with "negative studies" on a similar topic [8]. There appears to be a "publication bias" against "negative studies" [6–8]. The effect of this "publication bias" upon systematic reviews is obvious. If only "positive studies" are published, then only "positive studies" will be included in the systematic review and an overestimation about the benefits of a treatment may result. Systematic reviews based upon a few studies with small sample sizes are most susceptible to publication bias, and readers of these systematic reviews should be cautious about the conclusions from this type of systematic review. As Gordon Guyatt said, "Results that seem too good to be true may well not be true." Nevertheless, "negative studies" are frequently published as abstracts. In order to avoid "publication bias," the authors of a systematic review should seek out "negative studies" that were published as abstracts, but may not have been accepted for publication as a full manuscript. Therefore, the proceedings from national and international meetings should be reviewed in order to identify recently published abstracts that fit the study selection criteria.

When the authors of systematic reviews identify a topical abstract that has not been published in full manuscript form, they will need to obtain detailed study results from the authors of the abstract. It may be difficult to get the authors of these abstracts to assist you with your systematic review, and this is another area where your "content expert" may be helpful. If your "content expert" is well known in the field, then he or she may have personal relationships with top investigators in this field, or a reputation that makes it easier for him or her to pick up a phone and ask another investigator for assistance with your systematic review.

Assessing the validity of individual studies in your systematic review

Systematic reviews should assess the methodologic quality of individual studies included in the review. Epidemiologic studies describe the criteria for high-quality studies of therapy (Box 9.2), and evidence-based medicine articles provide guidelines to assess the quality of studies on therapy, diagnostic tests, prognosis, etc. These principles can be applied when assessing the methodologic quality of individual studies [9–12]. It is beyond the scope of this chapter to review these criteria in detail, although some basic points should be reviewed.

First, there is no single correct way to assess the methodologic quality of individual studies. Various systems have been utilized by different authors [13]. Using evidence-based medicine principles, you should define your system for assessing the methodologic quality of individual studies, describe this system in the "Methods" section of your systematic review, and apply it to the individual studies in your systematic review. The results of your methodologic quality assessment for each individual study should be reported in the "Results" section of your systematic review. Second, studies of therapy should generally be limited to randomized controlled trials because nonrandomized controlled trials are much more likely to provide biased evidence. There has been one validated scale to assess the

---

Box 9.2 Validated criteria for a well-designed study of a therapy

1 Was the study randomized? Did the study include randomization with concealed allocation?
If the study was described as randomized, then award one point. If the study was described as randomized and used concealed allocation and used computer generation of the randomization sequence, then award two points. If the study was described as randomization, but used inappropriate randomization (e.g., patients allocated alternately), then award zero points.

2 Was the study double-blinded?
If the study was described as double-blind, then award one point. If the study was described as double-blind and described use of identical placebo or active placebo, then award two points. If the study was described as double-blind, but used inappropriate blinding (e.g., comparison of tablet vs injection with no double dummy), then award zero points.

3 Did the study account for withdrawals and drop-outs of study patients?

(Adapted from Jadad *et al.* [14], with permission from Elsevier.)

---

validity of individual therapy studies [13,14]. This scale focuses on the use of randomization with concealed allocation, the use of double-blinding, and the complete follow-up of study patients as the criteria to identify a high-quality therapy study. Third, individual studies of a new diagnostic test should compare the new diagnostic test with a valid gold standard diagnostic test, which definitively rules in or rules out the diagnosis [11]. For example, a study about the utility of magnetic resonance cholangiopancreatography (MRCP, a "new" diagnostic test) for the diagnosis of choledocholithiasis might be compared with the gold standard of endoscopic retrograde cholangiopancreatography (ERCP). This comparison should be done in a blinded fashion where the physician performing the MRCP does not know the results from the "gold standard" diagnosis by ERCP [15]. Finally, the new diagnostic test should be studied in a patient population that is similar to the population where the new diagnostic test is likely to be used. Further discussions about techniques to assess methodologic quality of individual studies are referenced and should be reviewed by the interested reader [11,16].

Assessment of individual studies should be reproducible

When performing a systematic review, the data from individual studies need to be extracted and the methodology of these studies needs to be evaluated. This process requires some judgment because some studies do not provide adequate detail about study methodology (e.g., the process for blinding patients and physicians) or presentation of study results may not be straightforward. Consequently, data extraction about study results and assessment of study methodology is subject to mistakes (i.e., random errors) and bias (i.e., systematic errors).

In order to overcome this obstacle, two or more people should independently review each individual study. After data extraction is complete, the investigators can compare the results of their data extraction. If disagreement occurs, then the individual study may be reviewed by both authors in order to resolve this disagreement. This process reduces the potential for mistakes (e.g., random errors). If disagreement is common between two authors of the systematic review, then the reader should suspect that one author was biased in their data extraction process. Well-designed systematic reviews report the frequency of agreement between two investigators who have extracted data. Many systematic reviews will include this type of statement: "independent duplicate extraction of data was performed by two authors, and agreement between the two authors for data extraction was greater than 95%. Disagreements in data extraction were resolved by consensus between the two authors after review of an individual study."

Presenting the results

The next chapter in this book, concerning meta-analyses, will provide a more detailed discussion about the quantitative presentation of results from a systematic review. In a meta-analysis, numerical data from individual studies are combined to create a single summary statistic. In order for this quantitative summary to be valid, the results from individual studies should be similar, and this assumption may be tested with a statistical technique called the "test of heterogeneity."

Sometimes, individual studies use very different endpoints, and a quantitative summary of the data cannot be performed. The health services researcher on your systematic review team can help you decide if it will be impossible to combine the data quantitatively into a single summary statistic. If a quantitative analysis isn't possible, then a qualitative summary of the data should be performed. Generally, a systematic review contains multiple tables that provide a detailed description of all included study populations, study design, study intervention and results. By providing these data in a tabular form, the reader can easily assess differences and similarities between individual studies, and identify differences in study population, study design or study intervention that may account for the differences in individual study results.

Conclusion

Because the volume of published medical research is expanding exponentially, review articles provide a valuable resource for clinicians. Systematic reviews provide a tool to summarize comprehensively the data about a specific topic. The methodology of systematic reviews minimizes the potential for bias in the selection or assessment of individual studies included in the systematic review. Such reviews may identify the most appropriate patient population for a particular therapy or the most effective dosage for a particular therapy. Therefore, the results of a systematic review may facilitate your individual patient care. Systematic reviews are also a valuable research tool. Before beginning a new research study, investigators should ensure that they are not repeating studies that have already been conducted. Systematic reviews also provide investigators with a tool to generate hypotheses because these reviews may identify questions that have not been adequately addressed by published research.

References

1. Mulrow CD. The medical review article: state of the science. *Ann Intern Med* 1987;**106**:485.
2. Oxman A, Guyatt G. The science of reviewing research. *Ann NY Acad Sci* 1993;**703**:125.
3. Sackett DL *et al.* (eds) *Evidence Based Medicine: How to Practice and Teach EBM*. New York: Churchill Livingstone, 1993;13.
4. Guyatt G, Rennie D (eds) *Users' Guides to the Medical Literature: A Manual for Evidence-Based Clinical Practice*. Chicago: AMA Press, 2002;155.
5. Irwig L *et al.* Guidelines for meta-analyses evaluating diagnostic tests. *Ann Intern Med* 1994;**120**:667.
6. Dickersin K. The existence of publication bias and risk factors for its occurrence. *JAMA* 1990;**263**:1385.
7. Stern JM, Simes RJ. Publication bias: evidence of delayed publication in a cohort study of clinical research projects. *Br*

Med J 1997;**315**:640.

8. Ioannidis JP. Effect of statistical significance of results on the time to completion and publication of randomized efficacy trials. *JAMA* 1998;**279**:281.

9. Guyatt G *et al.* Users' guides to the medical literature. How to use an article about therapy or prevention. *JAMA* 1993;**270**:2598.

10. Schoenfeld P *et al.* An evidence based approach to gastroenterology therapy. *Gastroenterology* 1998;**114**:1318.

11. Schoenfeld P *et al.* An evidence based approach to gastroenterology diagnosis. *Gastroenterology* 1999;**116**:1230.

12. Laupacis A *et al.* Users' guides to the medical literature. How to use an article about prognosis. *JAMA* 1994;**272**:234.

13. Moher D *et al.* Assessing the quality of randomized controlled trials: an annotated bibliography of scales and checklists. *Control Clin Trials* 1995;**16**:62.

14. Jadad AR *et al.* Assessing the quality of reports of randomized clinical trials: is blinding necessary? *Control Clin Trials* 1996;**17**:1.

15. Chan Y *et al.* Choledocholithiasis: comparison of MR cholangiography and endoscopic retrograde cholangiography. *Radiology* 1996;**200**:85.

16. Egger M *et al.* (eds) *Systematic Reviews in Health Care: Meta-Analysis in Context.* London: BMJ Publishing Group, 2001.

10 Meta-analyses

Paul Moayyedi

Key points

- Meta-analysis is a statistical tool to derive a weighted average of study results.
- There is often heterogeneity between studies and it is not clear in this circumstance which statistical method should be used to pool results.
- It is important to explore reasons for heterogeneity.
- Heterogeneity can occur because of publication bias, methodologic differences or clinical characteristics of the study.
- Analysis can be conducted using subgroup analysis or meta-regression but results should be interpreted cautiously.

Introduction

Information technology has dramatically increased the speed at which data can be communicated to the scientific community and has also expanded choices for accessing and disseminating knowledge. The advantages of this are obvious, but physicians can become bombarded with information that is sometimes contradictory and difficult to assimilate. Systematic reviews can help to overcome this by rigorously identifying all available information on a specific research question. A good systematic review will then use methodology that minimizes bias in determining which studies are eligible and how the data are extracted. Systematic reviews have been applied mostly to randomized controlled trials of healthcare interventions, but there are many research questions where this design is not feasible or appropriate. In these situations observational designs such as cross-sectional, case series, case-control and cohort studies can be very helpful, and methods for conducting systematic reviews of these types of studies have been described [1]. Once all relevant information has been collected then researchers often attempt to combine the data statistically, and this is termed meta-analysis. It must be emphasized that it is only sensible to attempt to combine the data if all relevant studies have been identified and the data extracted appropriately as described in the previous chapter. Too often researchers will perform a meta-analysis on data that have not been rigorously identified and collected. This approach is likely to lead to erroneous conclusions and is akin to building an elaborate skyscraper without bothering to construct any founda-tions. Even if the systematic review is rigorous, the method of statistically pooling the data is not straightforward, particularly in the context of epidemiologic studies.

Synthesizing the data

The first step in synthesizing the data is to decide on the summary statistic that will be utilized [2]. These are usually odds ratio, relative risk, risk difference or another ratio such as a simple proportion. Continuous data (e.g., height or weight) can also be pooled but these will not be discussed further. The choice of the summary statistic is often decided by the type of study design. For example, case control studies should be summarized using odds ratios whereas the prevalence of disease will be described as a proportion. Co-hort studies are usually presented in terms of relative risk.

Once the summary statistic has been chosen, then this is calculated for each study in the systematic review. The overall result is then calculated by taking a **weighted average** of these summary statistics. The method of weighting varies but in practice this often relates to the **inverse variance of the outcome** being assessed, which in turn is correlated with the sample size.

There are two statistical approaches to meta-analysis. One approach is the **fixed effect** meta-analysis [3], which assumes that each study is measuring the same effect and any variation between studies is due to chance. This assumption can be tested statistically using a test for heterogeneity [4]. If the P value falls below a prespecified threshold (conservatively this is usually set at 0.1, 0.15 or

0.2 rather than the traditional $P < 0.05$) then there is statistically significant heterogeneity. The assumption that all the studies are measuring the same effect is therefore not fulfilled and a fixed effect model may give invalid results. The other approach is a **random effects** model [5], which does not make the assumption that each study is measuring the same underlying effect. This type of analysis **adds a constant** to the weighting of the studies that is **related to the between-study variance**. This has the effect of making the weighting of the studies more similar but also widens the confidence interval.

For example, a systematic review of bismuth salts in functional dyspepsia [6] identified five placebo-controlled randomized trials, and in the fixed effects meta-analysis there was a statistically significant effect in favor of the active treatment (Fig. 10.1a). However, there was statistically significant heterogeneity in the data, so the assumption made in the fixed effects analysis that all trials were measuring the same effect of bismuth is very unlikely. A random effects model was more conservative and did not find a statistically significant effect of bismuth salts in functional dyspepsia, although a trend was still apparent (Fig. 10.1b). This example also highlights the problem of random effects models. As studies are weighted more equally, the smaller negative study is weighted almost the same as the larger

positive study. Small randomized trials are often of poorer quality than larger trials so there is a danger that this analysis is putting more emphasis on inferior studies and this may bias the results. For this reason, there is no consensus on whether random or fixed effects models should be used to synthesize the data [7]. If there is little heterogeneity between studies then the constant that is applied to random effects models will be close to zero and both approaches will give very similar results. If there is important heterogeneity between studies then it will be unclear which approach is more valid. Indeed, some have argued that the results should not be synthesized at all in view of this uncertainty and more emphasis should be placed on exploring the reasons for variablity between studies [8].

Whilst clearly true of randomized controlled trials, this is even more relevant to observational studies. Epidemiologic studies are open to bias and confounding factors that can give rise to spurious associations. Study designs can attempt to minimize bias and control for confounding factors but ultimately these may still influence the overall result. In the case of randomized controlled trials, one of the main reasons to perform a meta-analysis is that individual studies are underpowered and synthesizing the data should give a more precise estimate of effect. This is not the case with epidemiologic data as large database studies

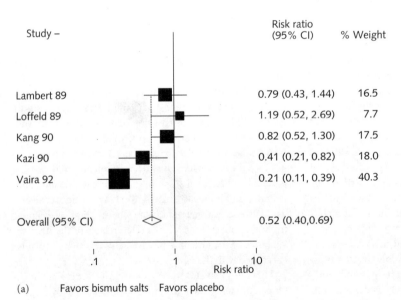

(a)   Favors bismuth salts   Favors placebo

Fig. 10.1* Meta-analysis of bismuth salts versus placebo in functional dyspepsia using (a) a fixed effects model *(Continued.)*

*How to read a forest plot: forest plots are a graphical representation of a group of studies. Each box represents an individual study. The size of the box represents the weight given to that study in the overall meta-analysis. The line running through the box is the 95% confidence intervals (CI) of that study. If the 95% CI cross the vertical axis then that study did not give a statistically significant result. The diamond at the bottom of the graph represents the pooled results. Again if the diamond crosses the vertical axis then the pooled data did not give a statistically significant result. In this example the diamond is to the left of the vertical line, suggesting bismuth salts have a statistically significant effect on dyspepsia.

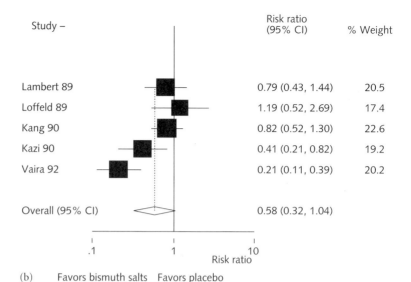

Fig. 10.1 *(Continued.)* (b) a random effects model [4]. In (a) the test for heterogeneity χ2 = 18.0, degrees of freedom = 4, P = 0.001. Note that in (b) the weight of a small negative trial (Loffeld, 1989) increases from 7.7% to 17.4% and the weight of a large positive trial falls from 40.3% to 20.2%.

can be performed relatively easily and cheaply. However, as they use routinely collected data they may be more prone to bias and may not capture all important confounding factors. The issue with epidemiologic studies is therefore often not lack of precision but concern whether the results are spurious. Combining all data to give one overall effect may simply magnify the methodologic weaknesses of each individual study, and in this case the increased statistical power of a meta-analysis can be irrelevant [9]. For this reason, some researchers suggest that meta-analysis of epidemiologic data should not be performed [10]. This is probably overstating the case but it is clear that the overall effect size should not be presented in isolation and often should not be the prominent component of the review. Instead, most emphasis should be placed on why there are variations in the study findings so a more measured conclusion can be reached.

Exploring reasons for heterogeneity

There are a various reasons why studies can give different results and these can broadly be categorized as small study effects, differences in study quality, and clinical variations between studies [11].

Publication bias and other small study effects

In randomized controlled trials small studies are more likely to be published if they are positive and are also more likely to be cited [12]. This publication bias can lead to a meta-analysis suggesting that there is a positive treatment effect, albeit one driven by only small positive trials being published and included in a systematic review. This possibility can be evaluated by assessing funnel plot asymmetry. Funnel plots are a graphical representation of the study effect size on the x-axis and a measure of the overall size of the study on the y-axis. There should be a large spread of treatment effects reported with small studies due to random variation but this should get less as the sample size gets larger. An ideal funnel plot should therefore be symmetrical around the overall effect size of the meta-analysis, with a lot of variation at the bottom of the plot (representing the small studies) and much less at the top of the plot. If the quadrant of 'negative' small studies is missing at the bottom right-hand corner of the plot, this suggests publication bias (Fig. 10.2). This asymmetry can be tested statistically [13].

Funnel plots can also be used to detect publication bias in epidemiologic studies but the interpretation of asymmetry is often more complex [14]. The assumption when evaluating funnel plots is that the smaller studies exaggerate the treatment effect. This is usually correct in randomized controlled trials but this is not the case with observational studies. For example, a small study that carefully avoids bias in the assessment of risk factors and disease outcomes and also adjusts for a wide variety of potential confounding factors may be more accurate than a large database study that collects very little information on a huge sample size.

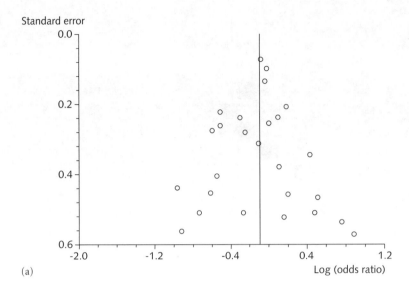

(a)

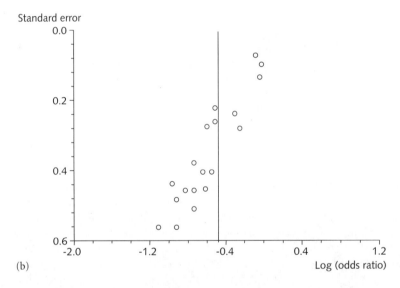

(b)

Fig. 10.2 Theoretical example of a Funnel plot. (a) Symmetrical plot; (b) asymmetrical plot.

Differences in study quality

The factors in study methodology that influence the outcome of randomized controlled trials and should be addressed in meta-analyses have been well characterized. Trials that are truly randomized, have concealment of allocation, and are double blind with almost complete follow-up provide the most rigorous assessment of treatment effect [15]. The factors that influence the meta-analysis of observational studies have been less well characterized [16]. Nevertheless, some general principles can be followed. There are numerous causes of bias in epidemiologic research [17]. For example, the investigator and subject may know whether or not a subject has the disease of interest. The investigator could therefore be biased in their assessment of the patient with disease, and cases may be more likely to recall exposures to a variety of putative risk factors compared with controls. Masking of investigators can reduce some biases, and meta-analyses of case-control studies that are not blinded can result in an exaggerated association between risk factors and disease [18].

Prospective cohort studies are less prone to some types of bias than case-control studies as the participants have not yet developed the disease. Cohort studies may therefore give a less biased estimate of whether a risk factor is associated with disease. A meta-analysis of observational studies evaluating coffee intake and colorectal cancer suggested that coffee reduced the risk of developing disease [19]. The authors separated out case-control and cohort studies, and the "protective" effect of coffee consumption was only seen in case-control studies, with no statistically significant association found in cohort studies (Fig. 10.3a,b). It is more likely that the cohort studies revealed the truth in this analysis and combining these study designs may produce spurious conclusions.

Clinical variations between studies

There are numerous clinical factors that can impact on study results. Demographic factors such as gender, age, ethnicity, social class and country of origin can influence outcomes. The accuracy of measurement of risk factor and outcomes is also important. If there is a lack of rigor in measuring these there will be random misclassification of subjects, which will bias the study results toward the null hypothesis [20]. Different approaches to measuring risk factors and disease outcomes can also increase heterogeneity between studies. For example, there are numerous general population surveys of the prevalence of dyspepsia, with results varying between 10% and 50% [21]. Such wide variation was not due to chance but much of it could be explained by the definition of dyspepsia used in the study. Those that included predominant heartburn in their definition had consistently higher estimates of prevalence than those that excluded this symptom from their definition of dyspepsia (Fig. 10.4).

Approaches to assessing reasons for heterogeneity

The two main approaches to assessing reasons for heterogeneity are subgroup analysis and meta-regression. Subgroup analyses are conducted by categorizing the factor that is thought to be important in causing heterogeneity and performing meta-analyses on each subgroup to assess whether overall results are different between the groups and whether heterogeneity is less within each group. The alternative approach is to use meta-regression [22], which is analogous to logistic regression but measures

Summary meta-analysis plot [random effects]

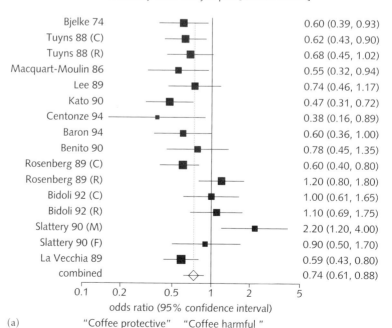

Bjelke 74	0.60 (0.39, 0.93)
Tuyns 88 (C)	0.62 (0.43, 0.90)
Tuyns 88 (R)	0.68 (0.45, 1.02)
Macquart-Moulin 86	0.55 (0.32, 0.94)
Lee 89	0.74 (0.46, 1.17)
Kato 90	0.47 (0.31, 0.72)
Centonze 94	0.38 (0.16, 0.89)
Baron 94	0.60 (0.36, 1.00)
Benito 90	0.78 (0.45, 1.35)
Rosenberg 89 (C)	0.60 (0.40, 0.80)
Rosenberg 89 (R)	1.20 (0.80, 1.80)
Bidoli 92 (C)	1.00 (0.61, 1.65)
Bidoli 92 (R)	1.10 (0.69, 1.75)
Slattery 90 (M)	2.20 (1.20, 4.00)
Slattery 90 (F)	0.90 (0.50, 1.70)
La Vecchia 89	0.59 (0.43, 0.80)
combined	0.74 (0.61, 0.88)

0.1   0.2   0.5   1   2   5

odds ratio (95% confidence interval)

"Coffee protective"   "Coffee harmful "

Fig. 10.3 Meta-analysis of (a) case-control studies. *(Continued.)*   (a)

Summary meta-analysis plot [random effects]

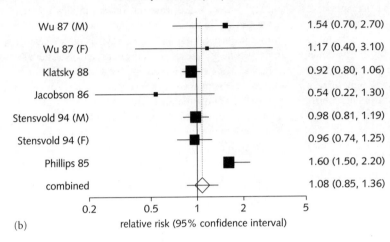

Wu 87 (M)	1.54 (0.70, 2.70)
Wu 87 (F)	1.17 (0.40, 3.10)
Klatsky 88	0.92 (0.80, 1.06)
Jacobson 86	0.54 (0.22, 1.30)
Stensvold 94 (M)	0.98 (0.81, 1.19)
Stensvold 94 (F)	0.96 (0.74, 1.25)
Phillips 85	1.60 (1.50, 2.20)
combined	1.08 (0.85, 1.36)

relative risk (95% confidence interval)

(b)

Fig. 10.3 *(Continued.)* (b) cohort studies evaluating the association between coffee intake and colorectal cancer [19].

study level characteristics in the model. This approach can allow multiple factors to be adjusted for simultaneously and will also give a quantitative estimate of the effect a given factor has on the overall result. For example, in a systematic review of *Helicobacter pylori* eradication in the prevention of peptic ulcer disease [23] there was statistically significant heterogeneity, which in part was explained by the efficacy of regimens used in the various studies in eradicating *H. pylori*. Meta-regression allowed

a quantitative estimate to be made of how this impacted on results. Although the average eradication rate achieved in the trials was only 72% from meta-regression, it could be predicted that there would be a 2 percentage point reduction in duodenal ulcer relapse for every 10 percentage point increase in eradication rate [23]. One of the disadvantages of meta-regression is that the factors measured are at the level of the individual study rather than the individual patient, and any positive result could be spurious and due to the ecological fallacy [24]. This can be avoided by obtaining individual patient data from each study and conducting an individual patient data meta-analysis [25]. This is a much more rigorous and powerful approach to meta-analysis, but is very laborious and is usually not possible for older studies.

There are countless factors that could influence results of studies. It may not be possible to evaluate reasons for variation as there are insufficient papers in the systematic review. On the other hand, if there are a large number of papers identified by the review then there is a temptation to exhaustively assess all possible reasons for heterogeneity. If this approach is taken then there will be differences between subgroups that are due simply to chance as multiple testing has been performed [26]. It is important therefore to write a protocol before conducting a systematic review and prespecify the analyses that are going to be performed to try to explain the variation between studies.

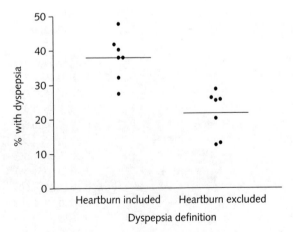

Fig. 10.4 Variation in dyspepsia prevalence in the general population depending on definition used [21].

Conclusions

Meta-analysis is a powerful tool to synthesize research findings from a systematic review. Usually there is heterogeneity in the results of studies and it is important to go beyond the grand mean [27] and explore why researchers reach different conclusions. Subgroup analyses in meta-analyses, like subgroup analyses in trials, can be prone to bias and need to be interpreted cautiously. Nevertheless, describing the data more fully can lead to greater understanding of the research question being addressed and provide new insights that can guide future studies.

References

1. Stroup DF *et al*. Meta-analysis of observational studies in epidemiolog y: a proposal for reporting. Meta-analysis Of Observational Studies in Epidemiology (MOOSE) group. *JAMA* 2000;**283**:2008.
2. Deeks JJ. Issues in the selection of a summary statistic for meta-analysis of clinical trials with binary outcomes. *Stat Med* 2002;**21**:1575.
3. McElvenny DM *et al*. Meta-analysis in occupational epidemiology: a review of practice. *Occup Med-Oxford* 2004;**54**:336.
4. Higgins JP et al. Measuring inconsistency in meta-analyses. *Br Med J* 2003;**327**:557.
5. Ades AE, Higgins JPT. The interpretation of random-effects meta-analysis in decision models. *Med Decis Making* 2005;**25**:646.
6. Moayyedi P *et al*. Pharmacological interventions for non-ulcer dyspepsia. *Cochrane DB Syst Rev* 2004;(4):CD001960; PMID:15495023.
7. Thompson SG, Pocock SJ. Can meta-analyses be trusted? *Lancet* 1991;**338**:1127.
8. Thompson SG. Why sources of heterogeneity in meta-analysis should be investigated. *Br Med J* 1994;**309**:1351.
9. Egger M *et al*. Spurious precision? Meta-analysis of observational studies. *Br Med J* 1998;**316**:140.
10. Shapiro S. Meta-analysis/Shmeta-analysis. *Am J Epidemiol* 1994;**140**:771.
11. Moayyedi P. Meta-analysis: Can we mix apples and oranges?. *Am J Gastroenterol* 2004;**99**:2297.
12. Sterne JA *et al*. Systematic reviews in health care: Investigating and dealing with publication and other biases in meta-analysis. *Br Med J* 2001;**323**:101.
13. Sterne JA *et al*. Publication and related bias in meta-analysis: power of statistical tests and prevalence in the literature. *J Clin Epidemiol* 2000;**53**:1119.
14. Sutton AJ *et al*. Empirical assessment of effect of publication bias on meta-analyses. *Br Med J* 2000;**320**:1574.
15. Juni P *et al*. Systematic reviews in health care: Assessing the quality of controlled clinical trials. *Br Med J* 2001;**323**:42.
16. Blettner M *et al*. Traditional reviews, meta-analyses and pooled analyses in epidemiology. *Int J Epidemiol* 1999;**28**:1.
17. Sackett DL. Bias in analytic research. *J Chron Dis* 1979;**32**:51.
18. Nelemans PJ *et al*. An addition to the controversy on sunlight exposure and melanoma risk: a meta-analytical approach. *J Clin Epidemiol* 1995;**48**:1331.
19. Giovannucci E. Meta-analysis of coffee consumption and risk of colorectal cancer. *Am J Epidemiol* 1998;**147**:1043.
20. Lyngbye T. Methodological problems in assessing health-related, neuropsychological effects of lead absorption in a very low-level exposed area. *Cent Eur J Pub Health* 1997;**5**:70.
21. Moayyedi P, Delaney BC. Dyspepsia. In: Stevens A, Raftery J (eds) *Health Care Needs Assessment*, 3rd edn. Oxford: Radcliffe Press (http://hcna.radcliffe-oxford.com/dysframe. htm).
22. Thompson SG, Higgins JP. How should meta-regression analyses be undertaken and interpreted? Stat Med 2002;**21**:1559.
23. Ford AC *et al*. Eradication therapy for peptic ulcer disease in Helicobacter pylori positive patients. *Cochrane DB Syst Rev* (2):CD003840, 2006.
24. Higgins JP, Thompson SG. Controlling the risk of spurious findings from meta-regression. *Stat Med* 2004;**23**:1663.
25. Simmonds MC *et al*. Meta-analysis of individual patient data from randomized trials: a review of methods used in practice. *Clin Trials* 2005;**2**:209.
26. Higgins J *et al*. Statistical heterogeneity in systematic reviews of clinical trials: a critical appraisal of guidelines and practice. *J Health Services Res Policy* 2002;**7**:51.
27. Davey Smith G *et al*. Meta-analysis. Beyond the grand mean? *Br Med J* 1997;**315**:1610.

11 Large Databases for Epidemiologic Studies

Jessica A. Davila and Hashem B. El-Serag

Key points
- Large databases can be a powerful source of information to examine the clinical epidemiology and outcomes of digestive and liver disorders.
- Research using large databases requires the same essential skills needed to conduct research studies using other data sources. These include a rigorous study design, expertise in analytic methods, and relevant research questions.
- The completeness and accuracy of information contained in the database must be assessed. Methods for improving the quality and completeness of this information should be considered.
- Despite similarities among large databases, gaining insight and experience into the structure and content of each database is essential.
- Examples of commonly used large databases are presented with a synopsis of information contained in the database, as well as strengths and limitations of using the database for research.

Introduction

Although a simple Excel spreadsheet containing information on a few subjects is technically a database, this discussion is restricted to large databases with thousands (or millions) of records. These databases are used primarily either for administrative purposes (e.g., healthcare claims), or for research purposes (e.g., disease registries or large health surveys).

"Database study" and "data mining" are terms often used to describe research that utilizes large datasets. We feel these terms inaccurately describe many studies that utilize large databases, and underestimate the complexity and rigor of the methods used to conduct these studies. We recommend a systematic approach to utilizing large databases to address research questions, which includes:

1 developing specific research questions and determining the best possible study design to answer the question;

2 evaluating all potential data sources, which may include a pre-existing database, cross-sectional survey, or medical record review, and;

3 selecting the most appropriate data source based on the study question and design.

Several types of studies have been performed using large databases, including the evaluation of temporal (secular) trends, geographic variations, economic burden of disease, outcomes of disease management, resource utilization, determinants of disease, and pharmacoepide-miologic studies. The most commonly used study designs include cross-sectional, cohort, case-control and ecologic studies.

Examples of commonly used databases

For each database, we will provide a brief description of the contents, highlight strengths and weaknesses, and provide links for more detailed information (see Table 11.1).

SEER program

The Surveillance, Epidemiology, and End-Results (SEER) program is an important source of population-based cancer incidence and survival in the US. It currently covers approximately 25% of the US population [1]. The SEER program of the National Cancer Institute (NCI) provides support for population-based tumor registries in seven metropolitan areas (San Francisco/Oakland, Detroit, Atlanta, Seattle, Los Angeles County, San Jose-Monterey Counties and the Greater California area) and eight states (Connecticut, Iowa, New Mexico, Utah, Hawaii, Kentucky, New Jersey and Louisiana).

The SEER database contains information on more than 2.5 million cancer cases, and approximately 160 000 new cases are accessioned each year. Routinely collected infor-

Table 11.1 Databases and their web links

Data source	Website
Surveillance, Epidemiology, and End Results Program (SEER)	www.seer.cancer.gov
Medicare	www.cms.hhs.gov
Department of Veterans Administration (VA)	www.virec.research.va.gov
SEER-Medicare	www.healthservices.cancer.gov/seermedicare
American Medical Association (AMA)	www.ama-assn.org
Healthcare Cost and Utilization Project (HCUP)	www.hcup-us.ahrq.gov
National Hospital Discharge Survey (NHDS)	www.cdc.gov/nchs
Behavioral Risk Factor Surveillance System (BRFSS)	www.cdc.gov/brfss
Medical Expenditure Panel Survey (MEPS)	www.ahrq.gov
United Network for Organ Sharing	www.unos.org
United Kingdom General Practice Research Database	www.gprd.com/home
National Health and Nutrition Examination Survey (NHANES)	www.cdc.gov/nchs/nhanes.htm
Medicaid	www.cms.hhs.gov

mation includes patient demographics, primary tumor site, tumor morphology, stage at diagnosis, first course of treatment and follow-up for vital status.

SEER registries hold the highest level of certification of data quality [1–3], including completeness of case ascertainment, accuracy of data recording, and reliability of data abstraction. The SEER program's standard for the completeness of case ascertainment is 98% [4]. SEER public use data can be accessed at no cost through the SEER website (http://seer.cancer.gov). In addition, reports on cancer statistics are available from the SEER website. SEER also offers two free software programs (SEER*Prep and SEER*Stat) that can be used to analyze SEER public-use datasets.

Several studies have examined digestive and liver malignancies using the public-use SEER database. For example, we examined temporal trends in the incidence and survival of hepatocellular carcinoma [5], cholangiocarcinoma [6], esophageal adenocarcinoma [7] and malignant gastrointestinal tumors [8].

Medicare claims files

The Medicare Claims Data System collects information on all services provided to Medicare beneficiaries under its hospital (Part A) and supplemental (Part B) insurance plans. All Medicare beneficiaries receive Part A benefits and 95% of beneficiaries subscribe to Part B coverage

[1,3]. The former covers inpatient hospitalizations and care in skilled nursing homes, whereas the latter covers physicians' services, hospital outpatient services, durable medical equipment, home health services, and other outpatient medical services such as diagnostic X-rays and laboratory tests.

Several individual files are included as part of the Medicare database. Denominator files contain data on enrollment information, demographics (date of birth, race, zip code of residence), month-by-month eligibility information, HMO membership and date of death.

The Medicare Provider Analysis and Review (MedPAR) File contains inpatient hospital and skilled nursing facility stay records. Information contained in this file includes dates of admission and discharge, up to ten diagnosis codes (ICD-9-CM), and up to ten procedure codes.

The Physician/Supplier File includes line item detail for 100% of physician and supplier data. Each claim record includes some beneficiary demographic information, dates of service, procedure provided (such as office visit, surgical procedure, administration of chemotherapy), place of service (e.g., office, home, outpatient hospital, skilled nursing facility, emergency room) and diagnosis codes in ICD-9-CM format.

The Outpatient Standard Analytic File (SAF) includes dates of outpatient hospital service, revenue center codes, and up to ten fields for diagnoses (ICD-9-CM) and procedures (CPT).

CMS routinely monitors and reports the accuracy of Medicare claims and payments. Public reports about data accuracy and quality are available at www.CERTprovider.org.

Medicare claims files have been utilized to examine issues in digestive disease. For example, a study was done to examine the polyp detection rate of colonoscopy using Medicare claims files [9].

Department of Veterans Affairs (VA) administrative databases

VA Patient Treatment File

Since 1970, the Patient Treatment File (PTF) has captured information about inpatient hospitalizations at approximately 127 VA facilities across the US. The PTF contains medical diagnoses as well as inpatient medical and surgical procedures. Diagnostic (ICD-9-CM) and procedure (CPT) codes are based on information contained in the medical record, such as healthcare provider progress notes, imaging studies and laboratory reports. The PTF does not contain information about pharmacy, pathology or laboratory results.

VA Outpatient Care File

In 1996, the Outpatient Care File (OPC) was established to track visits to VA outpatient clinics. This file contains information on clinic specialty, date of visit, provider type, ICD-9-CM diagnosis codes, and current procedural terminology (CPT) codes [10].

The Beneficiary Identification and Records Locator Subsystem Death File

The mini-Beneficiary Identification and Records Locator Subsystem Death File (BIRLS) has dates of death reported by the VA, the Social Security Administration, the Department of Veterans Affairs cemetery system, and funeral directors. Information on cause of death is generally not available [10]. Due to various incentives, up to 90–95% of deaths among veterans are captured by the BIRLS file as compared with the National Death Index [11–13].

VA-Medicare linked database

This database contains VA administrative data and Medicare claims files for all Medicare-enrolled veterans who use the VA system. Data are currently available for calendar years 1999–2003. Researchers with IRB approved protocols can request VA-Medicare linked data through the

Veterans Administration Information Resource Center (VIReC; www.virec.research.va.gov).

VA databases have been used to examine the temporal trends of cases of hospitalization as a result of gastroesophageal malignancies [14] and colorectal cancer [15], and to examine the outcomes of fundoplication [14,16,17].

SEER-Medicare linked database

Data from the SEER tumor registries for cancer cases diagnosed from 1973 through 2002 have been linked with Medicare claims data from 1986 through 2003. The SEER-Medicare linkage is updated every three years.

Several studies have been conducted using the SEER-Medicare database, including ones examining risk factors for hepatocellular carcinoma [18,19] and cholangiocarcinoma [20], as well as the extent, patterns and therapeutic outcomes of hepatocellular carcinoma (HCC) [21]. Other studies have examined the use of upper endoscopy prior to esophageal adenocarcinoma [22]. A complete list of published studies can be found on the National Cancer Institute website (http://healthservices.cancer.gov/seer-medicare/overview/publications.html).

SEER-Medicare data are not public use files, and therefore investigators must obtain approval prior to requesting the datasets. Research protocols and data requests can be submitted to the SEER-Medicare contact, listed on the National Cancer Institute website (http://healthservices.cancer.gov/seermedicare).

Healthcare Cost and Utilization Project (HCUP)

The Healthcare Cost and Utilization Project (HCUP) is a collection of healthcare databases supported by the Agency for Healthcare Research and Quality. Data are collected by state data organizations, hospital associations, private data organizations and the federal government to create a resource for patient-level healthcare data.

National HCUP databases include the Nationwide Inpatient Sample (NIS) and the Kids Inpatient Database (KID). The NIS contains inpatient data from a national sample of over 1000 hospitals and is currently available for the period 1988 to 2003. It contains data from approximately seven million hospital stays on all patients, regardless of payer. Data elements in the NIS include primary and secondary diagnoses, procedures, admission and discharge status, patient demographics, expected payment source, total charges, length of stay and hospital characteristics.

State-specific HCUP databases are also available for those states that have agreed to participate. These include the State Inpatient Databases, State Ambulatory Surgery Databases, and State Emergency Department Databases (http://www.hcup-us.ahrq.gov/sidoverview.jsp). HCUP databases are available for purchase through the HCUP Central Distributor. An online application is available at www.hcup-us.ahrq.gov.

The NIS database has been previously utilized for gastrointestinal (GI) research. One recently published study examined differences in risk factors between black people and white people for hepatocellular carcinoma [23].

National Hospital Discharge Survey

The National Hospital Discharge Survey (NHDS) is a national probability survey designed to collect information on inpatients discharged from non-Federal, short-stay hospitals in the US. The NHDS collects data from a sample of approximately 270 000 inpatient records acquired from a national sample of approximately 500 hospitals.

Two data collection procedures are used. One is a manual abstraction of data from the medical records performed by hospital or NCHS staff. The other is an automated system in which medical record data are purchased from commercial organizations, state data systems, hospitals or hospital associations. Patient characteristics contained in the database include age, sex, race, ethnicity, marital status and expected source of payment. Information about dates of inpatient admission and discharge, and discharge status, as well as diagnoses and procedure codes are also available. Quality control procedures and edit checks are used to maintain data quality. A detailed review is also conducted for most variables for each hospital.

Several studies have been conducted using NHDS data. For example, one published study using NHDS data examined perioperative risk of noncardiac surgery in patients with hypertrophic cardiomyopathy [24]. Other studies have examined trends in hemorrhoids and constipation [25,26].

Data from NHDS are released annually and can be obtained free of charge at the National Center for Health Statistics website (www.cdc.gov/nchs). Data files are available on public-use data tapes, data diskettes or CD-ROMs, or can be downloaded from the ftp (file transfer protocol) server.

Medical Expenditure Panel Survey

The Medical Expenditure Panel Survey (MEPS) has col-

lected information on healthcare use and costs in the USA. MEPS collects information, from civilian populations living in US communities, on health conditions, healthcare expenses, type of medical services used, how frequently they are used, the cost of services, how services are paid for, and health insurance availability and coverage.

The MEPS program conducts three separate but related surveys, including the Household Component Survey, the Medical Provider Survey and the Insurance Component Survey. The Household Component Survey collects information at the person and household level on health conditions, use of medical care services, charges and payments, access to care, satisfaction with care, health insurance coverage, income and employment. The Medical Provider Component Survey supplements and validates information on medical care events by contacting medical providers and pharmacies identified by household respondents. The Insurance Component Survey collects data on health insurance plans obtained through private and public-sector employees.

MEPS public-use data are available for download directly from the MEPS website or can be ordered on diskette or CD-ROM from AHRQ. MEPSnet is an interactive statistical for MEPS data and is available from the MEPS website (www.ahrq.gov/data/mepsweb.html).

Other databases

Other databases that have been used extensively for research purposes include the United Network for Organ Sharing (http://www.unos.org/), United Kingdom General Practice Research Database (UKGPRD; http://www.gprd.com/home/), National Health and Nutrition Examination Survey (http://www.cdc.gov/nchs/nhanes.html) and Medicaid (http://www.cms.hhs.gov/MedicaidDataSourcesGenInfo/).

Recommendations for the use of large databases for research studies

Most caveats described below are extensions of sound design and analysis of clinical or epidemiologic research studies irrespective of the data source (Box 11.1).

Because the information collected in most administrative databases was not collected with a specific research question in mind, the **completeness** and **accuracy** of information for exposures and outcomes of interest as well as potential confounders and effect modifiers should be evaluated.

Completeness of the database

The investigator has to ask the question: does this data source capture all patient encounters? For example, patients enrolled in an HMO are likely to receive all or most of their care within the constraints of their HMO as long as they are enrolled, and therefore the majority of their healthcare utilization is likely to be captured. Similarly, the great majority of individuals aged 65 and over will have their healthcare claims recorded in Medicare, and once enrolled, most persons remain in Medicare. Conversely, Medicaid is a less stable engagement where persons qualify based on income-related criteria and get reviewed periodically and therefore they may lose their Medicaid coverage periodically and more frequently.

Accuracy of information

The vast majority of administrative databases use ICD-9-CM and CPT codes to indicate diagnoses and procedures. These codes are selected based on information contained in the medical record. The presence and accuracy of codes that are specific for the condition of interest is a potential limiting factor of studies that use administrative databases and therefore should be evaluated prior to using these codes for research. Not all conditions have specific codes; for example the codes for pancreatitis (acute and chronic) do not distinguish between alcoholic and biliary causes. Moreover, the accuracy of these codes can vary depending on the disease as well as the database. Positive and negative predictive values can be calculated for each code to determine its accuracy. Positive predictive value refers to the presence of disease when the code is present, while negative predictive value refers to the absence of disease in the absence of the code. The accuracy of codes varies depending on the condition, even within the same database, and therefore has to be dealt with individually, one disease or procedure at a time. For example, rapidly symptomatic and easily diagnosed conditions, such as esophageal cancer, are unlikely to remain undiagnosed and therefore the negative predictive value of these conditions is likely to be high. Conversely, the positive predictive value, although intuitively high, may not be specific enough to distinguish between esophageal adenocarcinoma, esophageal squamous cell carcinoma and other gastroesophageal junction cancers.

To evaluate the accuracy of diagnostic and procedure codes, an advisable approach is to conduct a survey or chart validation study of subjects nested within the study cohort that was identified in the database. For example, in a study of esophageal peptic strictures, one would identify a randomly selected group of individuals in the database with and without the ICD-9-CM code 150.3 (esophageal stricture) [27]. The medical records for these subjects are then manually or electronically reviewed for the presence (or absence) of esophageal strictures. Agreement between the medical record "gold standard" and the databases can then be evaluated and estimates of accuracy reflecting both positive and negative predictive values for ICD-9-CM code 150.3 can be calculated. The investigator may then decide not to pursue the study question any further due to poor accuracy of crucial codes in the database. Alternatively, if accuracy is very high, the study can be conducted with great confidence. A likely scenario is that the accuracy is intermediate; in that case, algorithms can be constructed to improve the accuracy of those codes. For example, while codes for upper GI bleeding might be low if only these codes are examined, an algorithm using a logistic regression model that incorporates the presence of hospitalization, an endoscopy and blood transfusion into the definition is likely to increase the accuracy of the original codes. Such an algorithm also allows the investigator to conduct sensitivity analyses that account for possible miscoding.

It is the responsibility of the investigators to develop a comprehensive, accurate and updated list of codes to indicate a disease condition or a medical/surgical procedure because these codes change over time, with new codes appearing and old codes disappearing. The number of available fields per record in which diagnoses/procedures can be entered should also be considered. For example, a spurious increase in the rate of a disease condition (especially conditions that are unlikely to be the primary reason for the encounter with the healthcare system) may be seen as a result of increasing the number of fields per encounter in which diagnoses can be recorded.

Use of publicly available statistical calculators

For several databases described above (e.g., SEER), there

are publicly available calculators to perform statistical computations. Although these calculators are convenient to use, it is important to verify that data are being inputted properly into the software program and that calculations are being correctly performed. We advise investigators to emulate the calculation of previously known figures/rates, even if they do not pertain to the question of interest, to ensure that the program is being used correctly.

Determining patient comorbidity

Patient comorbidity can be captured and adjusted for by calculating one of several disease comorbidity indices. We recommend the use of an index that includes conditions recorded in both inpatient and outpatient files. Older indices have relied on inpatient diagnoses, but as hospitalizations for most conditions have steeply declined, the amount of comorbidity that can be captured through hospitalization records is relatively limited. Nevertheless, in most circumstances, only 20–40% of patients in studies that use a comorbidity index have a recorded comorbidity at all. Therefore residual unmeasured comorbidity may still be present and may confound the observed associations. Diagnosis-based measures, however, are subject to the many known limitations of administrative claims data, such as incomplete or inaccurate coding [28,29]. A growing body of literature has examined the use of pharmacy prescription-dispensing information to create comorbidity measures when the use of drugs indicates the disease condition of the patient [30–32]. The rationale for its use is that pharmacy prescription records may not have the same weaknesses as diagnostic information. For example, pharmacy measures are based on the actual fill record and are not subject to variations of coding diagnoses. However, this approach is subject to the availability of complete pharmacy data.

Robustness of findings

Given the various reasons for misclassification and incomplete recording of exposure and outcomes of exposures, outcomes and confounders, one has to be convinced that the results are consistent or robust. Therefore, we recommend performing sensitivity analyses to test the robustness of findings given different assumptions for accuracy and completeness of disease outcome and exposures. The source for assumptions included in the sensitivity analyses can be derived from the chart validation studies described in the previous section. Given that it is highly unlikely than any code or combination of codes will yield 100%

accuracy, one can define the variables using the worst- and best-case scenario for accuracy and then repeat or rerun the analysis using both assumptions. If the findings are consistent with the main analyses then confidence is given to the findings, otherwise the results should be interpreted cautiously.

Power and sample size considerations

An advantage of using administrative databases is the ability to examine a very large number of subjects using one data source. This large sample size enables the detection of small differences in rare outcomes. The potential disadvantage is that statistically significant differences can be detected that may not be clinically meaningful. One should not confuse large sample size with the number of outcomes of interest. For example, a study with a sample size of one million subjects that has only 30 outcome events (i.e., a rare cancer) is still underpowered. The ability to adjust for potential confounders and effect modifiers is dependent on the number of outcome events not on the entire underlying sample size. As a rule of thumb 15–20 outcome events are required to adjust adequately for one predictor variable.

In conclusion, large databases represent a potentially valuable source of information for research studies that examine the epidemiology and outcomes of a variety of digestive and liver disorders. Regardless of the data source, it is important to begin with an important research question and a study design that properly addresses that question. If the research question and study design lend themselves to utilizing a particular database as the data source, it is the responsibility of the investigator to consider the strengths (e.g., large sample size, long duration of follow-up, relative low cost and short time required to conduct the study) versus the weakness (issues related to accuracy and completeness of information, and the availability of appropriate expertise in the particular database and advanced computer programming skills) in deciding whether to use the database for their research.

References

1. Warren JL *et al.* Overview of the SEER-Medicare data: content, research applications, and generalizability to the United States elderly population. *Med Care* 2002;**40**(8 Suppl.): IV–18.
2. Edwards BK *et al.* Annual report to the nation on the status of cancer, 1975–2002, featuring population-based trends in

cancer treatment. *J Natl Cancer Inst* 2005;**97**:1407.

3. Potosky AL *et al.* Potential for cancer related health services research using a linked Medicare-tumor registry database. *Med Care* 1993;**31**:732.

4. Zippin C *et al.* Completeness of hospital cancer case reporting from the SEER Program of the National Cancer Institute. *Cancer* 1995;**76**:2343.

5. El-Serag HB *et al.* The continuing increase in the incidence of hepatocellular carcinoma in the United States: an update. *Ann Intern Med* 2003;**139**:817.

6. Shaib YH *et al.* Rising incidence of intrahepatic cholangiocarcinoma in the United States: a true increase? *J Hepatol* 2004;**40**:472.

7. El-Serag HB *et al.* Epidemiological differences between adenocarcinoma of the oesophagus and adenocarcinoma of the gastric cardia in the USA. *Gut* 2002;**50**:368.

8. Tran T *et al.* The epidemiology of malignant gastrointestinal stromal tumors: an analysis of 1,458 cases from 1992 to 2000. *Am J Gastroenterol* 2005;**100**:162.

9. Cooper GS *et al.* The polyp detection rate of colonoscopy: a national study of Medicare beneficiaries. *Am J Med* 2005;**118**:1413.

10. Boyko EJ *et al.* US Department of Veterans Affairs medical care system as a resource to epidemiologists. *Am J Epidemiol* 2000;**151**:307.

11. Fisher SG *et al.* Mortality ascertainment in the veteran population: alternatives to the National Death Index. *Am J Epidemiol* 1995;**141**:242.

12. Page WF *et al.* Ascertainment of mortality in the U.S. veteran population: World War II veteran twins. *Mil Med* 1995;**160**:351.

13. Page WF *et al.* Vital status ascertainment through the files of the Department of Veterans Affairs and the Social Security Administration. *Ann Epidemiol* 1996;**6**:102.

14. El-Serag HB, Sonnenberg A. Opposing time trends of peptic ulcer and reflux disease. *Gut* 1998;**43**:327.

15. Rabeneck L *et al.* Surgical volume and long-term survival following surgery for colorectal cancer in the Veterans Affairs Health-Care System. *Am J Gastroenterol* 2004;**99**:668.

16. Dominitz JA *et al.* Complications and antireflux medication use after antireflux surgery. *Clin Gastroenterol Hepatol* 2006;**4**:299.

17. Tran T *et al.* Fundoplication and the risk of esophageal cancer in gastroesophageal reflux disease: a Veterans Affairs cohort study. *Am J Gastroenterol* 2005;**100**:1002.

18. Davila JA *et al.* Hepatitis C infection and the increasing incidence of hepatocellular carcinoma: a population-based study. *Gastroenterology* 2004;**127**:1372.

19. Davila JA *et al.* Diabetes increases the risk of hepatocellular carcinoma in the United States: a population based case control study. *Gut* 2005;**54**:533.

20. Shaib YH *et al.* Risk factors of intrahepatic cholangiocarcinoma in the United States: a case-control study. *Gastroenterology* 2005;**128**:620.

21. El-Serag HB *et al.* Treatment and outcomes of treating of hepatocellular carcinoma among Medicare recipients in the United States: a population-based study. *J Hepatol* 2006;**44**:158.

22. Cooper GS, Payes JD. Receipt of colorectal testing prior to colorectal carcinoma diagnosis. *Cancer* 2005;**103**:696.

23. Yu L *et al.* Risk factors for primary hepatocellular carcinoma in black and white Americans in 2000. *Clin Gastroenterol Hepatol* 2006;**4**:355.

24. Hreybe H *et al.* Noncardiac surgery and the risk of death and other cardiovascular events in patients with hypertrophic cardiomyopathy. *Clin Cardiol* 2006;**29**:65.

25. Johanson JF, Sonnenberg A. The prevalence of hemorrhoids and chronic constipation. An epidemiologic study. *Gastroenterology* 1990;**98**:380.

26. Johanson JF, Sonnenberg A. Temporal changes in the occurrence of hemorrhoids in the United States and England. *Dis Colon Rectum* 1991;**34**:585.

27. El-Serag HB. Temporal trends in esophageal strictures among veterans. *Am J Gastroenterol* 2006;**101**:1727.

28. Black C, Roos NP. Administrative data. Baby or bathwater? *Med Care* 1998;**36**:3.

29. Iezzoni LI. Assessing quality using administrative data. *Ann Intern Med* 1997;**127**:666.

30. Clark DO *et al.* A chronic disease score with empirically derived weights. *Med Care* 1995;**33**:783.

31. Johnson RE *et al.* Replicating the chronic disease score (CDS) from automated pharmacy data. *J Clin Epidemiol* 1994;**47**:1191.

32. Von Korff M *et al.* A chronic disease score from automated pharmacy data. *J Clin Epidemiol* 1992;**45**:197.

12 Nutritional Epidemiology

Linda E. Kelemen

Key points
- The choice of dietary assessment depends on the research question and the pathophysiology of the disease.
- Long-term dietary patterns are most relevant to estimate chronic disease risk.
- Most risk models will need to adjust for total energy.
- Knowledge of potential sources of error in nutritional assessment is essential.
- Statistical methods exist to estimate and correct measurement error.

Introduction

One of the earliest applications of nutritional epidemiology was in the study of gastrointestinal diseases. In the late 1960s, Burkitt [1] observed differences in fecal bulk between individuals in rural Africa compared with industrialized Western countries and hypothesized that this was the result of the high fiber intake of the former. Subsequently, he hypothesized that dietary fiber protects against the development of colorectal cancer. To date, there are more than 400 published accounts on this topic.

Nutritional epidemiology is the assessment of diet and its relationship to the causes of diseases in populations. This includes the intake of essential nutrients (e.g., vitamins, minerals and amino acids), energy sources (protein, carbohydrate, fat and alcohol), naturally occurring food compounds (e.g., plant fiber, cholesterol and caffeine) or, for specific hypotheses, the intake of chemicals formed in cooking, such as heterocyclic aromatic amines formed in well-done or charred meats, or from food processing, such as *trans* fatty acids. An observed association between a nutrient and disease is complemented by statistical analysis of the nutrient's food source (e.g., food, food groups) with the disease, which strengthens the hypothesis under study.

The investigator's choice of dietary assessment method will depend on his or her knowledge of the disease pathology. Events that are acute and occur over a relatively short period, such as maternal dietary folate intake and risk of fetal neural tube defects, require methods that accurately and precisely assess an individual's intake over the course of days or weeks. In contrast, events such as cancer that are chronic and are complicated by exposure time, require methods that capture patterns of consumption among populations over a period of years, because measurement of diet several years prior to disease manifestation probably represents the more relevant exposure period for understanding these diseases. Diet–disease associations may be confounded or modified by several factors, including body size, physical activity, other dietary factors and genetic susceptibility. Understanding the interplay among these factors is crucial to derive unbiased estimates of disease risk.

Dietary assessment instruments

Two methods of dietary assessment typically used in clinical settings have been modified for use in epidemiologic studies. Both the 24-hour recall and the diet record assess short-term dietary intake, but when used as repeated measurements, can inform of usual patterns of intake over a longer period.

The **24-hour recall** interview is administered in person or by telephone. Subjects report their exact intake in the preceding 24 hours guided by the interviewer's standard questions, which may also use visual aids to assist with recall of portion size (these may be mailed to subjects in advance of unannounced 24-hour recalls undertaken by telephone). In its favor, memory of recent intake may be more precise and quantities may be estimated with greater accuracy with minimal participant burden. Well-trained interviewers are required, however, and the nutrient analysis of food intake can be laborious. Because individual diets vary greatly from day to day, a single day's dietary recall does not represent usual dietary intake.

The **diet record** is similar to the 24-hour recall, except that the subject records actual food and beverage intake prospectively over several days. Subjects are asked to provide detailed descriptions of preparation methods and food quantities, which are assessed by weighing, volume/dimension measurements or estimation assisted by the use of photographs. The prospective nature of diet recording reduces errors associated with recall and minimizes omission of foods consumed. However, the method requires a high level of subject literacy, motivation and training, and can be costly to analyze. Furthermore, consecutive days of dietary recording may result in food intake that is highly correlated from day to day (due to consumption of leftover meals or alteration of usual diet to include foods that are easy to record), possibly introducing bias. A trade-off is to collect fewer records per subject on a greater number of individuals. In the absence of objective assessments of long-term dietary intake, the diet record is considered the "alloyed" gold standard. Like the 24-hour recall, multiple days of records over several months or one year can reduce day-to-day correlation of intake, improve accuracy and precision of individual intake and capture seasonal variation in food intake.

For investigations of several hundreds or thousands of individuals, **food frequency questionnaires (FFQs)** are a viable option to assess long-term diet. These questionnaires consist of a list of foods and beverages that represent the major contributors to the macronutrient and micronutrient content of the diet of the population under study. Thus, they are population- or ethnic-specific [2,3]. For each food or beverage item, the subject selects one of several options that best defines their frequency of intake over the past year with or without a selection for a portion size option (Fig. 12.1). Photographs of different serving sizes assist with portion recall. FFQs are easily administered in person or by mail, provide information on the intake of a large number of foods, food groups and individual nutrients, and are substantially less expensive to analyze particularly if in scannable form. Repeated FFQ administrations over several years can capture dietary changes over time. Table 12.1 summarizes characteristics of some large, prospective studies employing FFQs.

In evaluating dietary assessment methods, it is worth commenting on two important dimensions that affect nutritional epidemiologic research. The first is the distinction between group and individual, and the second is between quantitative precision and classification or ranking of individuals [4]. A clinician might value a dietary assessment method that gives accurate results for each individual, in micrograms of folate or kilocalories of total energy; that is, patient A's dietary assessment accurately reflects patient A's intake. However, such accuracy at an individual level and in such precise quantities is not essential to produce valid and useful research on diet and disease at the group level, provided the dietary assessment instrument is valid for the population under study [4]. Indeed,

	Never	A few times per year	Once per month	2–3 times per month	Once per week	2 times per week	3–4 times per week	5–6 times per week	Every day		How much on those days See portion size pictures for A-B-C-D			
Green beans or green peas	○	○	○	○	○	○	○	○	○	▶	How much	○ A	○ B	○ C
Spinach (cooked)	○	○	○	○	○	○	○	○	○	▶	How much	○ A	○ B	○ C
Greens like collards, turnip greens, mustard greens	○	○	○	○	○	○	○	○	○	▶	How much	○ A	○ B	○ C
Sweet potatoes, yams	○	○	○	○	○	○	○	○	○	▶	How much	○ A	○ B	○ C
French fries, home fries, hash browns	○	○	○	○	○	○	○	○	○	▶	How much	○ A ○ B	○ C	○ D

Fig 12.1. Example of the format of the Block Food Frequency Questionnaire 2005. (Reproduced from www.nutritionquest.com, with permission from Block Dietary Data Systems.)

Table 12.1 Characteristics of prospective cohort studies utilizing validated Food Frequency Questionnaires

Study	Date initiated	Study characteristics	FFQ administration	Outcome ascertainment	Contact
Nurses' Health Study I	1976	~121 700 registered nurses aged 30–55 years from 11 US states	Every 4 years	Medical and pathology record review, linkage with national death index	http://www.channing.harvard.edu/nhs/
Nurses' Health Study II	1989	~117 000 registered nurses aged 25–42 years from 14 US states	Every 4 years	As above	As above
Health Professionals Follow-up Study	1986	~52 500 US male health professionals aged 40–75 years	Every 4 years	As above	http://www.hsph.harvard.edu/hpfs/
Iowa Women's Health Study	1986	~100 000 Iowa women aged 55–69 years	Baseline	Linkage with Iowa cancer registry, national death index	http://www.cancer.umn.edu/page/research/prevent6.html
European Prospective Investigation of Cancer	1992	~521 000 men and women aged 35–70 years from ten European countries	Baseline	Cancers reported by each country's cancer registries to a central IARC database	http://www.iarc.fr/epic/Sup-default.html
ACS Cancer Prevention Study II	1992	~184 000 men and women aged 50–74 years from 21 US states	Every 2 years	Linkage with state cancer registries, national death index	http://www.cancer.org/docroot/RES/content/RES_6_2_Study_Overviews.asp
Multiethnic Cohort Study	1993	~215 000 men and women aged 45–75 from Hawaii and Los Angeles of Caucasian, Latino, African-American, Native Hawaiian and Japanese-American ethnicities	Baseline	Linkages to cancer registries and death certificate files in Hawaii and California and to the national death index	Cancer Research Center of Hawaii, University of Southern California/Norris Comprehensive Cancer Center

ACS, American Cancer Society; IARC, International Agency for Research on Cancer.

John Snow did not need to know the exact dose of the organism necessary to cause cholera in order to produce a tremendous advance in public health. Valid but less precise methods that locate individuals on the distribution in broad categories of low, medium and high intake still permit the examination of nutritional hypotheses and the assessment of dose–response relationships [4], whereas invalid instruments will bias associations.

Study designs in nutritional epidemiologic research

The most common application of nutritional assessments using FFQs is for epidemiologic investigations utilizing case-control, prospective cohort and cross-sectional study designs. The characteristics of these study designs are discussed in detail in Chapter 3.

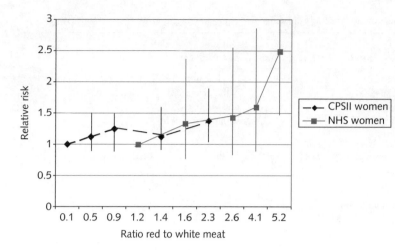

Fig 12.2. Ratio of red to white meat intake and risk of colon cancer among women in 2 national US cohorts. CPSII, Cancer Prevention Study II; NHS, Nurses' Health Study. Vertical bars represent 95% confidence intervals. (Source: Willett *et al.*, 1990 and Chao *et al.*, 2005.)

The reference period of dietary intake differs between study designs. For **case-control studies**, the disease process may alter the subject's dietary intake during the period leading up to diagnosis, through food intolerances or changes in appetite; therefore, the FFQ typically asks about usual eating habits "before one year ago" and not including any recent dietary changes. On the other hand, dietary assessment among disease-free subjects in a **prospective cohort study** is based on recollection of usual eating habits in the past year.

A major limitation of case-control studies is recall bias of exposure among the cases, who may over-report foods that they believe may have contributed to their diagnosis and under-report healthier foods that they believe may have prevented their disease. This biases relative risks further from the null value than would be observed in

a prospective study of the same association. Moreover, selection bias, driven by the eagerness of cases to find the "cause" of their disease, probably contributes to their higher participation than controls in epidemiologic studies [5]. Controls who participate may be more health conscious, for example, consume more fruits and vegetables and less fat. The effect of recall and selection bias is not trivial and could lead to apparent inverse associations with fruits and vegetables and positive associations with dietary fat [6].

Differences in findings even among cohort studies may be due to various reasons, including differences in the populations or in the endpoints studied (e.g., colon adenomas vs carcinomas), follow-up duration, the choice of nutrient database (discussed below), and the range of intake captured by the FFQ. For example, two national

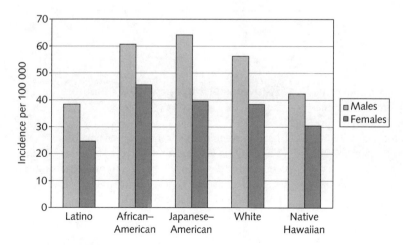

Fig 12.3. Incidence (1988–1992) of colorectal cancer in the Multiethnic Cohort Study by ethnicity, age-adjusted to the 1970 U.S. standard population. (Data from Kolonel *et al.*, 2000 [2].)

US cohorts examined the ratio of red to white meat intake with risk of colon cancer among women (Fig. 12.2). Higher intakes increased risk in both cohorts, which were similar in cohort size and duration of follow-up (6–9 years). The overlap in distributions, however, suggests the full extent of increased risk is observed only at very high intakes.

Identifying the role and extent of dietary stimuli in the development of disease is usually easier and more efficient when comparing and contrasting **culturally heterogeneous populations** (e.g., ethnic groups) who have differences in lifestyle practices. For example, the Multiethnic Cohort was established to study diet and cancer among 215 251

adult men and women living in Hawaii and Los Angeles, who showed baseline differences in incidence for common cancers according to ethnicity [2] (Fig. 12.3). The inclusion of multiple ethnic groups within a single study permits interethnic comparisons of diet–disease associations by using common data collection methodology in all groups and, where no heterogeneity exists among ethnic groups in the estimates of disease risk, allows the pooling of data for a wide range of dietary intakes to estimate the overall effect with disease. As the numbers of cancer cases accrue, this study promises to evaluate the extent to which dietary and other environmental exposures explain interethnic differences in disease incidence.

(a)

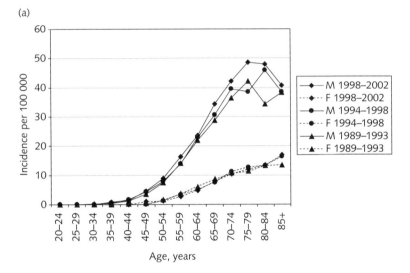

(b)

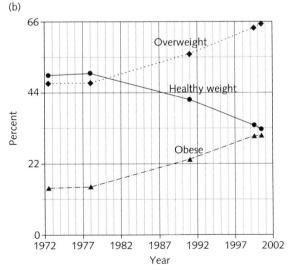

Fig 12.4. (a) Age-specific incidence of esophageal cancer per 100 000 in the US for 3 time periods, white males (M) and females (F). Source: Surveillance, Epidemiology and End Results registries (http://seer.cancer.gov/). (b) Percent of adults ages 20-74 years who were at a healthy weight, overweight or obese: 1971–74 to 2000–02. Data are age-adjusted to the 2000 population standard. (Source: National Cancer Institute Cancer Trends Progress Report 2005 Update (http://progressreport.cancer.gov/).)

Secular trends can also identify changes in incidence rates caused by environmental factors. Figure 12.4a shows the age-specific incidence for esophageal cancer per 100 000 of the US population among white males and females over three time periods. For all age groups over 40, the incidence increases sharply during the most recent period, 1998–2002. Similar trends are observed for African-American males and females. During this period, the number of overweight and obese individuals also increased (Fig. 12.4b), and vegetable intake decreased, suggesting possible links that require further investigation. Indeed, investigators recently explored the hypothesis that increased carbonated soft drink consumption is associated with this trend [7].

The hypothesis that an individual's genetic susceptibility to developing disease may be modified by diet is emerging as an active area of investigation. A well-known example of a **diet–genetic association study** is that of folate and the $677C{\rightarrow}T$ polymorphism in the gene encoding the folate-metabolizing enzyme, methylenetetrahydrofolate reductase (MTHFR), which impairs the conversion of 5,10-methylenetetrahydrofolate (5,10-mTHF) to 5-methyltetrahydrofolate (5-mTHF). 5,10-mTHF is involved in essential one-carbon transfer reactions that are important in DNA synthesis and replication whereas 5-mTHF functions in the methylation of many compounds including DNA, RNA, proteins and phospholipids [8] (Fig. 12.5). Folate deficiency is implicated in cancer development by either pathway [8]. On the basis of the functional effects of the polymorphism, and the inverse association between folate status and disease, it might have been expected that the variant would be associated with increased risk of colorectal cancer [9]. On the contrary, most studies showed that the variant (*TT*) genotype is associated with moderately reduced colorectal cancer risk, which may result from accumulation of 5,10-mTHF that serves as a cofactor for DNA synthesis and repair reactions. Alternatively, higher dietary folate can lower risk by stabilizing the MTHFR enzyme among individuals with the variant T allele. This favors 5-mTHF production, critical for methylation reactions [9].

Nutrient databases

Most software for analyzing the nutrient content of foods combines various sources, such as the US Department of Agriculture (USDA) database, with data provided by food manufacturers. These databases can contain upwards of 25 000 different foods and provide information on over 100 different nutrients. The nutrient value of foods varies by plant variety, soil mineral content, storage, processing and cooking conditions, and country-specific food fortification practices. Furthermore, the values of items such as dietary fiber can vary according to different definitions (e.g., plant lignin, cellulose, non-starch polysaccharides) and analytic techniques used for quantification, and could partly explain differences in risk estimates across studies. During the design of their studies, investigators interested in nutritional hypotheses are encouraged to involve personnel who are knowledgeable about these databases.

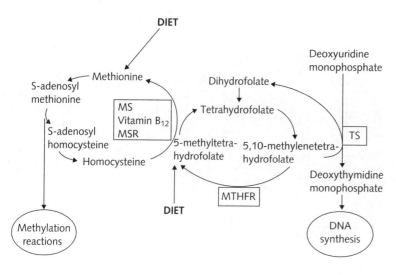

Fig 12.5. The role of folate in pathways of DNA synthesis and methylation reactions. MS, methionine synthase; MSR, methionine synthase reductase; MTHFR, methylenetetrahydrofolate reductase; TS, thymidylate synthase. (Reproduced from Sharp [9], with permission from Oxford University Press.)

Statistical issues in dietary analyses

Energy adjustment

Statistical adjustment for energy intake in models of diet and disease is important for several reasons. Because intakes of nutrients, particularly macronutrients, are correlated with total energy intake, these nutrients may be noncausally associated with disease from confounding by total energy intake [10]. Residual confounding from factors difficult to measure or measured with error that are associated with energy intake (including body size, physical activity and metabolism) can attenuate associations with disease risk. Failure to account for total energy intake can obscure associations between nutrient intakes and disease risk or possibly reverse the direction of the association. Several disease-risk models are described to control for energy intake in epidemiologic studies [10], although recent studies show the superiority of one or two statistical models over the others [11].

Measurement error correction

The recall of diet is associated with both random and systematic error. The former attenuates diet–disease risk estimates by introducing noise and reducing precision, whereas the latter biases risk estimates from overestimating or underestimating a person's "true" intake. Although neither error can be completely removed, the best safeguard against biased data is to evaluate the validity of a FFQ, described in detail elsewhere [10]. To reduce the effects of random measurement error, several statistical approaches exist to correct estimates of correlation coefficients and regression coefficients to produce approximate unbiased point and interval estimates from linear, Cox and logistic regression models [10]. These correction methods, however, rely on data from a validation study.

Conclusions

Nutritional epidemiology has contributed significantly to our understanding of the relationships between diet and disease over the past three decades. Ongoing investigations that further characterize important exposure periods (early life, *in utero*) and clarify associations within the context of genetic susceptibility will continue to elucidate our understanding of the pathophysiology of complex diseases, and support future recommendations for disease prevention.

References

1. Burkitt DP. Epidemiology of cancer of the colon and rectum. *Cancer* 1971;**28**:3.
2. Kolonel LN *et al.* A multiethnic cohort in Hawaii and Los Angeles: baseline characteristics. *Am J Epidemiol* 2000;**151**:346.
3. Kelemen LE *et al.* Development and evaluation of cultural food frequency questionnaires for South Asians, Chinese, and Europeans in North America. *J Am Diet Assoc* 2003;**103**:1178.
4. Block G. A review of validations of dietary assessment methods. *Am J Epidemiol* 1982;**115**:492.
5. Morton LM *et al.* Reporting participation in epidemiologic studies: a survey of practice. *Am J Epidemiol* 2006;**163**:197.
6. Willett WC. Diet and cancer: an evolving picture. *JAMA* 2005;**293**:233.
7. Mayne ST *et al.* Carbonated soft drink consumption and risk of esophageal adenocarcinoma. *J Natl Cancer Inst* 2006;**98**:72.
8. Choi SW *et al.* Folate and carcinogenesis: an integrated scheme. *J Nutr* 2000;**130**:129.
9. Sharp L *et al.* Polymorphisms in genes involved in folate metabolism and colorectal neoplasia: a HuGE review. *Am J Epidemiol* 2004;**159**:423.
10. Willett WC. *Nutritional Epidemiology*, 2nd edn. New York: Oxford University Press, 1998.
11. Michels KB *et al.* The effect of correlated measurement error in multivariate models of diet. *Am J Epidemiol* 2004;**160**:59.

13 Infection Epidemiology and Acute Gastrointestinal Infections

Sarah J. O'Brien and Smita L.S. Halder

Key points
- The epidemiologic approach to the investigation of gastrointestinal infection is influenced by the interaction between microorganisms and the host.
- The infection epidemiologist can draw on "standard" epidemiologic techniques and on special methods.
- Collaboration with microbiologists is essential for studying infection epidemiology.

The purpose of this chapter is to introduce the features of infection epidemiology that differentiate it from disease epidemiology in general. Epidemiologic concepts covered in other chapters will not be repeated here, but readers should bear in mind that those methods are also available to use in the study of infection.

What makes infection epidemiology different?

The epidemiologic approach to the investigation of infectious diseases uses similar methodology to so-called "chronic disease" epidemiology. Development of case definitions, detailed description of cases, formulation of hypotheses, and testing hypotheses using standard analytical techniques like case-control and cohort studies are all commonplace. However, there are five distinctive features of the epidemiologic study of infection [1]. These are:

1 A case can be a risk factor, i.e., transmission of infection can occur between individuals.

2 People develop immunity and are thus no longer at risk of becoming cases.

3 Asymptomatic or subclinical cases can be sources of infection.

4 Urgent investigation may be required, especially during large outbreaks where the timescale of the investigative process is compressed to hours or days, rather than months or years, whilst maintaining scientific rigour.

5 The scientific basis for intervention is well founded.

The infection process

To understand the epidemiologic approach to infection is it important to be familiar with the infection process, which depends on the properties of invading microorganisms as well as the host. Intrinsic properties of infectious agents that affect their propensity to cause disease include:
- morphology;
- size;
- chemical make-up;
- antigenic make-up;
- growth requirements;
- ability to survive outside a host;
- ability to produce a toxin;
- ability to acquire new genetic material [2].

The likelihood of infection depends upon host–agent interactions, which are described in the following terms:
- Infectivity, which is defined as the ability of an agent to invade and multiply (produce infection) in a host. A commonly used term is the median infectious dose (ID_{50}), which is the minimum number of agents required to establish infection in 50% of a group of hosts.
- Pathogenicity, i.e., the ability to produce clinically apparent illness.
- Virulence, which is the proportion of clinical cases resulting in severe clinical manifestations, including sequelae. A measure of virulence is the case fatality rate (CFR).
- Immunogenicity or the ability of the host to mount an immune response, either via humoral immunity (antibody production) or cell-mediated immunity.

- Environmental conditions.
- Dose of organisms to which the host is exposed.
- Route of infection.
- Intrinsic host factors such as age, sex, ethnic origin, nutritional status and presence of underlying medical conditions [2].

Transmission pathways

The next consideration is the route by which infectious agents cause infection. By convention transmission routes are usually classified as:

1 **Direct**, either via contact or via droplets.

2 **Indirect**, via:

- Vehicle, e.g., food, water, fomites (note that the agent may or may not multiply or develop in/on vehicle).
- Vector:
  –mechanical – simply transferring pathogens from one place to another, for example on the feet of insects;
  –biological – in this situation the agent has a life cycle inside the insect vector as well as inside the human host.
- Airborne:
  –droplets – in this instance respirable particles are usually less than 5 μm in diameter;
  –dust.

Infection can sometimes spread via more than one route.

Infection epidemiology definitions

In general, the terminology of infection epidemiology mirrors that of chronic disease epidemiology. However, there are some definitions that only really apply to infection epidemiology. These include:

- Index case – this is the first case to come to the attention of the clinician, i.e., the first recognized case. It may or may not be the same as the primary case.
- Primary case – the individual who brings infection into a population.
- Secondary cases are the people infected by the primary case.
- Attack rate is the proportion of the exposed population that becomes clinically ill.
- Generation time (or serial interval) – this is the period of time that elapses between acquisition of infection by a host and maximal communicability of that host. Strictly it is the time between the appearance of symptoms in suc-

cessive generations of cases. It is usually roughly equal to the incubation period unless a person is infectious before symptoms appear, in which instance the generation time will be shorter than the incubation period.

- Incubation period – this is the time interval between acquisition of infection and onset of illness/symptoms.
- Reproductive rate – describes the potential for an infectious disease to spread from person to person in a population. This, in turn, depends on four things:
  –the probability that transmission will occur in a contact between infected and susceptible individuals;
  –the frequency of contacts in the population;
  –the duration of communicability;
  –the proportion of immune individuals in the population [1].

How does illness severity affect the representativeness of cases?

Not all those who become infected with a microorganism will develop overt signs of clinical infection. The extent of subclinical and mild disease presentations affects the proportion of cases that are recorded in routine surveillance systems. Figure 13.1 shows how variations in the severity of illness affect the likelihood of a case being officially recorded. In England the extent to which the burden of acute gastroenteritis is hidden was ascertained by means of a national prospective cohort study, conducted between 1993 and 1996 [3]. This study showed that for every case of acute gastroenteritis recorded in national surveillance statistics there were 136 cases in the community (Fig. 13.2). The greatest loss of potential cases occurred right at the base of the reporting pyramid. Only 23 of the 136 cases presented to a primary care physician, and therefore had a chance of being recorded in local and national statistics. What the infectious intestinal disease (IID) study in England also demonstrated was that the proportion of cases recorded varied by pathogen. For every case of salmonellosis reported to national surveillance there were 3.2 in the community, whereas for every case of norovirus infection reported to national surveillance there were 1562 in the community [3]. Norovirus infection, though unpleasant, is a very short-lived illness and most cases have recovered before they are able to obtain an appointment with a primary care physician. Tam and colleagues [4] used data from the IID study to determine what influences patients to present to a primary care physician and found that perceived illness severity was the most important factor.

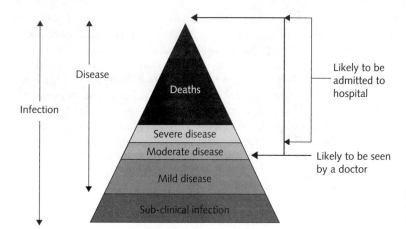

Fig. 13.1 How illness severity affects the likelihood of cases being recorded in surveillance statistics.

Spatial and temporal clustering

Infections spread from person to person, or those with an environmental reservoir may exhibit clustering in space and/or time. Shiga toxin-producing *Escherichia coli* (STEC) O157 is a serious zoonotic infection that affects children particularly badly. It can precipitate hemolytic uremic syndrome – the commonest cause of acute renal failure in children [5]. The incidence of STEC O157 in Scotland is the highest in the world. The majority of cases are sporadic, that is, not linked epidemiologically to others as part of outbreaks. Cattle are the main reservoir for STEC O157. Innocent and colleagues [6] have investigated the spatial epidemiology of STEC O157 infection in Scotland. Their methods enabled them to look separately at spatial and temporal components and at a space–time interac-

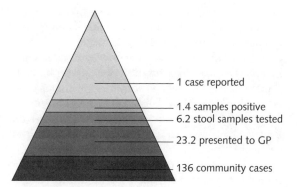

— 1 case reported

— 1.4 samples positive
— 6.2 stool samples tested

— 23.2 presented to GP

— 136 community cases

Fig. 13.2 The surveillance pyramid for acute infectious intestinal disease in England, showing how data are lost at many stages of the process.

tion component. They demonstrated significant variation in the spatial and temporal distribution of sporadic STEC O157 cases that were associated with human population density, cattle population density and the number of cattle per person. Similar findings have previously been reported in Canada [7].

Urban–rural gradients have been described for other zoonotic gastrointestinal pathogens. *Campylobacter* infection is the most common bacterial cause of acute gastroenteritis in the developed world. Consumption of contaminated poultry is widely accepted as a leading risk factor for sporadic disease, yet this does not fully explain the epidemiology of infection. In Sweden Nygard and colleagues [8] investigated associations between *Campylobacter* infection and environmental risk factors using a geographical information system. They found that *Campylobacter* incidence was independently associated with the average length of drinking water-pipe serving the household and with ruminant density, suggesting that drinking water and contamination from livestock may also be important risk factors for the human burden of campylobacteriosis. Intervention measures directed at controlling sporadic disease need to take account of urban/rural differences in the risk of acquiring infection.

Ecologic studies

One of the more controversial debates over recent years has revolved around the hypothesis that MMR (measles, mumps and rubella) vaccination increased an individual's risk of developing Crohn's disease. This hypothesis has been firmly refuted by a number of investigators, including Seagroatt [9], who conducted an ecologic analysis of national data on hospital admissions. She analyzed trends in age-specific admission rates for Crohn's disease in children and adolescents to see if the introduction of MMR vaccine in 1988 had increased rates in those populations that were vaccinated as infants. She found no increase in Crohn's disease rates associated with the introduction of MMR vaccine. The major drawback of ecologic studies, in which entire populations are compared, is the potential for confounding.

Case-case studies

A technique that is being used increasingly in infection epidemiology is the case-case comparison [10,11]. This has been enabled by advances in microbiological typing of infectious agents that enable cases with the same disease to be divided into etiologically meaningful subgroups. Cases in these subgroups can then be compared with each other, allowing a more refined analysis of factors associated with exposure to the infecting agent. The technique overcomes many of the biases inherent in selecting cases from sometimes highly inefficient surveillance systems and comparing them with controls not selected in a similar way.

However, there are also major drawbacks [10]. Firstly, exposures that are a risk for infection for both comparison groups will not be identified or might be underestimated. By using patients with the same infection, albeit with different subtypes, as "controls," there is a danger of obscuring an association with the infection of interest because the controls might share some of the risk exposures with the cases. Thus, exposures common to both infections are controlled for by the study design. Secondly, controls are traditionally selected to provide an estimate of the exposure prevalence that would be seen in the cases if there were no association between the exposure and disease. Because controls have been differentially selected by factors that are related to certain exposures, they might not be representative of the exposure prevalence of the population group from which the cases originated. Case-case comparisons cannot, therefore, be used to make statements about the magnitude or direction of population risk. They are, however, a very useful technique for generating hypotheses and for studying risk factors for antimicrobial resistance. For example, Gillespie et al. [12] conducted a case-case comparison of the two major *Campylobacter* species – *C. jejuni* and *C. coli*. Their findings showed that case-control studies of *Campylobacter* infection need to be conducted at the species level. Similarly, the Campylobacter

Sentinel Surveillance Scheme Collaborators [13] showed that the risk of acquiring a fluoroquinolone-resistant *C. jejuni* infection was strongly associated with foreign travel. Restricting the analyses by foreign travel showed that the risk of acquiring a resistant infection whilst abroad was independently associated with travel destination, and consumption of chicken and bottled water. These findings can be verified in additional microbiological and environmental studies.

Case-crossover studies

In case-crossover studies cases act as their own controls [14,15]. This type of study is ideal for focusing on exposures acting over a short period of time and lends itself to studying an infection where the incubation period is known and is relatively short. A history is obtained for the cases over at least two time periods. One of these covers the exposure window and is one incubation time before the onset of the infection. The exposures in this time period are then compared with those in other time periods. This method was used successfully in the investigation of an outbreak of salmonellosis in France [16]. Food exposures during a three-day risk period before onset of illness were compared with those of a control time-interval of the same duration that preceded the risk period by two days. Seventy-seven percent of the cases had consumed hamburgers in the three days preceding onset of illness compared with 29% during the control period (odds ratio = 5; 95% CI = 1.1–46.9). The epidemiological finding that hamburgers were the vehicle of infection was corroborated by environmental and laboratory investigations.

Collaboration is essential

One of the infection epidemiologist's most important professional allies is their microbiologist colleague. Improvements in typing techniques have helped the infection epidemiologist considerably, for example by increasing specificity in case definitions. Microbiological tools for confirming exposure to and/or presence of infection are being refined all the time.

Conclusion

In this brief introduction to infection epidemiology we have highlighted its unique features and described some of the special methods available to track infection to its source. However, other methods described elsewhere in this book can also be applied to the study of infection.

References

1. Giesecke J. *Modern Infectious Disease Epidemiology*, 2nd edn. London: Arnold, 2002.
2. Mausner JS, Kramer S. *Epidemiology – An Introductory Text*, 2nd edn. London: WB Saunders, 1985.
3. Wheeler JG *et al*. Study of infectious intestinal disease in England: rates in the community, presenting to general practice, and reported to national surveillance. The Infectious Intestinal Disease Study Executive. *Br Med J* 1999;**318**:1046.
4. Tam CC *et al*. The study of infectious intestinal disease in England: what risk factors for presentation to general practice tell us about potential for selection bias in case-control studies of reported cases of diarrhoea. *Int J Epidemiol* 2003;**32**:99.
5. Tarr PI *et al*. Shiga-toxin-producing *Escherichia coli* and haemolytic uraemic syndrome. *Lancet* 2005;**365**:1073.
6. Innocent GT *et al*. Spatial and temporal epidemiology of sporadic human cases of *Escherichia coli* O157 in Scotland, 1996–1999. *Epidemiol Infect* 2005;**133**:1033.
7. Michel P *et al*. Temporal and geographical distributions of reported cases of *Escherichia coli* O157:H7 infection in Ontario. *Epidemiol Infect* 1999;**122**:193.
8. Nygard K *et al*. Association between environmental risk factors and campylobacter infections in Sweden. *Epidemiol Infect* 2004;**132**:317.
9. Seagroatt V. MMR vaccine and Crohn's disease: ecological study of hospital admissions in England, 1991 to 2002. *Br Med J* 2005;**330**:1120.
10. McCarthy N, Giesecke J. Case-case comparisons to study causation of common infectious diseases. *Int J Epidemiol* 1999;**28**:764.
11. Kaye KS *et al*. The case-case-control study design: addressing the limitations of risk factor studies for antimicrobial resistance. *Infect Control Hosp Epidemiol* 2005;**26**:346.
12. Gillespie IA *et al*. A case-case comparison of *Campylobacter coli* and *Campylobacter jejuni* infection: a tool for generating hypotheses. *Emerg Infect Dis* 2002;**8**:937.
13. Campylobacter Sentinel Surveillance Scheme Collaborators. Ciprofloxacin resistance in *Campylobacter jejuni*: case-case analysis as a tool for elucidating risks at home and abroad. *J Antimicrob Chemother* 2002;**50**:561.
14. Maclure M. The case-crossover design: a method for studying transient effects on the risk of acute events. *Am J Epidemiol* 1991;**133**:144.
15. Maclure M, Mittleman MA. Should we use a case-crossover design? *Annu Rev Public Health* 2000;**21**:193.
16. Haegebaert S *et al*. The use of the case-crossover design in a continuous common source food-borne outbreak. *Epidemiol Infect* 2003;**131**:809.

14 Genetic Epidemiology

Yuri A. Saito and Gloria M. Petersen

Key points

- Genetic epidemiologic methods, based on traditional epidemiology and genetics, can be used to identify disease-susceptibility genes for common, complex genetic diseases.
- Study designs rely heavily on analysis of various family structures including twins or siblings, parent–offspring, nuclear families and even multi-generational families, but also include population-based patients.
- This methodology has resulted in the identification of several disease genes in the field of gastroenterology, including Crohn's disease.

Introduction

Genetic epidemiology is a relatively young but increasingly recognized field that represents the marriage of several disciplines including genetics, epidemiology and biostatistics. Its relevance as a field has increased with our growing knowledge and understanding of the human genome and the role of genetics in disease etiology. In the past, diseases were thought to be either exclusively genetic or environmental in origin. "Genetic diseases" were caused by one or a few highly penetrant mutations in select genes that typically presented at birth or early in childhood. Other diseases were the result of environmental exposures such as infection or radiation. However, increasingly, we are realizing that there are a number of chronic disorders with both genetic and environmental contributors, called "complex genetic diseases"

(Fig. 14.1). Complex genetic diseases are common in the general population, are thought to explain many chronic diseases, are due to multiple genes of modest effect, and may present in a clinically heterogeneous manner due to the presence or absence of various environmental and genetic risk factors and their gene–environment interactions. Because of these features, discovering the genetic susceptibility loci for common disorders is challenging, but is not futile when sound research methods are used. This chapter will provide an overview of genetic epidemiology and various study designs to provide an introductory but illustrative resource for those wishing to learn more about this field as applied to gastrointestinal (GI) disease.

Comparison of traditional epidemiology and genetic epidemiology

Genetic epidemiology shares many features with traditional epidemiology. For example, identifying risk factors for disease development and disease progression are at the heart of both types of epidemiology studies (Fig. 14.2) However, where traditional epidemiology has conventionally evaluated environmental risk factors and their interactions leading to disease in hosts, genetic epidemiology focuses on the evaluation of genetic risk factors and their interactions with environmental risk factors in the development of disease in susceptible individuals. Thus, the research questions are framed slightly differently between the two disciplines. In contrast to

Genetic Diseases	Complex Genetic Diseases	Environmental Diseases
Examples: Familial polyposis syndromes Hirschprung's disease	*Examples:* Crohn's disease Colon cancer	*Examples:* Radiation enteritis Viral hepatitis

Fig. 14.1 Spectrum of disease etiology.

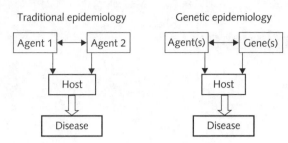

Fig. 14.2 A comparison of traditional epidemiology and genetic epidemiology.

classic epidemiology, which asks questions such as "Who gets the disease? Why does an individual get the disease? How does one prevent the disease or complications of the disease?," in genetic epidemiology, the question may be "What are the genetic factors that lead to the development of disease?"

There are many other inherent differences between the two fields. The focus of genetic epidemiology studies is not on studying incidence and prevalence, but rather genotype and phenotype frequencies. Similarly, rather than looking at epidemics in the general population or a clustering of disease in a community, genetic epidemiology focuses more on ethnic and geographic clusters and families. The study of families provides insight into both the genetic and environmental contributors to disease. It follows that factors such as age of onset, penetrance and carrier state, and expressivity are terms and concepts that may be of greater interest in genetic studies rather than traditional epidemiology. Nonetheless, genetic epidemiology studies need not be family-based, and as with epidemiologic studies, can be population-based.

An important difference between the two fields is the greater emphasis in genetic epidemiology on biospecimen collection and genetic, laboratory-based testing. Genetic epidemiologic techniques can be used to answer specific questions such as identifying where a gene is in the genome map, how much this gene can explain disease in the population, and determining the causal link between the gene and the disease. As a consequence, a greater understanding of the disease biology, of genetics, and of genotyping technologies is required for genetic epidemiology studies, and a team consisting of a clinical researcher, genetic epidemiologist, statistical geneticist and laboratory-based geneticist is usually required in order to conduct specific types of studies.

Study designs and approaches

The types of study designs that are commonly used in genetic epidemiology studies are summarized in Box 14.1.

Clinical and historical studies

Clinical and traditional epidemiologic studies may be required prior to proceeding with other lines of inquiry. Clinical studies may indicate features that suggest a genetic basis for the disease of interest, such as association with other known genetic diseases, racial differences in predisposition, or a family history of disease. Association with other diseases that have a known genetic basis certainly provides one form of evidence of a genetic basis for disease. If the disease of interest appears race-specific, additional migration or admixture studies may be helpful to determine whether the predisposition is due to genetics or cultural factors. Similarly, a positive family history of disease may indicate the need for further family-based studies, to determine whether the clustering is due to genetics or shared environmental exposures or lifestyle.

Family studies

Family studies may simply consist of comparing the frequency of cases that have a positive family history with the proportion of controls that have a positive family history of the disease of interest. The most basic type of this study collects family history data from affected cases, and compares the proportion with a positive family history with either the population prevalence rate or, more ideally, with age-, gender- and race-matched controls. This study design is no different from a conventional case-

---

Box 14.1 Genetic epidemiology study designs
- Clinical and historical studies
  Age-of-onset, race, geography, migration studies
- Descriptive family studies
  Familial aggregation studies
  Twin studies
  Adoption studies
- Segregation analyses
- Genome-wide studies
  Linkage analysis
  Genome-wide association studies
- Candidate-gene association studies

control study and is also referred to as the family history approach. However, collecting family medical data from cases and controls can be fraught with error, particularly if the disease of interest is not visible or easily recognizable by laypeople, has many causes, is in an early or mild stage, has a social stigma associated with it, or has an onset late in life when the individual is not sharing a household with siblings or children. For example, relatives are more likely to be aware of a diagnosis of cancer or cirrhosis in the family, but may be less knowledgeable about whether the cancer is primary or metastatic, or whether the liver disease is due to primary biliary cirrhosis or nonalcoholic fatty liver disease. Family members may also not feel comfortable discussing their bowel habits with others, and thus irritable bowel syndrome may be under-recognized by cases and controls alike. Thus, there is a danger of misclassification of the relative's affected/unaffected status based on proband report alone.

Rather than collecting the relatives' medical data from probands, a better approach for familial aggregation studies is referred to as a family case-control design or family study approach. This design consists of direct survey of the relatives themselves, and may involve review of their medical records, or even clinical evaluation and diagnostic testing. Therefore, misclassification of "affected" and "unaffected" status of relatives can be minimized. The disadvantage of this approach is that not all relatives may wish to participate in the study, not all relatives may be alive to participate in the study, and not all relatives may be able to participate in the study due to the presence of other medical comorbidities such as dementia. These factors may lead to much "missing" information. However, missing data can be minimized by asking the next of kin or those with power of attorney for deceased individuals or individuals unable to participate to provide consent and release of medical information for that relative.

With the data collected from family members, various analyses may be performed. First, pedigree construction – manually or using software such as Progeny (www.progeny2000.com) or Pedigree-Draw (www.pedigree-draw.com) – may be illustrative to identify interesting families worthy of greater study. Second, comparison of the proportions of positive family history of disease between cases and controls may also be illustrative of the risk that family members of cases have for the disease of interest given that there is an affected family member (i.e., recurrence risk). Third, because different relative types may have different patterns of risk, the risk or heritability for specific relationships may be calculated. Fourth, evaluation of and detection of relevant gene–environment interactions may

be performed using this study design. Thus, confirmation of familial aggregation represents an important line of investigation to determine whether additional genetic studies are merited in searching for disease etiology.

Twin studies represent a specific type of family study, with a classic gene versus environment approach whereby a genetic basis for disease is assumed if there is greater concordance of disease in monozygotic (identical) twins than in dizygotic (nonidentical) twins. Environment is thought to play a greater role if there is greater or equal concordance in dizygotic twins than monozygotic twins. If there is evidence for a genetic basis for disease, these studies can provide a quantitative estimate of general liability for disease by calculating the difference in concordance between monozygotic twins and dizygotic twins. However, twin studies have several limitations, including the inability to adjust for prenatal differences between twins (position *in utero*, manner of delivery, shared or non-shared placental circulation) and postnatal differences in upbringing; ultimately further study is warranted to identify disease gene loci. Nonetheless, twin studies often provide additional evidence supporting a genetic basis for disease.

Segregation analyses

Segregation analysis is a method that requires further in-depth study of families. Pedigrees are constructed and family members are assigned an affected or unaffected status. Segregation analysis compares the observed distribution of affected and unaffected individuals in a series of families under a specific genetic hypothesis (e.g., autosomal dominant model) with the distribution that would be expected under specific genetic or nongenetic models. Segregation analysis compares these multiple models to establish which model best fits the observed data, thereby enabling the likely model for the disease to be inferred. Segregation analysis studies thus answer questions such as whether or not a major gene contributes to disease expression, whether multiple genes with small effects can result, and whether nongenetic factors contribute to disease etiology. Segregation studies are most helpful not only in providing a genetic model for disease transmission but also in estimating the penetrance and attributable frequency required for parametric analysis in follow-up linkage studies.

However, special considerations regarding segregation analysis must be made. First, this method identifies the best-fitting model of the ones tested, but does not necessarily reject an incorrect model (type II error). Also, this method is not immune to type I errors (i.e., incorrectly rejecting the correct model). Furthermore, segregation analysis is particularly susceptible to a form of selection bias called ascertainment bias; that is, the families studied may not be representative of those in the general population. In this situation, while adjustments for ascertainment can be incorporated in the analysis, conclusions drawn may be distorted. Confounding by other factors, such as environmental exposures, must also be taken into account. Many of these points apply to any observational epidemiologic study, but this is particularly important because segregation analysis often provides the parameters and assumptions needed for linkage studies.

Linkage analysis

Linkage studies are performed if no gene has been firmly tied to disease causation and the investigator is trying to identify the region in the genome map where the disease gene may lie. Approximately 500–6000 genetic markers with known genomic location that span the human genome are selected; these markers are then genotyped in family members. Parametric or model-based linkage uses set penetrance estimates and an inheritance model (which may be derived from segregation analyses), and the observed transmission of each marker with disease status is compared to determine which genetic marker appears to be most closely linked to the disease of interest. Alternatively, linkage analysis can be performed without such estimates (model-free linkage or nonparametric linkage analysis). It is hoped that a genetic marker will identify a region of up to 10 Mb (megabases) in size; then additional markers can be used to narrow the region of interest further. The concept behind linkage is that genetic recombination is more likely between genetic loci that are far apart thus separating them during meiosis; so, by looking at the recombination rate between family members (who should share large regions of the genome inherited from the same recent ancestor), the position of the disease gene relative to the marker can be estimated. Linkage studies require the participation of families, which can be extended multigenerational families, nuclear families or specific subunits such as affected sibling pairs. Genetic markers of study include restriction fragment length polymorphisms (RFLPs), variable number of tandem repeats (VNTRs), microsatellites and single nucleotide polymorphisms (SNPs).

The main limitation of parametric linkage methods is that the genetic model must be specified, and if incor-

rect, may result in false positives as well as false negatives. Any error in the model leads to inconsistent parameter estimates and lack of power. For these reasons, nonparametric, model-free methods are also utilized. In addition, because of the low rate of recombination events within most families, linkage analyses may not be able to narrow the genomic region of interest below several megabases. Furthermore, although linkage studies have been immensely successful in identifying disease susceptibility loci for Mendelian diseases, these studies are less powerful when studying a complex, non-Mendelian genetic disease caused by multiple genes of modest genetic effect. In this situation, association studies may be a better alternative to identifying specific disease-causing gene or genes.

Genome-wide association studies

Genome-wide association studies (also referred to as whole-genome association studies) offer investigators the opportunity physically to localize areas of interest on the genome by analyzing genotyping data from genetic markers spanning the genome. Association studies typically use classic epidemiologic case-control designs to compare the allele frequency of a genetic marker in disease cases and unrelated healthy controls with the goal of identifying markers with allele frequencies that differ between the two groups. Association studies are thought to be advantageous when studying common alleles with modest disease risk, and do not require the assembly of pedigrees and collection of DNA from family members, and it is typically easier to collect DNA from a large series of unrelated cases and controls than it is to collect DNA from family members, as described above. However, because the number of markers shared between unrelated individuals will be fewer, more (thousands to possibly hundreds of thousands) high-density markers will need to be genotyped among thousands of study subjects. Although advances in high-throughput genotyping technology have decreased costs, this method is still resource intensive, and therefore remains expensive to conduct, limiting the number of these studies that can be performed.

Candidate gene-disease association studies

Similar to genome-wide association studies, candidate gene-disease association studies compare allele frequencies of a given polymorphic genetic marker between cases and controls; if an allele is found to be more common in cases, this finding suggests that this polymorphism may be contributing to the development of disease. These studies may involve studying only one to a few polymorphisms and using chi-squared analysis or Fisher's exact test, and thus, are fairly simple to perform and analyze. However, these studies require *a priori* knowledge of a putative candidate gene, and selecting the right polymorphism may not be easy with an estimated 30 000–40 000 genes in the genome, and over 25 polymorphisms in the form of SNPs, RFLPs, VNTRs, and insertions and deletions in an average 27 kb gene. Nonetheless, this method represents a direct test of association that may be powerful if the polymorphic marker is carefully selected on the basis of biological plausibility and linkage studies.

How the NOD2/CARD15 gene in Crohn's disease was discovered

Multiple studies evaluating family history in first-degree relatives of patients with Crohn's disease (CD) and ulcerative colitis consistently demonstrated familial aggregation of inflammatory bowel disease (IBD), although aggregation rates ranged between 3.5 and 22% [1]. A good example of a family history study was published by Orholm *et al.*, who interviewed 662 patients with IBD to collect data about first- and second-degree relatives and demonstrated that relatives of probands with CD were ten times more likely than the general population to have CD, and 3.85 times more likely to have ulcerative colitis [2]. Three twin studies demonstrated that the estimated genetic liability of CD ranged between 13.5% and 58% [3–5]. Thus, these family-based studies provided the foundation to identify a genetic basis for CD.

One segregation analysis of 265 probands with CD suggested the presence of a recessive gene with complete penetrance [6]. However, the probands selected for this study were recruited from a specialty clinic at a major university, raising the concern of ascertainment bias. The first population-based segregation analysis study of CD was also published by Orholm and colleagues in 1993 [7]. Focusing on CD, 133 patients with CD diagnosed in Copenhagen County before 1979 were mailed family history questionnaires, and positive responses led to telephone calls to collect names and dates of birth of relatives, and review of the affected relatives' medical records. The 133 CD pedigrees were split into 209 nuclear families with 549 children. Segregation analysis of these relatives demonstrated that the best-fitting model was a major recessive gene with complete penetrance, although this model was not significantly different from a multifactorial model.

Hugot *et al.* subsequently published a paper mapping a susceptibility locus for CD to chromosome 16 [8]. Initial study of 25 families using parametric linkage analysis of 270 markers and assuming a recessive mode of transmission resulted in exclusion of the whole genome. Only when the analysis was repeated using nonparametric methods were four markers in two regions identified, and further study of that genomic region resulted in the first "IBD1" locus being described on the pericentromeric region of chromosome 16. Thereafter, Hugot *et al.* and Ogura *et al.* published simultaneously their discovery of the *nod2* gene within the IBD1 locus using a positional cloning strategy and candidate gene approach, respectively [9,10] Subsequently, several genotype-phenotype correlation studies and protein structure, expression and function studies have been conducted supporting the role of this gene in CD pathogenesis [11], but the full details regarding interaction between a bacterial pathogen and the immune system resulting in disease remain unclear. Nonetheless, the story of how this gene and other susceptibility loci were discovered illustrates the progression of studies that led to successful gene identification.

Conclusion

Because many gastrointestinal diseases appear to aggregate in families, the question of how clinical and laboratory researchers can determine the genetic contributions to their disease of interest will arise frequently. Teasing out the genetic and environmental contributors to these complex genetic diseases is not easy, but unraveling the respective genetic etiologies for each disease can be performed using sound genetic epidemiology methods and techniques. The approaches taken will likely use a combination of family-based as well as population-based study patients, and more than one approach may be successful. The successful discovery of the *NOD2/CARD15* gene, and other disease susceptibility loci in Crohn's disease, provides a good example of the application of various methods to a gastrointestinal disease. Those interested in pursuing this line of investigation are encouraged to obtain additional training, and collaborate closely with genetic epidemiologists, biostatistical geneticists and laboratory-based geneticists to develop the approaches and resources needed for their field of study.

The Mayo Foundation retains copyright on all original artwork.

References

1. Russel MG *et al.* Familial aggregation of inflammatory bowel disease: a population-based study in South Limburg, The Netherlands. The South Limburg IBD Study Group. *Scand J Gastroenterol* 1997(Suppl.);**223**:88.
2. Orholm M *et al.* Familial occurrence of inflammatory bowel disease. *N Engl J Med* 1991;**324**:84.
3. Tysk C *et al.* Ulcerative colitis and Crohn's disease in an unselected population of monozygotic and dizygotic twins. A study of heritability and the influence of smoking. *Gut* 1988;**29**:990.
4. Thompson NP *et al.* Genetics versus environment in inflammatory bowel disease: results of a British twin study. *Br Med J* 1996;**312**:95.
5. Orholm M *et al.* Concordance of inflammatory bowel disease among Danish twins. Results of a nationwide study. *Scand J Gastroenterol* 2000;**35**:1075.
6. Kuster W *et al.* The genetics of Crohn disease: complex segregation analysis of a family study with 265 patients with Crohn disease and 5,387 relatives. *Am J Med Genet* 1989;**32**:105.
7. Orholm M *et al.* Investigation of inheritance of chronic inflammatory bowel diseases by complex segregation analysis. *Br Med J* 1993;**306**:20.
8. Hugot JP *et al.* Mapping of a susceptibility locus for Crohn's disease on chromosome 16. *Nature* 1996;**379**:821.
9. Hugot JP *et al.* Association of NOD2 leucine-rich repeat variants with susceptibility to Crohn's disease. *Nature* 2001;**411**:599.
10. Ogura Y *et al.* A frameshift mutation in NOD2 associated with susceptibility to Crohn's disease. *Nature* 2001;**411**:603.
11. Gaya DR *et al.* New genes in inflammatory bowel disease: lessons for complex diseases? *Lancet* 2006;**367**:1271.

15 A Career in GI Epidemiology

Linda Rabeneck

Key points
- It is important to define your goals, understand the measures of academic success and the requirements for promotion, and to have a mentor.
- Formal research training is essential.
- Develop a thematic research agenda that is externally funded.
- Career Development Awards are a key building block to a successful career.
- Having protected time to do research and being skilled at time management are key determinants of academic success.

A career in academic gastroenterology (GI) as a clinical researcher is intellectually stimulating and satisfying. However, many trainees and faculties do not know how to develop such a career. Whereas career development for basic science investigators in GI is well understood, the career path for clinical researchers is not so well worn. The purpose of this chapter is to describe how to develop a career in clinical research in GI for those who wish to become a principal investigator, defined as someone who develops the ideas, obtains funding, and who assumes responsibility for the conduct of the research and the publication of results. Although there is a body of published literature on the topic [1–6] that serves as a basis for this chapter, the content also reflects the opinions and experience of the author.

General principles for a successful academic career

Several principles can guide a person to career success in academic GI focusing on epidemiology and clinical research. First, it is important to define your goals. Second, you need to understand the measures of academic success and the requirements for promotion. Third, you need to have a mentor.

Defining goals

The overarching goal for a career in GI epidemiology is to conduct meaningful research that makes an important contribution to new knowledge. The research should be of sufficient caliber to enable the researcher to obtain external, federal, peer-reviewed funding, for example from the National Institutes of Health (NIH) or Veterans Affairs (VA). The research agenda comprises a body of linked studies in a topic area or theme, for example colorectal cancer screening. The research is published in the peer-reviewed literature – as much as possible in journals with higher impact factors. The researcher achieves peer recognition for this body of work. This is characterized by invitations to give presentations at the annual scientific meetings of the professional societies, such as the American Gastroenterological Association (AGA) at Digestive Disease Week.

Given this overarching goal, the next step is to identify two or three long-term (5-year) goals [1]. An example would be to achieve a grant from a federal funding agency to support a research project that forms part of the thematic research agenda. Short-term goals are important building blocks. An example of a short-term (6–12-month) goal is to conduct a pilot study to support a funding application. Another example would be to submit a manuscript that reports research results that relate to the overall thematic research agenda and provide evidence of feasibility of the research to be proposed in the funding application.

It is important to review your short- and long-term goals annually, at a minimum, with your Division Chief to ensure that your goals are aligned with your Chief's expectations, and that she or he has the opportunity to provide guidance, support or course correction if that is needed.

Measures of academic success

The first measure of success is peer-reviewed publication – for which there is no substitute. Original articles, which report the results of your own research, are the academic "coin of the realm" [1]. Note that book chapters are not considered peer-reviewed, and do not carry the same "weight" as original articles. Therefore, early in a career, in general, you would undertake to write a book chapter only if it clearly supported the long-term goal of achieving peer-reviewed funding. Too often a junior researcher agrees to write a book chapter on a topic unrelated to his or her research agenda when the time would be more profitably spent writing an original article. This is a common pitfall that arises when a senior – and often overextended – researcher is asked to undertake a book chapter and seeks to delegate this to a junior colleague.

The second measure of success is research support. Federal support (NIH, VA) is given more "weight" than support from foundations (e.g., Crohn's and Colitis Foundation of America) and professional disease societies (e.g., AGA), which in turn are given more weight than industry support. The reason for this is that federal funding applications undergo the most formal and rigorous peer review process, and therefore this type of funding is more difficult to obtain. Moreover, industry support is often not peer-reviewed.

Getting promoted

Know the "rules of the game" [1]. The criteria for promotion from Assistant to Associate Professor are defined **locally**, by each institution. This means that the criteria for promotion cannot be precisely compared across institutions. Institutions have different career tracks. The career tracks for a gastroenterologist who takes a position in a Division of Gastroenterology will be the career tracks for that institution's Department of Medicine. Typically there are several tracks. The number of tracks and their descriptors will be described and available in a faculty handbook. Examples of typical tracks would be: Clinician Scientist (75% research, 25% patient care and teaching), Clinician Investigator (50% research, 50% patient care and teaching) and Clinician Teacher (>75% patient care and teaching). The job descriptions – and therefore the expectations to meet criteria for promotion – differ among these tracks. The first two tracks are relevant for a junior researcher who intends to pursue a career in GI epidemiology. It is important to be appointed to the appropriate track from the outset, to be clear what the track entails, and what the expectations are for promotion. It is important that you and your Division Chief agree on your track. Compared with the Clinician Investigator, the bar is set higher for the Clinician Scientist in terms of research productivity, as measured by publications and grant funding. However, this is offset by the greater amount of time that one has to devote to research. Some institutions will have established a number of years during which an individual has to achieve promotion, for example 7 years. Find out whether your institution has such a rule and what the implications are for you.

To achieve promotion to Associate Professor in the Clinician Scientist track requires a record of peer-reviewed publications, external peer-reviewed funding and an emerging national reputation. It is unlikely that the faculty handbook will identify the number of publications that are expected; clearly this depends on the journals in which the papers are published. This is for the Promotions Committee at the institution to judge. A smaller number of papers in the very top journals – as measured by impact factor – will be viewed more favorably than a larger number in lower impact journals. A good number to aim for is 25 publications. Not all will be first-author papers, but a reasonable proportion should be.

If you are in a Clinician Scientist track, it would be a mistake to focus solely on publications and grant funding. Virtually all institutions expect contributions to patient care and teaching, and the quality and quantity of these will be assessed. Superb achievement in research will not offset poor teaching evaluations when it comes to meeting the criteria for promotion.

Letters of support are an important part of the "package" to support promotion. The faculty handbook at your institution will generally indicate how many are needed. The letters should be from senior experienced researchers in your field at other institutions, who know of your work, and are able to judge your contributions. Letters from peers who are at the same stage of career as you are not generally helpful. The corollary to this is that you need to achieve visibility in the field. You do this by presenting your work at national scientific meetings so that senior researchers will get to know you and your work.

Having a mentor

Given what we have discussed thus far, it makes sense to have a mentor to guide you in matters such as promotion. Researchers who are mentored are more likely to achieve career success. What are the characteristics of a good mentor? First, if your goal is to be a Clinician Scientist with all that entails – especially external grant support – you need a mentor who has the skill set. Successful grant writing is a skill set; you need a mentor who has achieved peer-reviewed funding. A common pitfall among junior investigators is to select a mentor who may be recognized in the field, but who has not written or cannot write a successful federal grant application. Second, your mentor needs to be at a career stage when he or she is willing to devote the time and energy required to assist you. This means that not only is your mentor more senior in terms of academic rank, but also has reached a stage of maturity when she or he has a desire to give assistance and see others flourish and succeed. Not all senior researchers achieve this stage of maturity – something to keep in mind in selecting a mentor.

Research training

This is essential. Your clinical training in GI has taught you the principles and practice of gastroenterology, including how to function as a consultant, and how to perform endoscopic procedures. In the course of your clinical training and clinical practice, you will have formulated clinical questions for which you cannot find answers in the literature. What you do not have are the skills needed to address your research questions. In other words, your clinical training has not provided you with the skills needed to conduct independent research if your intended career is a Clinician Scientist or Clinician Investigator. You need formal training in clinical investigation. This is completely analogous to the situation in laboratory research, in which it is mandatory for a trained gastroenterologist who seeks a career as a Clinician Scientist to acquire research training in the laboratory [2,4].

Training in clinical investigation generally consists of formal coursework and conducting one or more research projects under the guidance of a mentor. The research project should lead to peer-reviewed publication. The coursework encompasses study design, biostatistics, and the principles of classical epidemiology and clinical epidemiology. Additional topics include decision sciences, health economic analysis and health services research. A minimum 2-year period of training, leading to a master's degree is desirable. Researchers who have formal training in clinical investigation are more likely to achieve external funding than those who are not trained [3].

One of the oldest and most successful programs for formal training is the Robert Wood Johnson Clinical Scholars Program in the USA. Formal training can also be acquired at a School of Public Health or in a formal degree-granting curriculum within a Department of Medicine. The choice of formal coursework will be in part determined by your interest and by the requirement for the master's degree. Formal training is essential.

Developing a research agenda

The goal is to develop a thematic research agenda that is externally funded. In general, when beginning a career, it is important to focus on one or at most two topic areas. For example, you may want to develop a research agenda focused on colorectal cancer screening. Within that topic area, there are many possible research questions that could be developed, for example, what are current screening rates, what screening tests are used, what are the determinants of use of the various screening tests, etc. Try to develop a series of linked projects centered on a theme. An advantage of this is that when you are preparing grant proposals for external funding to support your research, you will need preliminary data. The more focused you have been in your research activities the likelier it is that you will have done studies to generate these data. In addition, by being focused you are more likely to develop a research team of co-investigators and collaborators to assist you with your grant proposals and studies. A common pitfall among junior investigators is lack of focus.

How do you choose a research theme? The first criterion is that it should interest you [1]. There will be setbacks along the way as you develop your research, and a deep and sustained interest in the topic will help you as you navigate the challenging times in which your manuscripts and grant proposals are rejected by reviewers. The second criterion is that it is preferable that the topic is important in terms of prevalence of disease, disease burden (morbidity, mortality) and use of healthcare resources. The more important the topic is to the field, the more likely you are to obtain funding to support the work. In addition, you will have the satisfaction of working in an area in which your research findings will have a larger impact. Finally, although not a criterion *per se*, be alert to research questions that are considered "hot" as you execute your studies. In any topic area, periodically a research question will arise that is considered the next key issue to be addressed. If you are already working in that area, you may be well positioned to address it. But do not switch from one "hot" topic to another – this is not the way to develop a thematic research agenda in the long term.

While it is important to have a research theme, you should diversify your studies and projects within that area. Try not to put all your eggs in one basket. An example would be a study that requires long-term follow-up and requires primary data collection. For such a study, a larger amount of funding will be needed, which will take some time to achieve, and the results will not be available soon. Try to develop a group of studies, some of which will provide results in the short term, such as an analysis of existing data.

Finally, seek feedback on your proposed research agenda. Having a mentor is crucial, because he or she would have the experience and judgment to advise you on what you propose. Your mentor will help you assess:

- is the project feasible?
- will it answer an important question?
- will it lead to further studies in the same area?
- is the topic area fundable?
- are the research questions interesting, i.e., do they pass the "so what" test?

Funding

Just as carefully as you and your mentor plan your thematic research agenda, you will also need to consider where to obtain funding. There are two types of funding: investigator-initiated research funding, also known as operating funds (to support your research projects), and career development awards (to provide salary support for you).

Operating funds

In terms of investigator-initiated funding, at the outset it is better to begin with small pilot projects to support your subsequent grant proposals (see above). You should be able to obtain local funds for this pilot work. Your mentor can help you identify these funds. For example, if your institution has an NIH-funded Digestive Disease Center, a Program Project grant, or is a participating site in a large collaborative group or consortium, often there are specific funds set aside to be used to support pilot studies. Funding may also be available from your Department of Medicine or Dean's Office. The latter funding mechanisms are intended to support the research of junior investigators to help them get started.

The second step is to seek external funding to support your research, for example from one of the gastroenterology or hepatology professional societies (e.g., AGA, ACG, ASGE, AASLD) or disease foundations (e.g., Crohn's and Colitis Foundation of America). Details about funding opportunities can be found on these organizations' websites.

The third step is federal funding to support your research, most commonly from the VA or the NIH. A common pitfall among junior investigators is to start here. Because federal funding is more difficult to obtain, you should do this when you are well prepared to be competitive. In general this means that you have completed preliminary studies and have some pilot data, and have published in the area, or at least have a manuscript that has been submitted and is under review. Do not attempt to obtain federal funding without good guidance. Your mentor can help you determine when it is time to compete for federal funds, and also help you determine whether you satisfy the eligibility criteria for VA funding if you practice at a VA Medical Center. Your mentor should help you prepare your grant proposal so that it is competitive. Keep abreast of NIH funding announcements, such as RFAs, by signing up for the electronic distribution list.

Career development awards

Nowadays, all gastroenterologists in the USA who hold an academic position must generate their own salary. For a Clinician Teacher, the salary is generated by the reimbursements from payers for patient care. A Clinical Scientist is not able to generate an entire salary in patient care. This means that funding for the 75% of the position that is devoted to research must be generated by other means. In general, at the time of the first faculty appointment, the Clinician Scientist will receive a guarantee in the contract of a specific minimum salary amount that will be provided, with the expectation that the remaining 25% be generated by income from patient care. The key to note is that the provision of the minimum salary guarantee will be time limited (generally 2–3 years), after which time it is the responsibility of the Clinician Scientist to establish this salary support.

The Clinician Scientist can generate this support from the salary component of a research grant, such as an NIH R01 or a Career Development Award (CDA). Obtaining a CDA is key at this crucial time in beginning a career as a Clinician Scientist. Two main sources for CDAs include the NIH K23 Award and the VA Health Services Research & Development (HSR&D) Career Development Award. Additional sources include the professional societies and disease-specific foundations.

CDAs differ in terms of the amounts of salary support and period of the award. The way in which they are judged, however, is similar. In general, an application for a CDA has four components on which it is judged. The first component is the candidate. Is there evidence of research productivity, such as a manuscript submitted or published? Does the candidate have formal training in research – or have a plan to obtain this training? The second component is the mentor. Does the mentor have a record of peer-reviewed federal funding? Is the mentor sufficiently senior to have the experience to undertake the mentoring? Does the mentor have a track record of successful research mentoring? How strong is the mentor's statement of commitment? A common pitfall for junior investigators is for a strong candidate to have selected a mentor who does not have the skills or track record to mentor the candidate to achieve peer-reviewed federal funding as a Principal Investigator. In this instance, a reasonable approach would be to identify two mentors: one who is an expert in the topic of the research (e.g., hepatocellular carcinoma), and a second who has the skills to teach successful grant writing. The latter need not be a gastroenterologist if there is no individual in the Division with this expertise. The third component is the proposed research. Is it feasible? Has the candidate thought through the issues carefully, and assembled a team that can pull it off? The fourth component of the application is the institution. Are there sufficient resources available? This could include the necessary patient population, a clinical database, co-investigators, a core facility, a tissue biorepository, etc. Are the Division Chief and Department Chair committed to supporting the career plans and development of the candidate? Is there tangible evidence of this support, such as protected time? How strong are the letters of support?

One of the tasks of the mentor is to assist the candidate in achieving a CDA within the first 3 years of faculty appointment. In doing so, the mentor is responsible – working with the candidate – to help to develop the candidate's research ideas and to identify co-investigators and resources, so that the research application is compelling and competitive.

Publishing

Getting published is much easier if you enjoy writing and want to do it. Most well-published researchers schedule a time to write. Find out when you prefer to write – for some this is early in the morning, for others it is late at night – and guard this time carefully [1]. Set a deadline, do an outline, and begin. If you have inertia because the task seems too large, break it up into chunks. For example, start with the Methods section of the manuscript, and begin by describing the study population, and do as much as you can. Or start with the Results section. It really does not matter where you start. Don't attempt to have a perfect draft before circulating it to co-authors, but focus on keeping the writing moving forward. Do a reasonable draft, then when you circulate the draft to co-authors you can indicate where you need their input.

Physicians tend to have undergraduate training in the sciences, rather than the arts, so that writing may not be a skill that they have developed. Writing skills can be acquired, however. Take a writing course. Also, having others, who may not be co-authors but who write well, to critique your drafts can be very instructive as you develop your own writing skills.

Time

You need time to do research. When you negotiate your first faculty position, if you already have formal training in research and your intention is to be a researcher, at a minimum you should be on the Clinician Investigator, but preferably the Clinician Scientist track. Note that the greater the proportion of your time that is spent in non-research activities, the lower the chance of obtaining external funding [3]. A common pitfall among junior faculty who seek to become independent researchers is not to obtain formal training in research, which means their Division Chief has no option other than to appoint them on the Clinician Teacher track.

An often neglected aspect of career development is a discussion of time management. Know when you are most productive and guard these times. Ensure that you schedule regular time slots for writing. This means that – as much as possible – you have to learn to say "no" to activities that take away your writing time [1,5]. This may mean finding a location other than your office, where you go to write. Discipline yourself to check emails at times that do not interfere with your writing time.

Characteristics of productive researchers

Previous work has identified at least six characteristics of productive researchers [1].

1 In-depth knowledge of the research topic. This underscores the point about the need to develop a focused research agenda. You are more likely to be up to date in

your own knowledge if you are not trying to keep abreast of multiple topic areas.

2 Productive researchers are well socialized. To do this you need to present your work at scientific meetings, where you will interact with others working in the same field, keep up to date, and develop a network of colleagues and potential collaborators.

3 Productive researchers are well mentored. This is key, for all the reasons discussed above.

4 Productive researchers have scholarly work habits. They guard their writing times carefully and stay focused on their goals.

5 Productive researchers have a supportive local environment, including a mentor, co-investigators, collaborators and the opportunity to compete for local funding.

6 Productive researchers tend to have multiple projects underway, within a thematic research area. Having a portfolio of small and larger projects, with a spectrum of short-term and longer-term results, at different stages of completion, will ensure that you always have work "in the pipeline."

Conclusions

An academic career in GI epidemiology is a challenging, stimulating, satisfying and very enjoyable endeavor. The principles outlined here are intended to serve as a guideline to enhance the chance of success for those who seek to become independent researchers. Good luck!

References

1. Applegate WB, Williams ME. Career development in academic medicine. *Am J Med* 1990;**88**:263.
2. Goldman L. Blueprint for a research career in general internal medicine. *J Gen Intern Med* 1991;**6**:341.
3. Lee TH *et al.* Correlates of external research support among respondents to the 1990 American Federation for Clinical Research survey. *Clin Res* 1991;**39**:135.
4. Lee TH, Goldman L. Models of postdoctoral clinical research training. *J Investig Med* 1995;**43**:250.
5. Sackett DL. On the determinants of academic success as a clinician-scientist. *Clin Invest Med* 2001;**24**:94.
6. Lewis JD. The pathway to academic success starts during fellowship. *Gastrointest Endosc* 2005;**61**:587.

16 Funding Opportunities at the National Institutes of Health

James E. Everhart and Judith M. Podskalny

Key points

- The National Institutes of Health (NIH) fund intramural and extramural research in digestive disease epidemiology.
- Funding opportunities exist, based on career stage, for training grants, career transition grants and independent investigator grants.
- Numerous resources regarding study funding are available at the NIH that are accessible by phone or online.

This chapter is a guide for investigators seeking training, career development and research support from the National Institutes of Health (NIH) of the USA to study the epidemiology of gastroenterological diseases. The chapter begins with early postdoctoral research training opportunities and proceeds through obtaining independent investigator initiated research grants. This path to independent investigator can be seen in Fig. 16.1. Table 16.1 provides the codes and internet resources used to support training and research applicable to gastroenterological epidemiology.

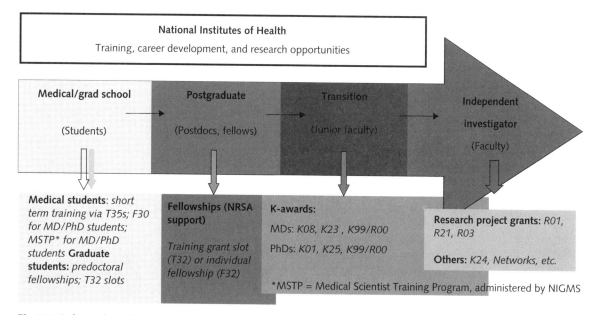

Fig. 16.1 Path to independent investigator through support by the National Institutes of Health.

Table 16.1 National Institutes of Health Grant Programs for Training, Career Development and Research. For entire list, see Types of Grant Programs (http://grants2.nih.gov/grants/funding/funding_program.htm) under the NIH Office of Extramural Research (http://grants2.nih.gov/grants/oer.htm)

Activity code or acronym	Title	Website
Training		
NRSA	National Research Service Award	http://grants.nih.gov/training/nrsa.htm
T32	Institutional Research Training Award (NRSA)	http://grants2.nih.gov/grants/guide/pa-files/PA-02–109.html
F30	Individual predoctoral awards for MD/PhD fellowships	http://grants2.nih.gov/grants/guide/pa-files/PA-05–151.html
F31	Individual predoctoral fellowship	http://grants2.nih.gov/grants/guide/pa-files/PA-04–032.html
F32	Individual postdoctoral fellowship (NRSA)	http://grants2.nih.gov/grants/guide/pa-files/PA-03–067.html
LRP	Loan Repayment Program	http://www.lrp.nih.gov/
Career development awards		http://grants2.nih.gov/training/careerdevelopmentawards.htm
K01	Mentored Research Scientist Development Award	http://grants2.nih.gov/grants/guide/pa-files/PA-06–001.html
K08	Mentored Clinical Scientist Development Award	http://grants2.nih.gov/grants/guide/pa-files/PA-00–003.html
K23	Mentored Patient-Oriented Research Career Development Award	http://grants2.nih.gov/grants/guide/pa-files/PA-05–143.html
K24	Mid-Career Investigator Award in Patient-Oriented Research Award	http://grants2.nih.gov/grants/guide/pa-files/PA-04–107.html
K99/R00	Pathway to Independence Award	http://grants.nih.gov/grants/new_investigators/index.htm
K25	Mentored Quantitative Research Development Award	http://grants.nih.gov/grants/guide/pa-files/PA-06–087.html
Research grant programs		
R01	Research Project Grant Program	http://grants2.nih.gov/grants/funding/r01.htm
R03	Small Grant Program	http://grants2.nih.gov/grants/funding/r03.htm
R21	Exploratory/Developmental Research Grant Award	http://grants2.nih.gov/grants/funding/r21.htm
R34	Clinical Trial Planning Grant Program	http://grants2.nih.gov/grants/funding/r34.htm
Other resources		
CRISP	Computer Retrieval of Information on Scientific Projects	http://crisp.cit.nih.gov/
NIH Guide	NIH Guide to Grants and Contracts	http://grants1.nih.gov/grants/guide/index.html
New Investigators		http://grants2.nih.gov/grants/new_investigators/

Background

Twenty years ago, it would have been difficult to find the breadth and depth of expertise to write this book. Fewer than a dozen persons in North America would have characterized themselves as digestive disease epidemiologists. Since that time, there has been an increasing recognition of the value of epidemiological methods applied to the clinical problems of gastroenterology. As a result, major contributions have been made to our knowledge of many important disorders. Government support in the USA and many other countries has contributed to much of this progress. In the USA the majority of public funding for biomedical research comes from the NIH. Nearly 20 of the expert authors of this book have received NIH funding for training or for clinical and epidemiological research.

Twenty-four of the 27 institutes and centers that make up the NIH fund research, as detailed on the NIH website (http://www.nih.gov/icd/). Many of the institutes provide funding for gastroenterological or for epidemiological research, or for both. For example, liver disease research is funded by 18 institutes (http://www.niddk.nih.gov/fund/divisions/ddn/ldrb/ldrb_action_plan.htm). The institutes that provide substantial support for gastroenterological epidemiology (including clinical trials) include the National Cancer Institute (NCI), the National Institute of Diabetes and Digestive and Kidney Diseases (NIDDK), the National Institute of Allergy and Infectious Diseases (NIAID) and the National Institute on Alcohol Abuse and Alcoholism (NIAAA).

The NIH funds what is termed intramural and extramural research. Intramural research is conducted at the laboratories and offices of the NIH and constitutes about 10% of the research budget. The National Cancer Institute funds much of the intramural research conducted on the epidemiology of gastroenterology, which focuses on gastrointestinal malignancies. The extramural NIH budget is much larger and provides funding for training and research across the USA and internationally. The bulk of funding goes toward investigator-initiated research (described below). Essentially all extramurally funded training and research proposals undergo peer review, by study sections organized by either the Center for Scientific Review (CSR) or by the funding institute.

Training opportunities

Individual predoctoral (**F30** and **F31**) and postdoctoral (**F32**) fellowships and institutional training grants (T32)

are available as part of the National Research Service Awards (NRSA) program. Only US citizens or permanent residents are eligible for NRSA support. At the predoctoral level, this program provides opportunities for students to obtain up to 5 years of funding toward a graduate research degree (F31) or the combined MD/PhD degree (F30). The fellowship award provides an annual stipend to help meet the fellow's living expenses, an allowance for tuition and fees and health insurance in accordance with NIH policy, and an annual institutional allowance. At the postdoctoral level, up to 3 years of mentored postdoctoral support is allowed. The first year of postdoctoral NRSA support is subject to a service payback obligation, while months 13 and beyond serve to fulfill the payback requirement. This payback system was adopted because studies have shown that fellows who participate in two or more years of postdoctoral research training are more likely to continue in a research career. Predoctoral students do not incur any payback obligation. Peer review of predoctoral fellowship applications focuses on the potential of the applicant for a research career, the quality of the doctoral program in which the applicant is enrolled, the experience and suitability of the sponsor and the environment, and the quality of the proposed dissertation project. Peer review of individual postdoctoral fellowship applications focuses on the following elements: the applicant, the mentor(s), the research project and the training potential. Many institutes use the F31 for students who are from minority groups that are underrepresented in the biomedical sciences. Fewer institutes use the F30 mechanism, which is for combined MD/PhD training.

Appointments of predoctoral students, postdoctoral fellows or both to an institutional training grant (**T32**) are made at the discretion of the training grant director, who is also its Principal Investigator. T32 applications are competitively reviewed and awarded for five-year periods for a set number of pre- and/or postdoctoral positions. As for the individual awards, NRSA positions on institutional awards are only available to US citizens or permanent residents. The review criteria for T32s include:

• the availability of a high-quality faculty to provide mentors;
• the past record of the faculty in successfully training fellows;
• a strong pool of potential trainees;
• a plan for organizing and overseeing the training program;
• the training environment.

The National Institute of General Medical Sciences (NIGMS) supports the vast majority of predoctoral training for the NIH via institutional training grants, as detailed by the NIGMS website (www.nigms.nih.gov/training), while most postdoctoral programs are supported by the other institutes and centers whose missions are more focused on specific organ or disease areas. For more information on training awards see the NIH Office of Extramural Research website (http://grants1.nih.gov/training/extramural.htm) and for electronic submission of all grants see the relevant webpage (http://era.nih.gov/ElectronicReceipt/).

Career development awards

Several career development, or K-series, awards are available. The purpose of most K awards is to protect the time of the applicant in order to further his or her career from the postdoctoral or, for physicians, postclinical training period to the independent stage of his or her research career. The awards most used at the NIH for early career development, providing 3, 4 or 5 years of salary and research support to individuals with a doctoral degree, are the **K01** (Mentored Research Scientist Development Award), **K08** (Mentored Clinical Scientist Development Award), **K23** (Mentored Patient-Oriented Research Career Development Award), and **K25** (Mentored Quantitative Research Development Award). The **K24** (Mid-career Investigator Award in Patient-Oriented Research) targets clinical or translation researchers at the associate professor, or higher, level. Only US citizens or permanent residents are eligible for most K awards, and only US institutions are eligible. The exception is the **K99/R00** (Pathway to Independence) Award. This award, begun in 2005, is aimed at shortening the time a research scientist spends in a postdoctoral position by providing a two-phased funding period: the first (K99) with mentor(s) and the next (R00) independently after securing a faculty appointment. Non-US citizens are eligible to apply for the K99/R00, but all work for both phases must be done in the USA.

All K awards are peer-reviewed with the following general categories included: qualifications of the candidate; the suitability and credentials of the mentor(s); and the quality of the research plan, the career development plan and the environment.

The support provided by training and career development awards has proven useful for funding coursework in epidemiology and biostatistics that would qualify the trainee for a master's or higher degree, even if an official degree is not granted. There are essentially two converging training paths for researchers in gastroenterological epidemiology. Physicians require the statistical and epidemiological training that is available from departments within schools of public health or within other academic divisions or centers devoted to these quantitative methodologies. PhD or equivalent candidates who are not physicians will usually go further in methodological coursework. They also need exposure to anatomy, physiology, mechanisms of disease, nutrition and other areas necessary to grasp the clinical aspects of digestive diseases. A dissertation that focuses on a digestive disease is most helpful in such training. Successful training in either path should confer a high level of competency in biostatistics, epidemiology and research design.

Loan repayment

The NIH encourages applications for educational loan repayment from qualified health professionals and researchers who have made a commitment to pursue a research career. The Loan Repayment Program is an important component of the NIH's efforts to recruit and retain the next generation of researchers by providing for the potential for developing a research career unfettered by the burden of student loan debt. Since 2002, the NIH has provided more than $20 million a year to repay educational debts for promising clinical and pediatric researchers who can demonstrate a commitment to pursuing a research career in these areas. To be eligible, an applicant must owe more than 20% of his or her yearly salary as a bona fide educational debt, agree to pursue 2 years of research for at least 50% of their time while the loan is being repaid, and be a US citizen or permanent resident working in the USA. Applications are submitted electronically via the Loan Repayment website (www.lrp.nih.gov) each fall and decisions reported after external, as well as program staff, reviews are completed in the following summer.

Research project grants

The largest portion of the NIH budget goes to investigator-initiated research, commonly known as the "R-series" grants. Institutions eligible for investigator-initiated research funding may be public (but not federal), private or commercial. Application is not limited to US institutions, although applications that propose to conduct research in other countries must discuss why that research cannot be conducted in the USA and may require clearance by the US Department of State before funds can be released.

Principal Investigators for R-series grants are usually not required to be US citizens. Generally, awards are limited to $500 000 direct research costs per year for a maximum of 5 years. The most common R-series grant is the **R01**. The purpose of an R01 is straightforward: to support a hypothesis-driven, circumscribed project in an area representing the investigator's specific interest and competencies, based on the mission of the NIH, as detailed on the NIH R01 webpage (http://grants2.nih.gov/grants/funding/r01.htm). R01s require that the applicant be considered, by virtue of past research productivity, training and reputation, an "independent investigator." Writing a successful R01 requires more than a sound and innovative research idea. Insight into the complexity of creating an R01 application can be obtained from the annotated example posted on the NIAID website (http://www.niaid.nih.gov/ncn/grants/app/default.htm.)

In recent years, three smaller and shorter-duration "R" awards of particular interest to epidemiologists and clinical researchers have grown in popularity. The **R03**, or Small Research Grant, provides 2 years of support for projects that can be carried out in this period of time, with the allowable maximum of $50 000 per year in direct costs. Two of the common uses of the R03 award of interest to digestive disease epidemiologists are to fund pilot or feasibility studies and to support secondary analysis of existing datasets. Not all NIH institutes accept unsolicited R03 applications; see the NIH Small Grant Program webpage (http://grants2.nih.gov/grants/funding/r03.htm). The **R21**, or Exploratory/Developmental Grant, provides support for the early, conceptual stage of a research idea. The research proposed should test a hypothesis and thus provide preliminary data that can be used for a subsequent R01 application. R21 support is limited to 2 years with a combined budget for direct costs for the 2-year project period of no more than $275 000. Some institutes only accept R21 applications in response to their specific program announcements; see the NIH Exploratory/Developmental Research Grant Award webpage ((http://grants2.nih.gov/grants/funding/r21.htm). Introduced in 2003, the clinical trial planning grant, or **R34**, provides support for the development of phase III clinical trials; see the NIH Clinical Trial Planning Grant Program webpage (http://grants2.nih.gov/grants/funding/r34.htm). This program supports the establishment of the research team, the development of tools for data management and oversight of the research, the definition of recruitment strategies, and the finalization of the protocol and other essential elements of the study included in a manual of operations/procedures. The R34

is not designed for the collection of preliminary data or for the conduct of pilot studies to support the rationale for a clinical trial. A project period of one year and a budget for direct costs of up to $100 000 per year are permitted.

Other resources and opportunities

There are additional online resources available to investigators interested in research funding. The Computer Retrieval of Information on Scientific Projects (CRISP) system is a searchable database (http://crisp.cit.nih.gov/) that provides the abstracts of grants funded by NIH, and several other government entities, such as the Food and Drug Administration and the Centers for Disease Control and Prevention. The NIH Guide for Grants and Contracts is the repository for all NIH program announcements (PAs), requests for applications (RFAs), requests for proposals (RFPs) and Notices that provide relevant information for current or potential grantees. Each PA, RFA and RFP lists the institute contacts most knowledgeable about the specific funding opportunity. The Guide for Grants and Contracts maintains a list-serve available to any investigator – see the Funding Opportunities and Notices webpage (http://grants1.nih.gov/grants/guide/index.html) – which supplies a weekly listing of newly released PAs, RFAs and Notices. Also, each NIH institute maintains its own website where unique resources for researchers can be found.

In addition to investigator-initiated research awards, the NIH also funds multi-institutional networks that are grounded in epidemiologic principles, including clinical trials and observational cohort studies. These networks originate through RFAs for cooperative agreements or through RFPs for contracts. Cooperative agreements and contracts involve NIH staff members in a substantive way as regards organization and technical assistance. Networks are supported by a data coordinating center that provides overarching data management and biostatistical expertise. Participation of junior researchers through attendance at investigator meetings and serving on study committees provides on-the-job training in the design, methodology and execution of large-scale clinical studies.

Another opportunity that all investigators should consider is serving as a reviewer for grant applications. A number of NIH study sections require and welcome investigators with clinical and epidemiological expertise in gastrointestinal diseases. Often an investigator will be asked to serve as an ad hoc reviewer for one or more grants during a given review cycle. Because all NIH-funded research passes through peer review, this is a unique opportunity to learn what constitutes successful research applications. It is also a service to the research community that does not go unnoticed by one's peers.

Finally, it should be noted that a main function of NIH program staff is to see that the best research gets funded. They are here to help investigators, and consultation with the appropriate program staff is strongly encouraged prior to submitting any application.

Part 3

Epidemiology of Specific GI Diseases

17 GERD, Barrett's Esophagus and Esophageal Cancer

Yvonne Romero and G. Richard Locke III

Key points

- Gastroesophageal reflux disease (GERD) is very common, with one out of five people having symptoms at least once a week.
- Obesity and family history of reflux are important risk factors for GERD.
- Barrett's esophagus and esophageal adenocarcinoma are complications of GERD.
- The incidence of esophageal adenocarcinoma has risen and continues to rise exponentially in developed countries.
- Early identification of patients with Barrett's esophagus holds the greatest promise for diminishing the mortality rate of esophageal adenocarcinoma.

Introduction

Gastroesophageal reflux disease (GERD) is the term currently used to describe all of the symptoms and signs associated with the abnormal reflux of gastric contents into the esophagus. In the past, GERD was typically thought of as erosive esophagitis and treated as an acute self-limited condition with short-term therapies similar to the treatment of peptic ulcer disease. Over time, our thinking regarding GERD has changed. GERD is now recognized as a chronic condition. Although there is an effective therapy for GERD, we need to recognize that we still do not know why people develop GERD. Among the complications of GERD, cancer is the most worrisome. At present, the incidence of esophageal adenocarcinoma is increasing significantly. Barrett's esophagus is the intermediate step between GERD and cancer. Understanding the epidemiology of GERD, Barrett's esophagus and adenocarcinoma of the esophagus is critical to developing an effective approach to ending this epidemic.

Epidemiology of GERD

The typical symptoms of GERD are heartburn and acid regurgitation [1]. Approximately 40% of the population will report having intermittent episodes of heartburn [2]. Twenty percent, or one in five, will report having heartburn once a week, and 7% will report having heartburn once a day [2]. Acid regurgitation is also reported by 20% of the population, but most people with frequent acid regurgitation also have frequent heartburn [2]. Not everyone with heartburn and acid regurgitation will have gastroesophageal reflux, and not everyone with GERD has these two symptoms. In an effort to estimate the prevalence of GERD, ambulatory pH monitoring was offered to a random sample of the population [3]. As expected, the response rate was poor; nonetheless, the estimated prevalence of GERD was 34.5% [3]. In another study, upper endoscopy was offered to a random sample of the population [4]. The prevalence of esophagitis was 12%, but interestingly, the prevalence of esophagitis in the asymptomatic control group was 8% [4]. The key is to note that each of these studies reports prevalence figures that are percentages of the population. Many conditions affect 10 or 100 people per 100 000. In GERD, the prevalence is two to three orders of magnitude higher.

Incidence is much more difficult to measure. People without GERD must be identified and followed over time to see if they develop GERD. Because symptoms fluctuate, a person may not have GERD symptoms at one point in time only to have GERD subsequently, and thus many of the reports of "incidence" are actually reports of symptom onset rates. In addition, many people with GERD never seek care. The best estimate for the incidence of GERD is 4.5 per 1000 person-years, or 450 per 100 000 [5].

Why people develop GERD remains unclear. When evaluating risk factors, one must distinguish between risk factors for a reflux event and those that predispose a person to have GERD. For example, people with GERD frequently note that if they eat a large meal late at night they will experience reflux symptoms. However, many people can eat the same meal and not have symptoms. This meal has caused a reflux event but has not caused GERD. Smoking and alcohol have long been implicated as risk factors for GERD. However, more recently the attention has focused on obesity. Increasing body mass index is clearly a risk factor for having GERD [6,7]. The impact of the obesity epidemic on the epidemiology of GERD is still under evaluation. Another key risk factor is family history. GERD aggregates in families, and this appears to be a risk factor independent of diet and obesity [6,8]. Whether a gene predisposes to GERD is a question of great interest [9].

Being a common condition, GERD has significant economic impact. In a recent study by the American Gastroenterological Association (AGA), GERD was the most costly digestive disease, with an annual cost of $10 billion [10]. Forty-one percent of people with GERD report loss of work productivity [10]. There is need for physician visits, diagnostic tests, and therapies. Finally, there is significant impact on quality of life [11,12]. In one study, the decreased quality of life in GERD was similar to that in depression [11].

Epidemiology of Barrett's esophagus

Barrett's esophagus is defined as the "displacement of the squamocolumnar junction proximal to the gastroesophageal junction with the presence of intestinal metaplasia" [13]. At present, standard upper endoscopy with biopsy is the most reliable method to diagnose Barrett's esophagus. Unfortunately the technique is prone to error as biopsies from the proximal stomach (cardia) can be mistakenly collected instead of tissue from the anatomic esophagus [14]. Thus, Barrett's esophagus requires endoscopic and histologic criteria to be met for diagnosis [1,13,15].

Most epidemiology studies, particularly those published before 1985, have reported results on long-segment Barrett's esophagus, defined as greater than 3 cm in length. However, subsequent studies have demonstrated that patients with short-segment Barrett's esophagus (<3 cm in length) have a neoplastic risk [16–18]. Histologic confirmation of intestinal metaplasia consistent with Barrett's is particularly important in patients who appear to have short-segment Barrett's. The border between the stomach and the esophagus can be ill-defined. Intestinal metaplasia of the cardia has been deemed a normal variant without significant neoplastic risk [18–20].

The incidence of Barrett's esophagus remains unknown. On average Barrett's esophagus is clinically diagnosed at age 63; however, the age at which patients actually develop Barrett's segment is not known [21].

The prevalence of Barrett's esophagus among White people of European background in developed countries has not significantly changed over the past 20 years. Two population-based studies have estimated the prevalence of long-segment Barrett's esophagus to be 0.34% and 0.5% [22,23]. The prevalence of intestinal metaplasia of any length has been estimated to be 1.6% [23].

The diagnosis of Barrett's esophagus is increasing (Fig. 17.1); however, this does not necessarily mean that the prevalence is increasing. The increase in diagnosis can be explained by two phenomena: increased detec-

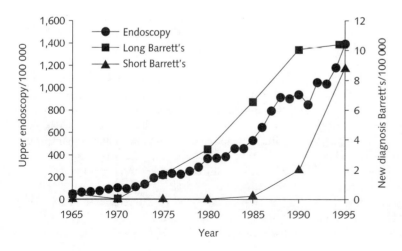

Fig. 17.1 The increasing number of persons diagnosed with short-segment (triangles) and long-segment (squares) Barrett's esophagus strongly correlates with the increase in number of endoscopies performed in residents of Olmsted County, MN, from 1965 to 1997. (Reproduced from Conio *et al.* [65], with permission from BMJ Publishing Group Ltd.)

tion due to higher utilization of diagnostic endoscopy, and increased physician recognition, especially in regard to short Barrett's. Figure 17.1 shows that the first case of short-segment Barrett's esophagus was diagnosed in Olmsted County in 1985 – because it was not recognized as a disease prior to 1985.

Risk factors for Barrett's esophagus include advanced age, male sex, frequent GERD symptoms of prolonged duration, White ethnicity, and to a lesser extent, tobacco and alcohol use [1,13]. More recently the roles of obesity and genetics have come under investigation.

Barrett's esophagus is rare in infants, children and even adolescents, with an estimated prevalence of 0.12% [24]. The presence of a hiatal hernia and older age were the best predictors of Barrett's esophagus even in this young cohort [24]. Patients are typically diagnosed with long-segment Barrett's esophagus in their sixth decade [21]. This reflects a bias introduced by clinical practice: older persons are more likely to seek medical attention, and to undergo upper endoscopy. Nonetheless, advancing age is a risk factor.

Population-based studies suggest that the ratio of males to females with biopsy-proven Barrett's segments of >2 cm length ranges from 1.5:1 to 2:1 [22,23]. The higher rates reported in the past appear to have been biased. Although multiple potential explanations for the difference among the sexes have been proposed, no definitive explanation has been found.

From a population perspective, GERD symptoms are strong risk factors for Barrett's esophagus [7]. In one study, 80% of persons with Barrett's esophagus had reflux symptoms, but 40% of people who were endoscopically normal had symptoms as well [23]. Thus GERD symptoms did not meaningfully help to distinguish those patients with Barrett's from those without. Therefore, although on a population level GERD symptoms are a strong risk factor for Barrett's esophagus; at the individual level, GERD symptoms have limited utility to determine who has Barrett's. GERD symptoms are common, cancer is rare, and many patients who develop esophageal adenocarcinoma are asymptomatic (Fig. 17.2).

A relationship between ethnicity, GERD symptoms and Barrett's esophagus may exist. About 3.5–7% of White people with GERD symptoms have long-segment Barrett's esophagus, compared with 1% of asymptomatic White people [22,25]. Despite a similar prevalence in GERD symptoms and, commonly, a higher body mass index, persons of African American descent have one-twentieth the risk of long-segment Barrett's esophagus than their White counterparts [26].

Epidemiology of GERD

- 100 000 adults
- 40 000 with infrequent reflux symptoms
- 20 000 will have weekly reflux symptoms
- 10 000 will have esophagitis
- 400 will have a Barrett's esophagus
- 2 per year will develop cancer

Fig. 17.2 The epidemiology of gastroesophageal reflux disease (GERD).

Studies assessing the association between obesity and Barrett's esophagus have met with divergent results, likely based upon the timing of the measurement and the proxy used to assess obesity. Studies that suggest an association collected weight data based on recall; studies refuting this association have used objective prospectively collected data [27–29].

Family history of Barrett's esophagus and/or esophageal adenocarcinoma have been proposed to be risk factors for Barrett's esophagus [8,30–32]. Based upon on a Swedish twin registry study, the heritability of GERD symptoms has been estimated as 31% [33]. There have been numerous case reports in the literature of families in which at least two members have hiatal hernia, Barrett's esophagus and, in some cases, esophageal adenocarcinoma – ranging from twins to four-generation families [34–41]. GERD symptoms have been shown to aggregate in families, as have reflux esophagitis and Barrett's esophagus [8,30–32,42]. Linkage analyses aimed at identifying the genetic loci that predispose to these GERD phenotypes have shown striking preliminary results, with further genotyping in progress [43].

Progression from Barrett's esophagus to adenocarcinoma

Patients with long-segment Barrett's esophagus have a 30–125-fold increased risk for esophageal adenocarcinoma [44–46]. The annual individual risk of transforming from Barrett's esophagus to esophageal adenocarcinoma is about 0.5% [46]. In other words, only one person of 200 with Barrett's will progress to cancer every year. Although there is an increased risk of cancer, most patients with Barrett's esophagus die of other causes, with a similar 10-year survival rate as the general population (>80%) [47].

To date, neither surgery nor medications have been shown to diminish the neoplastic transformation rate of Barrett's esophagus to cancer [48–50]. In a large retrospective Swedish cohort study the standardized incidence ratio of esophageal adenocarcinoma did not statistically differ among 11 077 persons who underwent fundoplication for reflux disease compared with 66 965 persons who were hospitalized for GERD but did not have fundoplication [48]. In a separate prospective, randomized trial, participants with severe reflux were randomized to antireflux surgery vs the antireflux medications of the time (ranitidine, metoclopramide, carafate and antacids) [49]. After a mean 7 years' follow-up, 2.4% of the participants randomized to medications had progressed to esophageal cancer compared with 1.2% of those randomized to fundoplication, a statistically nonsignificant difference [49].

Epidemiology of esophageal cancer

Esophageal adenocarcinoma, now the most prevalent form of esophageal cancer in developed countries, is a highly lethal malignancy – principally due to the late stage at which it is commonly diagnosed [51]. Its strongest risk factor is Barrett's esophagus, which in turn is caused by GERD. Over the past 10 years, adenocarcinoma has become the predominant form of esophageal cancer in the USA and is hence the focus of this chapter [52–54] (http://www.cancerresearch.uk/). Over a span of 20 years, the incidence of esophageal adenocarcinoma increased by 400% in White males; from 0.72/100 000 in 1974–78 to 3.7/100 000 in 1994–98 [52,53]. The incidence of esophageal adenocarcinoma arising in patients with Barrett's esophagus is even greater, at 500/100 000, or 0.5% [54]. In contrast, the incidence of esophageal squamous cell carcinoma, once the predominant type of esophageal cancer, has progressively declined over the past 30 years, becoming less common than adenocarcinoma in the USA in 1994 [29,53]. This epidemiologic change in cancer incidence over the past 30 years has been even more striking in Europe (http://www.cancerresearch.uk).

Risk factors for esophageal adenocarcinoma are very similar to those in Barrett's. In fact many studies assessing risk factors for cancer might merely be identifying risk factors for Barrett's. Fewer studies have evaluated the risk factors for cancer in those known to have Barrett's esophagus. Advanced age, male sex, frequent GERD symptoms of prolonged duration, White ethnicity, obesity and genetics have all been under investigation.

The prevalence of neoplasm in patients with Barrett's esophagus is remarkably higher among males than females, with a male:female ratio ranging from 3:1 to 8:1 [55,56]. GERD symptoms, particularly frequent symptoms of >20 years' duration, are strongly associated with esophageal

adenocarcinoma [7]. However, 40% of persons with esophageal adenocarcinoma are completely asymptomatic [7,57]. Although the age-adjusted incidence of esophageal adenocarcinoma has been fairly stable and low among Black and Asian/Pacific Islander males and females, and White females, over the past 10 years, it has continued to increase exponentially in White males [58,59]. Obese persons have a 2–16-fold increased risk for esophageal adenocarcinoma compared with their normal weight counterparts [7,60].

Unfortunately, the prognosis of esophageal adenocarcinoma remains quite poor, with an overall 5-year survival rate of 13%, attributed to late stage of presentation [51]. The main factors negatively impacting on prognosis are advanced tumor depth and/or nodal involvement [61,62]. At present, most patients with adenocarcinoma developing in a segment of Barrett's are diagnosed with both conditions at their first endoscopic examination [63,64]. This is a tragic situation. Most people with Barrett's esophagus are not diagnosed in advance of the development of cancer, and hence miss the opportunity potentially to benefit from chemoprevention and/or surveillance. The protective factors associated with being female or being of African American or Hispanic descent have not been elucidated. Although the incidence of esophageal adenocarcinoma is low in American Black persons, there is evidence to suggest disparities in survival, particularly for males [58].

Early identification of patients with Barrett's esophagus holds the greatest promise for reducing the mortality rate of esophageal adenocarcinoma. In 1987 only one of every 17 (6%) community residents with long-segment Barrett's esophagus had been diagnosed [22]. Therefore, 16 of 17 persons with Barrett's esophagus were unaware of their neoplastic risk and did not have the opportunity to participate in a surveillance program. By 1999, due in large part to open-access endoscopy, one of seven (14%) Olmsted County residents with Barrett's esophagus had been diagnosed [65]. Although these data reflect improvement, six of seven community residents with a preneoplastic risk for esophageal adenocarcinoma remain unaware of their risk. Only 5% of patients with adenocarcinoma in their Barrett's esophagus segments had been diagnosed with Barrett's at least 6 months in advance of the cancer [63]. A remarkably similar estimate was reported by Dulai *et al.*, who found only 4.7% of 1503 patients undergoing surgical resection of adenocarcinoma were aware of a previous diagnosis of Barrett's esophagus [64]. These data suggest that at the present time, with our current tools, we miss the opportunity to find those at risk for esophageal adenocarcinoma 90–95% of the time. We cannot adequately judge the impact of chemoprevention and/or surveillance on the mortality rate of esophageal adenocarcinoma until everyone with Barrett's esophagus is aware of their diagnosis.

Issues/gaps in epidemiology knowledge

Several key questions demand our attention if we are to gain a fuller picture of the epidemiology of Barrett's esophagus and esophageal adenocarcinoma.

• There are no data on the incidence of Barrett's esophagus. Once we know when Barrett's actually begins, we may be able to adjust our screening algorithms, and attempt to identify mechanisms whereby we might interrupt its occurrence. In theory, chemoprevention would begin at its onset. Surveillance would be initiated early in order to identify those making the transformation to cancer at a curable stage, preferably before esophagectomy was required.

• Why do men get esophageal adenocarcinoma more than women? Why is the risk so much greater in White people than among other ethnic groups? Understanding the genetic and environmental factors that lower the risk of Barrett's esophagus and esophageal adenocarcinoma in females and in Hispanic, Asian, Pacific Islander and Black people may help to identify factors that can be modified to lower the risk in White males.

• Should first-degree relatives of patients with long-segment Barrett's esophagus undergo screening endoscopy? Would confirmation of this finding make screening algorithms more cost-effective than they are currently?

Recommendations for future studies

The above listed gaps in knowledge suggest that further study is warranted in preventing symptoms and the complications of the common disorder, GERD. Furthermore, although esophageal adenocarcinoma is relatively uncommon, the late stage of diagnosis and poor survival thereafter argue that greater emphasis needs to be placed on early detection of the premalignant disorder, Barrett's esophagus. However, the high prevalence of GERD, the low incidence of cancer, and the high invasiveness and cost of screening with endoscopy suggest that greater emphasis needs to be placed on identification of biomarkers for cancer development. Because family history appears to be a strong risk factor for development of Barrett's and cancer, genetic epidemiology studies may be helpful to determine to what extent a genetic background predisposes to GERD

and its complications, Barrett's esophagus and esophageal adenocarcinoma.

Conclusions

Heartburn and acid regurgitation are common symptoms. Fortunately for most people with GERD, symptom management is the only issue. However, some people with GERD will get Barrett's esophagus, and some people with Barrett's will get esophageal cancer.

As the incidence of esophageal adenocarcinoma continues to rise exponentially in developed countries for unknown reasons, understanding Barrett's esophagus becomes increasingly more relevant. The majority of persons with Barrett's esophagus will not progress to cancer; however, because Barrett's esophagus is a fairly accessible premalignant lesion, a concerted collaborative effort should be made so that we can identify factors that can be modified in order to disrupt the neoplastic transformation and decrease the mortality of esophageal adenocarcinoma.

References

1. Vakil N *et al.* The Montreal definition and classification of gastroesophageal reflux disease: a global evidence-based consensus. *Am J Gastroenterol* 2006;**101**:1900.
2. Locke GR *et al.* Prevalence and clinical spectrum of gastroesophageal reflux: A population-based study in Olmsted County, Minnesota. *Gastroenterology* 1997;**112**:1448.
3. Andersen LI, Jensen G. Prevalence of benign oesophageal disease in the Danish population with special reference to pulmonary disease. *J Intern Med* 1989;**225**:393.
4. Johnsen R *et al.* Prevalence of endoscopic and histological findings in subjects with and without dyspepsia. *Br Med J* 1991;**302**:749.
5. Ruigomez A *et al.* Natural history of gastro-oesophageal reflux disease diagnosed in general practice. *Aliment Pharmacol Ther* 2004;**20**:751.
6. Locke GR 3rd *et al.* Risk factors associated with symptoms of gastroesophageal reflux. *Am J Med* 1999;**106**:642.
7. Lagergren J *et al.* Symptomatic gastroesophageal reflux as a risk factor for esophageal adenocarcinoma. *N Engl J Med* 1999;**340**:825.
8. Romero Y *et al.* Familial aggregation of gastroesophageal reflux in patients with Barrett's esophagus and esophageal adenocarcinoma. *Gastroenterology* 1997;**113**:1449.
9. Romero Y, Locke GR III. Is there a GERD gene? *Am J Gastroenterol* 1999;**94**:1127.
10. Goodman C *et al. The Burden of Gastrointestinal Diseases.*

Bethesda, MD: American Gastroenterological Association, 2001:20.

11. El-Serag HB *et al.* Health-related quality of life among persons with irritable bowel syndrome: a systematic review. *Aliment Pharmacol Ther* 2002;**16**:1171.

12. Revicki DA *et al.* The impact of gastroesophageal reflux disease on health-related quality of life. *Am J Med* 1998;**104**:252.

13. Sharma P *et al.* A critical review of the diagnosis and management of Barrett's esophagus: the AGA Chicago Workshop. *Gastroenterology* 2004;**127**:310.

14. Eloubeidi MA, Provenzale D. Does the patient have Barrett's esophagus? The utility of predicting Barrett's esophagus at the index endoscopy. *Am J Gastroenterol* 1999;**94**:937.

15. Practice Parameters Committee ACG, Sampliner RE. Updated guidelines for the diagnosis, surveillance and therapy of Barrett's esophagus. *Am J Gastroenterol* 2002;**97**:1888.

16. Schnell TG *et al.* Adenocarcinomas arising in tongues or short segments of Barrett's esophagus. *Dig Dis Sci* 1992;**37**:137.

17. Nandurkar S, Talley NJ. Barrett's esophagus, the long and short of it. *Am J Gastroenterol* 1999;**94**:30.

18. Spechler SJ *et al.* Prevalence of metaplasia at the gastro-oesophageal junction. *Lancet* 1994;**344**:1533.

19. Morales TG *et al.* Intestinal metaplasia of the gastric cardia. *Am J Gastroenterol* 1997;**92**:414.

20. Wallner B *et al.* The Z-line appearance and prevalence of intestinal metaplasia among patients without symptoms or endoscopic signs indicating gastroesophageal reflux. *Surg Endosc* 2001;**15**:886.

21. Cameron AJ. Epidemiologic studies and the development of Barrett's esophagus. *Endoscopy* 1993;**25**:635.

22. Cameron AJ *et al.* Prevalence of columnar-lined (Barrett's) esophagus. *Gastroenterology* 1990;**99**:918.

23. Ronkainen J *et al.* Prevalence of Barrett's esophagus in the general population: an endoscopic study. *Gastroenterology* 2005;**129**:1825.

24. El-Serag HB *et al.* The prevalence of suspected Barrett's esophagus in children and adolescents: a multicenter endoscopic study. *Gastrointest Endosc* 2006;**64**:671.

25. Winters C *et al.* Barrett's esophagus. A prevalent, occult complication of gastroesophageal reflux disease. *Gastroenterology* 1987;**92**:118.

26. El-Serag HB *et al.* Gastroesophageal reflux among different racial groups in the United States. *Gastroenterology* 2004;**126**:1692.

27. Kubo A, Corley DA. Body mass index and adenocarcinomas of the esophagus or gastric cardia; a systematic review and meta-analysis. *Cancer Epidemiol Biomarkers Prev* 2006;**15**:872.

28. Lagergren J *et al.* Association between body mass and adenocarcinoma of the esophagus and gastric cardia. *Ann Intern Med* 1999;**130**:883.

29. Crane SJ *et al.* The changing incidence of esophageal and gastric adenocarcinoma by anatomic sub-site. *Aliment Pharmacol Ther* 2007;**25**:447.

30. Trudgill NJ *et al.* Familial clustering of reflux symptoms. *Am*

31. Chak A *et al.* Familial aggregation of Barrett's oesophagus, oesophageal adenocarcinoma, and oesophagogastric junctional adenocarcinoma in Caucasian adults. *Gut* 2002;**51**:323.

32. Chak A *et al.* Familiality in Barrett's esophagus, adenocarcinoma of the esophagus, and adenocarcinoma of the gastroesophageal junction. *Cancer Epidemiol Biomarkers Prev* 2006;**15**:1668.

33. Cameron AJ *et al.* Gastroesophageal reflux disease in monozygotic and dizygotic twins. *Gastroenterology* 2002;**121**:55.

34. Everhart CW Jr *et al.* Occurrence of Barrett's esophagus in three members of the same family: first report of familial incidence [abstr.]. *Gastroenterology* 1978;**74**:A1032.

35. Gelfand MD. Barrett esophagus in sexagenarian identical twins. *J Clin Gastroenterol* 1983;**5**:251.

36. Crabb DW *et al.* Familial gastroesophageal reflux and development of Barrett's esophagus. *Ann Intern Med* 1985;**103**:52.

37. Prior A, Whorwell PJ. Familial Barrett's esophagus? *Hepatogastroenterology* 1986;**33**:86.

38. Jochem VJ *et al.* Familial Barrett's esophagus associated with adenocarcinoma. *Gastroenterology* 1992;**102**:1400.

39. Fahmy N, King JF. Barrett's esophagus: an acquired condition with genetic predisposition. *Am J Gastroenterol* 1993;**88**:1262.

40. Eng C *et al.* Familial Barrett's esophagus and adenocarcinoma of the gastroesophageal junction. *Cancer Epidemiol Biomarkers Prev* 1993;**2**:397.

41. Poynton AR *et al.* Carcinoma arising in familial Barrett's esophagus. *Am J Gastroenterol* 1996;**91**:1855.

42. Romero Y *et al.* Family history doubles Barrett's esophagus risk. *Gastroenterology* 2002;**122**(Suppl. M1388):A-292.

43. Romero Y *et al.* Evidence from linkage analysis for susceptibility genes in familial Barrett's esophagus and esophageal adenocarcinoma. *Gastroenterology* 2006;**130**:A106.

44. Cameron AJ *et al.* The incidence of adenocarcinoma in columnar-lined (Barrett's) esophagus. *N Engl J Med* 1985;**313**:857.

45. O'Connor JB *et al.* The incidence of adenocarcinoma and dysplasia in Barrett's esophagus: report on the Cleveland Clinic Barrett's Esophagus Registry. *Am J Gastroenterol* 1999;**94**:2037.

46. Drewitz DJ *et al.* The incidence of adenocarcinoma in Barrett's esophagus: a prospective study of 170 patients followed 4.8 years. *Am J Gastroenterol* 1997;**92**:212.

47. Eckardt VF *et al.* Life expectancy and cancer risk in patients with Barrett's esophagus: A prospective controlled investigation. *Am J Med* 2001;**111**:33.

48. Ye W *et al.* Risk of adenocarcinomas of the esophagus and gastric cardia in patients with gastroesophageal reflux diseases and after antireflux surgery. *Gastroenterology* 2001;**121**:1286.

49. Spechler SJ *et al.* Long-term outcome of medical and surgical therapies for gastroesophageal reflux disease: follow-up of a randomized controlled trial. *JAMA* 2001;**285**:2331.

50. Csendes A *et al.* Long-term results of classic antireflux surgery

in 152 patients with Barrett's esophagus: clinical, radiologic, endoscopic, manometric, and acid reflux test analysis before and late after operation. *Surgery* 1998;**123**:645.

51. Sampliner RE *et al.* Temporal trends (1973–1997) in survival of patients with esophageal adenocarcinoma in the United States a glimmer of hope? *Am J Gastroenterol* 2003:**98**:1627.

52. Brown LM, Devesa SS. Epidemiologic trends in esophageal and gastric cancer in the United States. *Surg Oncol Clin N Am* 2002;**11**:235.

53. Pera M *et al.* Epidemiology of esophageal adenocarcinoma. *J Surg Oncol* 2005;**92**:151.

54. Sharma P *et al.* Dysplasia and cancer in a large multicenter cohort of patients with Barrett's esophagus. *Clin Gastroenterol Hepatol* 2006;**4**:566.

55. Caygill CPJ *et al.* Characteristics and regional variations of patients with Barrett's esophagus in the UK. *Eur J Gastroenterol Hepatol* 2003;**15**:1217.

56. Blot WJ *et al.* Rising incidence of adenocarcinoma of the esophagus and gastric cardia. *JAMA* 1991;**265**:1287.

57. Chow WC *et al.* The relation of gastroesophageal reflux disease and its treatment to adenocarcinomas of the esophagus and gastric cardia. *JAMA* 1995;**274**:474.

58. Baquet CR *et al.* Esophageal cancer epidemiology in blacks and whites: racial and gender disparities in incidence, mortality, survival rates and histology. *J Natl Med Assoc* 2005;**97**:1471.

59. Wu X *et al.* Incidence of esophageal and gastric carcinomas among American Asians/Pacific islanders, whites and blacks. Subsite and histology differences. *Cancer* 2006;**106**:683.

60. Hampel H *et al.* Meta-analysis: obesity and the risk for gastroesophageal reflux disease and its complications. *Ann Intern Med* 2005;**143**:199.

61. Gu Y *et al.* The number of lymph nodes with metastasis predicts survival in patients with esophageal or esophagogastric junction adenocarcinoma who receive preoperative chemoradiation. *Cancer* 2006;**106**:1017.

62. Hosch SB *et al.* Esophageal cancer: the mode of lymphatic tumor cell spread and its prognostic significance. *J Clin Oncol* 2001;**19**:1970.

63. Corley DA *et al.* Surveillance and survival in Barrett's adenocarcinomas: a population-based study. *Gastroenterology* 2002;**122**:633.

64. Dulai GS *et al.* Preoperative prevalence of Barrett's esophagus in esophageal adenocarcinoma; a systematic review. *Gastroenterology* 2002;**122**:26.

65. Conio M *et al.* Secular trends in the epidemiology and outcome of Barrett's esophagus in Olmsted County, Minnesota. *Gut* 2001;**48**:304.

18 Helicobacter pylori Infection, Peptic Ulcer Disease and Gastric Cancer

Olof Nyrén

Key points
- Approximately half of all humans harbor *Helicobacter pylori*.
- Persistent *H. pylori* infection is a cause of peptic ulcer, gastric adenocarcinoma and MALT lymphoma.
- *H. pylori* prevalence in each birth cohort reflects the risk of acquisition that prevailed during the cohort members' childhoods.
- Peptic ulcer may affect, at some point in life, 4–12% of the adult population, and the population attributable risk (PAR) for *H. pylori* has been estimated to be 48%.
- Due to its poor prognosis, stomach cancer (adenocarcinoma) ranks number two among all causes of cancer death (more than 10% of all cancer deaths), with almost two-thirds of the cases occurring in developing countries.
- There has been a steep downward trend for distal stomach cancer in White men and women, but this decline does not seem to include cardia cancer.

Helicobacter pylori infection

Clinical microbiology and expression

Helicobacter pylori infection is an established cause of both peptic ulcer disease and gastric cancer. The *Helicobacter* genus consists of over 20 recognized species, including *H. pylori*. The latter is a curved bacterium, 2.5–4.0 µm long, that produces urease, which is thought to make short-term survival possible in the highly acidic intragastric environment. In contrast to many other bacterial pathogens, *H. pylori* is genetically heterogeneous, a result of several mechanisms for DNA rearrangement, including introduction and deletion of foreign sequences. The genetic heterogeneity is thought to reflect the microorganism's extraordinary ability for adaptation, both to the inhospitable acidic environment and to various attacks from the host's immune system. Some regions of the 1.7-Mbp bacterial genome are more variable than others. A striking example is the *cag* pathogenicity island (*cag* PAI), a 37–40-kb genetic element that contains the *cagA* gene [1]. It is present in approximately 50–70% of *H. pylori* strains and was early linked to a higher inflammatory response and to a particularly elevated risk of manifest diseases such as peptic ulcer or cancer in the host [2]. The entire island may be restored or lost through transformation [3]. The genes on the *cag* PAI encode 27–31 proteins, among them CagA and the components of a type IV secretion system (TFSS). The latter injects CagA into the host's epithelial cells [4],

where it is phosphorylated and interacts with a range of host signaling molecules. This, in turn, leads to morphologic changes and proliferation of the epithelial cells. The intimate interaction of the microorganism with the host cells results in the induction of potent proinflammatory cytokines such as interleukin 8 (IL-8) through the activation of the intracellular innate immune receptor Nod1 and nuclear factor kappa B (NF-κB) [5]. The *cag* PAI may be incomplete, and thus not fully functional. Comparisons between cancer or precancer-related *H. pylori* strains and non-cancer strains have indicated that the cancer-related ones tend to have more complete *cag* PAIs [6,7].

The primary lesion caused by *H. pylori* is gastritis. As opposed to the acute gastritis that follows initial colonization and that tends to be associated with transient nonspecific symptoms, the ensuing chronic gastritis is essentially symptomless in most individuals.

Persistent *H. pylori* infection may lead to peptic ulcer, gastric adenocarcinoma and mucosa-associated lymphoid tissue (MALT) lymphoma. Although several known and yet unidentified cofactors may be required for these respective outcomes, the causal relationships with the infection are widely accepted [8–10]. In the case of peptic ulcer and MALT lymphoma, the causality is supported by eradication studies demonstrating disease control after *H. pylori* eradication [11,12]. It is estimated that *H. pylori*-positive patients have a 10–20% lifetime risk of developing peptic ulcer disease and a 1–2% risk of developing gastric cancer [13]. Hence, the overwhelming majority of infected individuals will never develop any clinically manifest *H. pylori*-related disease. Numerous studies have explored possible associations between the infection and a variety of extragastric conditions, but with the possible exception of iron deficiency anemia [14], no conclusive evidence has emerged.

Distribution of *H. pylori* infection in the general population

Approximately half of all humans harbor *H. pylori* [15], but the prevalence shows large geographic variations. Whilst generally less than 40% of people in industrialized countries are *H. pylori* positive [16], the prevalence of the infection in various developing countries is more than 80% [17]. The range is even greater among child populations, with prevalence rates varying from below 10% to over 80% in high-income and low-income countries, respectively [18]. This means that children in many impoverished countries rapidly – typically before adolescence – reach the prevalence prevailing in the adult population. In several such populations, a prevalence of 50% is reached by the age of 5 years [19–23]. However, pediatric studies need to be interpreted with caution. Serology is problematic because young children with this infection often do not have detectable antibodies [24], and uninfected children may carry passively transferred antibodies from the mother. Furthermore, longitudinal studies have unveiled complex dynamics; in a US-Mexican cohort of infants, who were followed with ^{13}C-urea breath tests during the first 2 years of life, the initial acquisition of detectable *H. pylori* infection occurred at a rate of 20% per year, but most of these infections did not persist [25].

Whereas in developing countries the prevalence ceiling is reached before or during adolescence, *H. pylori* prevalence continues to rise with age in the adult population of industrialized countries. At the same time, there are strong indications that the overall prevalence in the latter countries is rapidly declining over calendar time [26]. Studies on stored sera suggest that this fall in prevalence is mainly explained by a birth cohort-wise decline in early acquisition of the infection [27,28]. Accordingly, the *H. pylori* prevalence in each birth cohort (generation) reflects the risk of acquisition that prevailed during the cohort members' childhood. Because this risk seems to have fallen dramatically in developed countries during the 20th century, the subsequent prevalence in any given calendar year is expected to be inversely related to year of birth and, consequently, positively related to age. The seroconversion

rate, marking the incidence of new *H. pylori* infections in these adult populations, has been estimated to be 1–2 per 200 persons and year [15,29], thus contributing little to the age effect. There are also seroreversions, that is, serologic indications of *H. pylori* disappearance. This rate was approximately 3 per 200 persons and year in both Sweden and Japan [29,30]. Hence, spontaneous disappearance of *H. pylori* will tend to balance the addition of new infections in adult populations.

Transmission of *H. pylori*

The mode of transmission of the infection has remained elusive, as have the mechanisms involved. Decades of intense research have failed to identify any important reservoir for the microorganism other than the human stomach. This implies that direct human-to-human transmission is the principal – perhaps the only – way by which the *H. pylori* species secures its continued existence. However, although challenged in some more recent studies [31,32], the infectivity in adulthood seems to be limited [15]. Most infected individuals, no doubt, have contracted their infection during childhood [33], but a Swedish study revealed strain concordance upon molecular typing in approximately one-fifth of married couples [34]. Moreover, the cumulative reinfection rate 18 months after successful *H. pylori* eradication was reportedly as high as 30% in a Peruvian adult high-prevalence population [35]. *H. pylori* has been detected in saliva, vomitus, gastric refluxate and feces. There is no conclusive evidence for predominant transmission via any of these vehicles [13]. Thus, it appears that the transmission can occur via both the oral-oral and fecal-oral route.

The family stands out as the most important framework for transmission, at least in developed countries [36]. Family size (both while growing up and as an adult), presence of infected family members, familial connections to high-prevalence regions, and residential crowding are all factors that are associated with an increased risk of being infected [20,37–40]. Clustering of *H. pylori* infection in sibships is consistent with transmission between siblings [20,34,37]. In a recent Swedish study, presence of infected siblings was an independent strong risk factor for infection among 11–13-year-old children, even after control for parental infection status [40]. Furthermore, in a molecular typing study from Sweden, siblings were frequently infected with the same strains [34]. However, in these families, it was common that the mother also carried the same strain. Thus, it is still possible that the mother might have been the common source. An *H. pylori*-infected mother is a much stronger risk factor for the child than an infected father [37–40], suggesting that close contacts are more important than possible genetic predisposition. Interestingly, close contacts with infected children outside the family, such as with peers at day-care centers or at school, were not associated with an increased risk of infection in studied index children in Sweden [38], while day-care attendance was a risk factor in urban Sardinia [41] (Fig. 18.1).

Although exposure opportunity in the form of close contacts with an infected family member may be more important than genetic factors, this does not mean that the host's genetic predisposition is unimportant. The concordance within adult twin pairs with regard to *H. pylori* seropositivity was considerably greater in monozygotic (81%) than in dizygotic (63%) twins [42], suggesting that genetic mechanisms in the host may be involved. The exact nature of these mechanisms remains to be clarified. Although not universally confirmed, studies in Japan and Sweden have demonstrated that presence of the *0102 allele of the human leukocyte antigen (HLA) class II *DR-DQA1* locus is inversely and significantly associated with *H. pylori* seropositivity [43,44]. An Italian study of polymorphisms in the interleukin (IL) gene cluster (*IL1B*, *IL1RN*), interleukin-10 gene (*IL10*), tumor necrosis factor alpha gene (*TNF-A*), and interferon gamma gene (*IFNG*) found the *TNF-A* –308AG genotype to be associated with

an increased overall prevalence of *H. pylori* infection, and the *IFNG* +874AA genotype to be linked specifically to *cagA*-positive infections, while the other studied polymorphisms were unrelated to *H. pylori* status [45]. The *Hinf*1 1622A/G SNP of the interleukin-1 receptor-1 has been linked to the infection in another study [46]. As these studies were all of a cross-sectional nature and conducted among adults, the genetic predisposition could equally well pertain to persistence of the infection as to initial acquisition. Because blood group antigens mediate bacterial adhesion to the gastric mucosa, and *H. pylori* strains may have adapted their binding affinity in accordance with the blood group antigen expression of different human populations [47], the blood group phenotype of the host is potentially of interest. However, the results of a handful of studies on Lewis genotypes and phenotypes, as well as ABO phenotypes, are inconsistent.

Risk factors for *H. pylori* infection in the adult population

The literature on risk factors for *H. pylori* seropositivity in adult life is large but generally cross-sectional and therefore unable to distinguish between effects on *H. pylori* acquisition and persistence. The possibility of reverse causation must also be borne in mind, for instance when anthropometric measures and dietary habits are

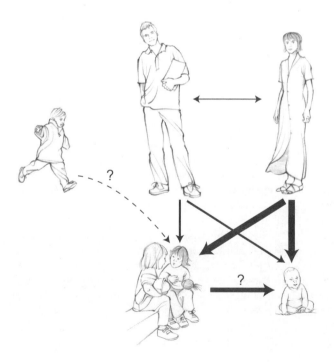

Fig. 18.1 Data from affluent Western populations point to the family as the most important framework for *H. pylori* transmission. An *H. pylori*-infected mother is a much stronger risk factor for the child than an infected father. As uninfected adults rarely contract the infection, transmission between spouses is rare. Clustering of *H. pylori* infection in sibships is often observed and siblings are frequently infected with the same strains, but the mother may be the common source. However, presence of infected siblings seems to be an independent strong risk factor for infection even after control for parental infection status. Close contacts with infected children outside the family, such as with peers at day-care centers or at school, do not seem to be associated with an increased risk of infection in well-developed countries.

considered as risk factors. Among the studies that can be characterized as population-based, there is overwhelming consensus about the importance of **age** (or, indirectly, birth year) and **socioeconomic status** (including various indices of domestic crowding and/or underprivileged home during childhood). In the USA, young African-Americans have more than a threefold increased *H. pylori* prevalence compared with their Caucasian peers [48]. It also appears that **men**, when compared with women, generally have a slightly higher risk of being infected, at least in Western populations [49–51]. Although not confirmed by all investigators, **family size** during childhood may be important, but data on the significance of birth order are conflicting. **Smoking** has generally been found to be unrelated to *H. pylori* status, but a few exceptions exist. Some investigators have found that a moderate **alcohol intake** may be associated with a decreased *H. pylori* seroprevalence [52–55], while others found no association, or even an increased seroprevalence [56]. Low intake of **fruit and vegetables** tended to be a risk factor in a number of studies [57–60], but the strength of the relationships varied widely, from small, nonsignificant associations to up to 19-fold risk gradients. As ascorbic acid inhibits the growth of *H. pylori* in animal models [61,62], the link between serum ascorbic acid levels and *H. pylori* seroprevalence has attracted much attention, but most clinical studies were unable to establish a clear relationship.

Peptic ulcer

Clinical outline

Peptic ulcers in the stomach or duodenum are defined as benign mucosal lesions that penetrate deeply into the gut wall, beyond the muscularis mucosae, and form craters surrounded by acute and chronic inflammatory cell infiltrates. Criteria for size of the lesion vary, but ≥5 mm is a common cutpoint. **Duodenal ulcers** are located in the upper portion of the duodenum (the duodenal bulb) and are generally associated with antrum-predominant gastritis, which contributes to a high and somewhat dysregulated acid output from the stomach. **Gastric ulcers** are located in the stomach proper, frequently along the lesser curvature and, in particular, in the transition zone from corpus to antrum mucosa. As opposed to duodenal ulcer disease, gastric ulcer tends to be preceded by pangastritis (affecting the entire stomach), often atrophic in character, resulting in low acid production.

Peptic ulcers tend to have a chronic remitting course; the ulcers come and go, often with imperfect correla-

tion between symptoms and presence of an open crater. Among 224 community-based Australian patients with duodenal ulcer followed for up to 7 years, dyspepsia was present during 20% of the time if untreated, and during 15% if they were on antiulcer treatment [63]. Asymptomatic ulcer occurrences are quite common, and complications may arise without any forewarning.

H. pylori eradication is the preferred treatment when definite cure and elimination of ulcer recurrence is the goal. Such treatment is associated with 3–5-fold higher success rates compared with placebo for both duodenal and gastric ulcer recurrence, and it is superior to pharmacologic acid suppression in duodenal ulcer healing [11].

Bleeding and perforation are the main complications. Gastric outlet obstruction is an increasingly rare complication, mainly restricted to duodenal ulcers. While the overwhelming majority of ulcer patients do not die of their disease, it has been estimated that the cure of active peptic ulcer increases life expectancy by 2.3 years in persons aged 40–44 years and 121 days in persons aged 70–74 years [64]. Among cases with newly diagnosed uncomplicated peptic ulcer in Funen County, Denmark, during 1993–2002, the standardized mortality ratio (SMR), which can be seen as the cases' relative risk of dying in comparison with the matching general population, was 2.5 (95% confidence interval (CI) 2.3–2.7) during year 2–10 after initial diagnosis [65]. The corresponding SMR among new cases with complicated ulcer (bleeding or perforated) was 2.6, suggesting that if a patient only survives the acute phase of the complication, the survival is similar to that among patients with uncomplicated disease.

Occurrence of peptic ulcer in the general population

There are a number of problems involved in the assessment of incidence and prevalence of peptic ulcer. In particular, many ulcers are asymptomatic. What is observed in healthcare may only be the tip of an iceberg. Moreover, dramatic changes in the management of peptic ulcer in the past decades have imposed calendar period-dependent selection forces that complicate comparisons of hospitalizations or outpatient visits over time. Mortality from peptic ulcer is low and confounded by age distribution among affected individuals, comorbidity and changes in management practices. Because only a minority of individuals with dyspepsia suggestive of peptic ulcer do in fact have the disease, and invasive tests in the form of radiology or gastroscopy are needed for a reliable diagnosis, self-reports form a shaky basis for calculations of incidence and prevalence. The superior way of investigating these matters is by means of population-based endoscopic surveys. Such surveys, on the other hand, may be severely biased unless a high participation rate is attained. The only such study that reasonably fulfills high-level quality requirements was conducted in northern Sweden [66]. The prevalence of peptic ulcer was 4.1%, with an equal contribution of gastric and duodenal ulcers. Interestingly, epigastric pain/discomfort was not a significant predictor of peptic ulcer disease. It should be noted that the accumulated nonparticipation rate corresponded to 46%. The final participants were, on average, older and were more likely to have symptoms, compared with the initial sample. Therefore, the prevalence may have been somewhat overestimated, but the proportion of all ulcers that were asymptomatic was presumably underestimated.

Secular trends in peptic ulcer occurrence

To summarize the secular trends as reflected by statistics of complications and mortality, the rates of peptic ulcer increased among successive birth cohorts in the 19th century to reach a peak among people born in around 1870–1920 (somewhat varying between populations),

with an earlier peak among men than among women, and with the peak for gastric ulcer preceding that for duodenal ulcer (Fig. 18.2). The subsequent calendar time-wise occurrence of ulcer deaths and complications is largely consistent with the birth cohort pattern, with falling rates among younger age groups, irrespective of gender and ulcer type, and a general – albeit not universal – tendency for downward trends also among elderly men, while the rates among women do not yet seem to diminish (Fig. 18.3). This has also shifted the much-cited 2:1 male:female ratio towards unity. However, increasing overall death rates, particularly attributed to complicated ulcer among women, in several populations in which the most risky birth cohorts are expected to be disappearing, suggest that another trend is superimposed on the pure birth-cohort pattern. This trend could tentatively reflect external exposures that were introduced or increased during the last decades of the 20th century; implicated factors include aspirin and other nonsteroidal anti-inflammatory drugs (NSAIDs), estimated to account for one-third of the overall risk of bleeding ulcer and its complications [67], selective serotonin reuptake inhibitors (SSRIs) [68] and oral anticoagulants [69]. Smoking among women may also be added to this list [70].

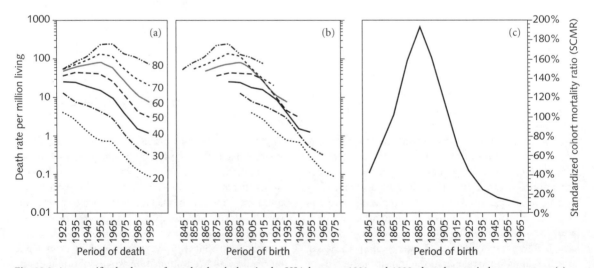

Fig. 18.2 Age-specific death rates from duodenal ulcer in the USA between 1921 and 1998 plotted as period-age contours (a), as cohort-age contours (b) and as standardized cohort mortality ratios (c). Every point of the standardized cohort mortality ratio curve represents an average (standardized) death rate among individuals of different ages born during the same time period. Thus (c) shows how successive birth cohorts during the early and mid-19th century showed increasing duodenal ulcer mortality up to the birth cohort born around 1885. Subsequent birth cohorts experienced successively falling mortality. The different lines (full, dashed, dotted, etc.) refer to the same ages in both (a) and (b). (Reproduced from Cucino C, Sonnenberg A, *Am J Gastroenterol* 2002;**97**:2657, with permission from Blackwell Publishing.)

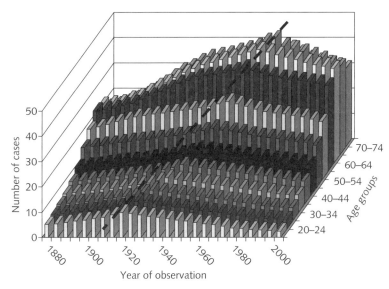

Fig. 18.3 Hypothetical distribution of peptic ulcer cases across calendar years and age groups in a Western male population. There has been a peak among men born around 1900. These birth cohorts have accounted for the peak in all subsequent years, but for each consecutive year, the peak shifted towards older age groups as the high-risk birth cohorts grew older. The birth cohort phenomenon is visible as an oblique ridge in the 3-D chart, marked with a dashed line. The occurrence increased with age in each consecutive year of observation, but declined in the oldest age groups because the oldest were dying off. However, because of the birth cohort effect, with declining rates in younger age groups and a shift of the high-risk birth cohorts into older ages, combined with a general increase in life expectancy, elderly people are presently much more dominating in the peptic ulcer population than they were in the distant past. Because the birth cohorts with the highest risk came approximately 20 years later in women than in men, the "peptic ulcer epidemic" does not yet seem to have culminated among elderly women, and there are so far no certain indications of a downward trend.

Incidence and prevalence of peptic ulcer from the healthcare perspective

Studies of peptic ulcer incidence, that is, the frequency of new disease occurrences among individuals without a previous history, have been based on self-reports of physician-diagnosed ulcers [71,72], searches in healthcare archives [65,73–75], or a combination of both [76]. The information is typically obtained through follow-up of defined cohorts/populations, but one study used 1-year retrospective self-reports to estimate incidence [72]. With a few exceptions, the overall peptic ulcer rates cluster between 1 and 3 per 1000 person-years, with higher rates among men than among women. The variable sources of information may have contributed at least as much to the variation in study results as the genuine geographic variability.

Prevalence rates – mostly lifetime period prevalence – of peptic ulcer tend to be higher when based on self-reports than when the information is obtained through searches in medical archives. This may reflect a higher sensitivity of self-reports, but it is also conceivable that their specificity is poorer. In investigated Western populations [71,76–81], peptic ulcer seems to have affected, at some point in life, 4–12% of the adult population.

Healthcare utilization

Rates of hospitalizations and outpatient visits may only partly mirror the true epidemiology of the disease but are nonetheless of interest because they are indicators of the burden falling on healthcare. In 1995, 4 million US patients visited a physician because of peptic ulcer, corresponding to a rate of 1500 per 100 000 of the US population per year [82]. Between 1958 and 1995, physician visits for duodenal ulcer showed a marked decline, while visits for gastric ulcer remained largely unchanged. Hospitalization rates for all ulcer types have fallen noticeably in the USA [83,84]. This downward trend is evident also in the UK [69,85], but among the oldest, admission rates for complicated peptic ulcer are going up. In Denmark, admission rates have fallen for men, while they have increased for all ulcer types among women [86].

Peptic ulcer in Asian populations

Most of the literature on peptic ulcer epidemiology emanates from Western countries, but the disease occurs at an approximately equal rate also in the East. It appears that the rapid rise that was seen in the West around the turn of the century (when the birth cohorts with the highest risks came into their "ulcer ages") occurred simultaneously in the East. However, the decline in the East appears to have started considerably later than in the West [87]. The male:female ratio is higher and the duodenal-to-gastric ulcer ratio exhibits a greater variation in the East, compared to the West.

Risk factors for peptic ulcer – environmental exposures

A large body of literature concerns risk factors for peptic ulcer. Increasing age, male gender and low socioeconomic status/income/educational attainment or underprivileged race/ethnic group are consistently linked to a higher risk, suggesting that factors linked to these circumstances, like *H. pylori* infection and smoking, may be etiologically important. Indeed, *H. pylori* infection, smoking and aspirin/NSAID use are the overshadowing risk factors for both gastric and duodenal ulcer. In an excellent systematic review and meta-analysis of the literature up to 1995, Kurata and Nogawa [88] reported that the overall risk ratio for total peptic ulcer among *H. pylori*-infected individuals relative to uninfected was 3.3 (95% CI 2.6–4.4). The risk ratio for serious upper GI events (bleeding, perforation or other GI events related to peptic ulcer disease resulting in hospitalization or death) among NSAID users relative to non-users was 3.7 (95% CI 3.5–3.9) with little variation between sexes and across age groups. The smoking-related overall risk ratio for peptic ulcer was 2.2 (95% CI 2.0–2.3), again remarkably similar among men and women and among younger and older people. Using exposure prevalence rates from US populations, Kurata and Nogawa estimated population attributable risk percent (PAR) for *H. pylori* at 48%. PAR expresses the percent of the studied outcome disease that can be attributed to the exposure under study, or in other words, the percent of all cases that might be prevented by eliminating this risk factor. The corresponding statistics for NSAID use and smoking, respectively, were 24% and 23%. Taken together,

these three risk factors were thus deemed to be responsible for 89–95% of the total peptic ulcer-related risk in the US general population [88]. The studies published after 1995 do not materially change the risk ratio estimates, but due to decreasing rates of *H. pylori* infection and smoking, at least among men, the PARs for these exposures are likely to be falling.

Some patients with ulcer disease exhibit no evidence of current or previous infection. In a large Italian study [89], patients with *H. pylori*-negative ulcer disease constituted 7.6% of duodenal and 8.3% of gastric ulcer cases. Such patients were, on average, 9 years older than the *H. pylori*-positive cases, more than three times more likely to use NSAIDs, and 3.5 times more likely to have current or previous ulcer-related complications. These differences were mainly confined to the duodenal ulcer group. Accordingly, the relative risk of having duodenal ulcer among infected people, relative to uninfected, was 53 in the age category <40 years but fell rapidly with increasing age. In the age bracket 40–60 years, the relative risk was 8.4, and among those above 60 years of age the relative risk was 2.9. In this Italian study, the PAR for *H. pylori* infection was 98% among persons under 40 years, 88% among those who were 40–60 years, and 66% among people older than 60 years [89]. Thus, it appears that the importance of *H. pylori* in the etiology of peptic ulcer decreases with increasing age – the ages where the ulcer complications tend to cluster. Consequently, the *H. pylori* prevalence is reportedly particularly low in complicated ulcer disease [90].

Associations of duodenal and gastric ulcer with liver cirrhosis and pancreatic diseases suggest that alcohol may be a common underlying risk factor [91]. A similar link with high blood pressure and stroke indirectly implicates salt intake [71]; although difficult to quantify on an individual level, studies with direct assessment of salt intake support the importance of salt in the etiology of gastric ulcer [92,93]. No association between self-reported alcohol intake and risk of duodenal ulcer was found in a Swedish population-based case-control study [94], nor could alcohol intake be confirmed as a risk factor for any peptic ulcer type in a cohort of American men of Japanese ancestry in Hawaii [92].

Diet

An association between duodenal ulceration and a low fiber intake and a high refined carbohydrate diet has been reported, but the association with fiber intake was attenuated after control for confounding in a British study [95]. In a Swedish cross-sectional study with careful dietary assessment [96], the presence of verified peptic ulcer was associated with a low intake of fruit and vegetables and consequently a low fiber and vitamin C intake, but no adjustments were made for potentially confounding factors. The latter study, further, found a positive association with regular intake of milk, possibly an expression of reversed causation. Intake of fermented milk, on the other hand, was associated with a reduced prevalence of peptic ulcer [96]. The consumption of fermented milk is relatively high in Sweden, and it could be speculated that lactobacilli in these products might have suppressed *H. pylori* growth. Analyses of the possible association of peptic ulcer with intake of fat and essential fatty acids have yielded conflicting results.

Psychological factors

Is psychological stress an important cause of peptic ulcer as has been widely believed? The evidence remains meager [78,97]. A population-based Swedish case-control study was unable to confirm any links with psychiatric morbidity, marital status, personal worries, type-A behavior, or experience of a hectic or psychologically demanding job in either sex [94]. Results from a Danish occupational cohort study indicated that low employment status and non-daytime work were associated with an increased risk of gastric ulcer [98], but confounding from socioeconomic status, particularly during childhood with possible consequences for *H. pylori* status, is difficult to rule out.

Genetic predisposition

Possible genetic components in the etiology of peptic ulcer disease have been addressed in several ways. A Finnish twin study found no more than modest familial aggregation but unveiled a significantly higher concordance among monozygotic than among dizygotic twin pairs [78]. Thirty-nine percent of the liability to peptic ulcer disease was explained by genetic factors and 61% by individual environmental factors. Very little of the liability was explained by shared environmental factors. Thus, the familial aggregation was attributable almost solely to genetic factors, while environmental effects not shared by family members were dominating predictors of disease. Investigators of associations between genetically determined phenotypic expressions and presence of peptic ulcer disease noted in the 1950s a modest excess ulcer prevalence among subjects with the ABO blood group O, and among subjects with ABH non-secretor status. A more recent Danish study [99] showed that car-

riers of ABO blood group A have a risk elevation that is comparable to that among individuals with blood group O. These investigators, and a Finnish group alike [100], found that people with the Lewis (a⁺b⁻) phenotype also have an increased risk of the same magnitude. The role of functional polymorphisms in genes that code for various cytokines involved in the inflammatory response to *H. pylori* infection has attracted considerable attention in recent years, but published studies have yielded mixed and partly contradictory results. Therefore, it appears that the relationship between polymorphisms of the *IL1* gene cluster and risk of peptic ulcer is incompletely understood at present. With the need for confirmation in rigorous epidemiologic studies in mind, it is worth mentioning that two studies have shown a positive association of carriage of the variant *A* allele of the *IL8* –251 locus with prevalence of gastric [101] and duodenal ulcer [102]. The gene product, IL-8, a major host mediator inducing neutrophil chemotaxis and activation, plays an important role in the pathogenesis of *H. pylori* infection.

Gastric cancer
Clinical outline

This section will only discuss adenocarcinoma, which is the dominating gastric neoplasm. Other types, such as lymphomas, carcinoids and leiomyosarcomas account for less than 5%.

There are several classifications of gastric adenocarcinoma, but the one most used in epidemiologic research is that proposed by Laurén [103]. It distinguishes between two main histologic types: (i) the intestinal type, with glandular epithelium composed of absorptive cells and goblet cells; and (ii) the diffuse type, with poorly differentiated small cells in a dissociated noncohesive growth pattern. In addition, mixed and unclassifiable tumors occur. Adenocarcinomas occurring in the gastroesophageal junction or immediately below are referred to as gastric cardia cancers. There is no unanimous agreement about which cancers to include in the latter category, and the definitions of cardia cancer vary between authors. The cardia cancers seem to behave differently compared with noncardia gastric cancer, both in terms of secular trends and risk factor pattern. This may be at least partly explained by heterogeneity among the cardia cancers; the cardia cancer category likely consists of a mix of genuine cardia cancer emanating from cardia epithelium (in view of the typical length of the segment occupied by such epithelium, the proportion of genuine cardia cancer is likely to be small), proximal non-cardia gastric cancers that invade the gas-troesophageal junction from below, and low esophageal adenocarcinomas that invade the same area from above. Unfortunately, there are no good morphologic or biochemical markers to help us distinguish between these tentative subgroups.

Stomach cancer has long belonged to the most deadly cancers. Five-year relative survival (i.e., survival adjusted for expected normal life expectancy) varied between 10% and 20% among patients diagnosed during the 1980s in the USA and Europe. This means that the survival at 5 years was no more than 10–20% of the survival among the age-, sex- and calendar period-matched general population. Despite the lack of major therapeutic breakthroughs, there has been a noticeable improvement in the past 20–30 years [104]. In the USA, the 5-year relative survival has increased from 15% in 1974–76 to 23% in 1995–2001 [105]. This increase was statistically significant.

A disappearing disease?

As opposed to peptic ulcer, the incidence of stomach cancer is relatively easy to study thanks to the existence of well-functioning cancer registration in several countries or regions. In the USA it is easy to get the impression that stomach cancer is disappearing entirely. After having been the most common cancer until the 1940s, stomach cancer now ranks number 11 among men and number 14 among women as far as incidence is concerned [105]. Approximately 13 400 men and 8800 women were diagnosed with stomach cancer in the USA in 2006. In terms of deaths, stomach cancer ranks number 13 and 12 among US men and women, respectively, with 6690 and 4740

deaths. Falling rates have been noted in most populations (Fig. 18.4). The decline in the age-specific incidence of stomach cancer seems to have begun in the early 1930s in the Western Hemisphere and thereafter spread eastward. The secular trend seems to fit well with a log-linear model, that is, the incidence decreases by a fixed percentage each year [106]. As for peptic ulcer, the decline is best explained by a marked fall in incidence in successive birth cohorts [106,107]. Notwithstanding this remarkable spontaneous global decline, stomach cancer, with an estimated 934 000 new cases in 2002, is still the fourth most frequent cancer worldwide, surpassed only by cancer of the lung, breast and colorectum [108]. Due to its poor prognosis stomach cancer ranks second among all causes of cancer death. In fact, with approximately 700 000 deaths annually, it accounts for more than 10% of all cancer deaths. Almost two-thirds of the cases occur in developing countries. The worldwide estimates of age-adjusted incidence (22.0 per 100 000 person-years in men and 10.3 per 100 000 person-years in women in 2002) are about 15% lower than the values estimated in 1985. Due to the aging of the world's population and the steep age gradient in incidence among the elderly, stomach cancer continues to claim an increasing number of victims: 800 000–900 000 per year, corresponding to a 6% increase between 1985 and 1990.

Geographic distribution

With reservations for possible differences in the availability of medical services, diagnostic methods and registration practices, the national incidence rates of stomach cancer vary approximately 10-fold, with the lowest reliable rates observed among North Americans (age-stan-

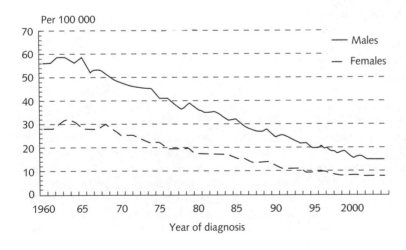

Fig. 18.4 Swedish data on gender-specific incidence of stomach cancer 1960–2004. There is an unabated decline among both men and women. The secular trend seems to fit well with a log-linear model, that is, the incidence decreases by a fixed percentage each year. (Reproduced from *Cancer Incidence in Sweden 2005*. Centre for Epidemiology. National Board of Health and Welfare. Official statistics of Sweden. Health and diseases 2005:9. Published at http://www.socialstyrelsen. se/Publicerat/2005/9042/2005-42-9.htm [January, 2006].)

dardized incidence of 7.4 per 100 000 person-years in men and 3.4 per 100 000 person-years in women, 2002) and the highest in Japan, where screening is ongoing [108]. The age-standardized incidence in Japan was 62.1 per 100 000 person-years in men and 26.1 per 100 000 person-years in women. With few exceptions, the incidence among women is approximately half that among men, regardless of geographic area, culture and religion. While the risk of stomach cancer seems to covary with socioeconomic conditions, there is no clear correlation between national level of economic development and national incidence rates. However, suspected underreporting may have deflated figures from poorly developed countries. Although the highest rates are observed in East Asia, low rates (<10 per 100 000 person-years) are reported from South and Southeast Asia. High incidence rates also are found in tropical Central and South America and in Eastern Europe [108].

Demographic distribution

In the USA the incidence is twice as high in African-Americans as in White people, and three to six times higher among Japanese-Americans than among US-born White people [109]. Immigrant Koreans have an incidence that is eightfold higher than that among White people [110], while the incidence among Filipino men, regardless of birthplace, is only 60% that of US-born White males [109]. Another example of marked differences within a limited geographic area comes from Singapore, where the incidence rates among men of Malay and Chinese descent vary more than threefold. When people move between populations with different risks of stomach cancer, their risk patterns are usually retained or only slightly modified, regardless of their country of origin and country of destination. In the succeeding generation, the rates adjust to that prevailing in the new environment, but this adaptation appears to be somewhat slower for stomach cancer than for colorectal and some other cancers. Though the patterns of risk in relation to migration are complex and defy simple dietary or other interpretation, it appears that early-life exposures are important for the future risk of gastric cancer.

Opposing secular trend for cardia cancer?

While the decline in incidence of gastric carcinoma overall has abated in the USA [111], a closer look at the data reveals two coinciding trends: the steep downward trend seems to persist for distal stomach cancer in White men

and women, but this decline is balanced by an increase in the incidence of cardia cancer. Increasing incidence rates of cardia cancer have been noted in a number of cancer registers in Europe and the USA in the past 20–30 years. However, considerable misclassification of the site within the stomach has been demonstrated [112]; following careful classification of all tumors, no increasing trend could be confirmed for cardia cancer [113]. Some other studies have also failed to verify any upward trend, and even in the USA, the trend seems to have leveled off in the 1990s [111]. Regardless of whether the incidence curve for cardia cancer is flat or turning up, it clearly differs from the descending one for distal gastric cancer.

Risk factors for stomach cancer
Helicobacter pylori

In the past 15 years, numerous observational studies of various designs have demonstrated a positive association between presence of anti-*H. pylori* antibodies and risk of stomach cancer. A recent review of published meta-analyses [114] showed that serologic evidence of *H. pylori* infection is associated with pooled odds ratios of stomach cancer ranging between 1.92 and 2.56, with little heterogeneity. In other words, carriers of antibodies to *H. pylori* allegedly run a risk for stomach cancer that is 2–3 times higher than among people without such antibodies. However, because some infections disappear spontaneously due to changes in the gastric microenvironment during the precancerous stages, it looks as if the strength of the association with stomach cancer risk may be underestimated [115,116]. Moreover, it appears that the association is confined to non-cardia gastric cancer, whereas the infection might even be inversely related to the risk of cardia cancer [117,118]. In studies that restricted the outcome to non-cardia stomach cancer and that took measures to overcome the misclassification of exposure, the relative risk linked to the infection was 20-fold or greater [116,119,120]. According to such studies, the PAR may be 70% or higher even in Western populations [116], while an American case-control study with conventional serotesting reported a PAR of 10.4% [121]. The risk seems to be particularly elevated among carriers of CagA-positive strains (and among carriers of CagA-positive strains in those with strains having the "A-B-D-type" CagA typically seen in Asian high-risk populations [122]), although CagA-negative strains are not without risk [123]. The *vacA* gene of *H. pylori*, encoding a vacuolating cytotoxin, comprises two variable regions; the s (signaling) and the m (mid) regions. *H. pylori vacA* type s1 and m1 strains appear to be more carcinogenic than strains with other *vacA* types [124]. Although the ultimate proof of causality is still missing, a growing number of randomized trials have either shown trends towards reduced gastric cancer incidence or indications of slowing progression of precancerous lesions after *H. pylori* eradication [125–130], thus gradually adding to our confidence in a causal inference.

Smoking

A relationship between smoking and risk of stomach cancer is well established [131,132]. The excess risk among current smokers is 1.5–2.5-fold and increases with higher doses and/or longer duration of cigarette smoking [133,134]. It appears that the risk returns to baseline relatively soon after quitting smoking [135], but in a pooled analysis of two Japanese cohorts, a significant risk elevation remained for up to 14 years after cessation [134]. While some studies suggest that smoking is more strongly related to cardia cancer risk [133,136,137], others indicate that the link with distal stomach cancer is not appreciably weaker, and in Japan it might even be stronger [134]. The PAR for smoking varies with the exposure prevalence, and thus between men and women, but within sexes the variation between American and European data is surprisingly small; thus, the PAR among men varied between 21.5% and 28.6%, and among women between 11% and 14% in three recent studies emanating from the US and Europe [121,133,138].

Alcohol

The most authoritative review of the literature published up until the mid-1990s [139] noted that the bulk of evidence weighed against the possibility of a substantial effect of alcohol consumption on the risk of stomach cancer. A meta-analysis in 2001 [140], however, arrived at a modestly increased summary relative risk estimate (1.15, 95% CI 1.09–1.22; and 1.32, 95% CI 1.18–1.49, for intake of 50 g and 100 g alcohol per day, respectively, relative to no intake). The literature on specific relationships between different types of alcoholic beverages and stomach cancer risk was recently reviewed [141] but no consistent pattern emerged.

Diet

Until recently, the most consistent nutritional epidemiology finding in relation to stomach cancer has been inverse associations with fruit and vegetable intake. In 1997, an international expert panel at the World Cancer Research Fund-American Institute for Cancer Research concluded that there was convincing evidence that high intake of vegetables, particularly raw vegetables and allium vegetables, reduces the risk of stomach cancer [139]. A similar conclusion was also drawn with regard to high fruit intake. A more recent meta-analysis, however, noted that the protective effect seemed to be weaker in cohort investigations than in case-control studies [142], suggesting that recall bias might have pushed the relative risk estimates away from the null value in the latter. The estimated overall relative risks that were based on all study types were 0.81 (95% CI 0.75–0.87) and 0.74 (95% CI 0.69–0.81) per 100 g intake per day of vegetables and fruit, respectively. Although heterogeneity was observed in essentially all analyzed substrata, the estimates for both fruit and vegetables were always less than unity [142]. The most recent addition to the literature, a large European multinational cohort study with careful dietary assessments and a fairly wide range of exposure [143], failed to verify any overall association of stomach cancer risk with total or category-specific vegetable or fruit intake. Even though the estimation of portion size and frequency of consumption of a wide range of vegetables is rather difficult and nondifferential misclassification may bias the relative risk estimates toward the null value, it is reasonable to assume that the more recent studies, particularly the cohort studies with increasingly sophisticated dietary assessments, are less affected by such bias compared with earlier studies. Therefore, it must be suspected that previous research may have overestimated the protection conferred by these plant foods.

Moreover, whereas there is almost total consensus among case-control studies that vitamin C intake is strongly protective, only one [144] out of four prospective studies [144–147] reported a significant inverse association between estimated vitamin C intake and stomach cancer. The summary estimate of relative risk in a meta-analysis, however, was still statistically significant (relative risk among subjects with the highest intake, relative to those with the lowest, was 0.77 (95% CI 0.61–0.97) [148]. A similar meta-analysis of the three prospective studies concerned with pre-disease blood levels of vitamin C [147,149,150] yielded a summary estimate that was also statistically significant (relative risk 0.64, 95% CI 0.41–0.98) [148].

Vitamin E (tocopherol), another important antioxidant in plant foods, has been investigated with regard to its relationship with stomach cancer risk in at least 18 case-control studies, close to half of which reported a statistically significant inverse association while the others were unable statistically to confirm any relationship at all. Among four prospective studies that related estimated dietary vitamin E intake with stomach cancer risk, only one – conducted among Finnish smokers [146] – showed a significantly reduced risk of non-cardia stomach cancer among individuals with the highest intake, but this study also noted an **increased** risk for cancer of the gastric cardia. Six prospective studies that proceeded from pre-disease blood levels of tocopherols yielded mixed results; a recent large European study reported a strong and statistically significant inverse relationship with stomach cancer risk, albeit seemingly limited to the diffuse histologic type [151], while a Chinese study showed a **positive** association with non-cardia cancer risk but no relationship with cardia cancer [152]. Thus, the effect of vitamin E on risk of stomach cancer remains uncertain.

At least 15 case-control studies have addressed the relationship between intake of total vitamin A (retinol and provitamin A carotenoids) and risk of stomach cancer, and the overwhelming majority of them have shown a trend towards an inverse association (in five such studies this trend was statistically significant) [148]. The results of prospective studies, particularly those that examined associations specifically with retinol or β-carotene, have been somewhat less persuasive [148].

Unfortunately, not even randomized intervention trials have been able to provide an unambiguous answer regarding the protective effect of the antioxidative vitamins in plant foods. Two such studies argue in favor of a protective effect; a Chinese study, performed in subjects who were likely to be vitamin deficient, showed a reduced incidence of gastric cancer mortality after administration of a combination of β-carotene, vitamin E and selenium [153]. In the other study, carried out in South America [126], treatment with either β-carotene or ascorbic acid significantly increased the rates of regression of atrophic gastritis and intestinal metaplasia. However, two other randomized intervention studies, conducted among Finnish male smokers [154,155] and American male physicians [156], respectively, showed no effect on prevention of stomach cancer incidence during or after supplementation with either β-carotene or α-tocopherol, the most active form of vitamin E. Moreover, two additional randomized Chinese intervention studies did not observe any significant reductions in stomach cancer incidence or mortality after daily supplementation with 14 vitamins and 12 minerals for 6 years [157,158] or a combination of vitamin C, vitamin E and selenium every second day for 7.3 years [130].

FIBER AND CARBOHYDRATES
Several investigators have found a decreased risk of stomach cancer among people with a high consumption of fiber. A particularly strong inverse association has been demonstrated between cereal fiber intake and risk of cardia cancer [159], possibly attributable to the nitrite scavenging properties of wheat fiber. However, the only prospective study addressing the relationship between intake of whole-grain foods and stomach cancer mortality was negative [160]. High-starch/carbohydrate diets, on the other hand, were reportedly linked to an increased risk of stomach cancer in some studies, but others showed no association. It is conceivable that the association noted in the positive studies may be explained by residual confounding by socioeconomic status.

SALT
Most textbooks list salt intake as an established risk factor for stomach cancer. Ecological studies provide support for a relatively strong correlation between urinary salt excretion and stomach cancer mortality [161–163]. Further, there are abundant case-control and cohort data on intake of salt or salty foods and risk of stomach cancer. Although the results are somewhat divergent, the bulk of evidence weighs towards a positive association, albeit not particularly strong. However, confounding is a major concern; in some of the studied populations, consumption of salted foods may have correlated inversely with socioeconomic status, access to refrigeration and consumption of fruits and vegetables, and positively with the prevalence of *H. pylori* infection. Moreover, salted foods tend to contain significant amounts of *N*-nitroso compounds (NOCs), which may be the true culprits. The relative risk estimates in cohort and case-control studies are mostly in the range where undetected confounding might well explain the association. It should also be noted that there is no laboratory evidence that salt *per se* is a carcinogen for any site of the body [164].

N-NITROSO COMPOUNDS
N-nitroso compounds (NOCs) have been found to be carcinogenic in multiple organs in at least 40 animal species. Humans are exposed to NOCs from diet (processed meats, smoked preserved foods, pickled and salty preserved foods, and foods dried at high temperatures such as the constituents of beer, whisky and dried milk), tobacco smoke and other environmental sources, but a large proportion (typically more than 50%) comes from

endogenous synthesis. The results of epidemiologic investigations addressing the possible association between estimated nitrite exposure (the precursor substance) and stomach cancer risk have been mixed. Similarly, studies of estimated NOC intake in relation to stomach cancer risk have yielded discrepant results, although the majority of case-control studies suggested a positive association. A recent analysis of data from the European Prospective Investigation into Cancer and Nutrition (EPIC) study [165] estimated exposure to endogenously formed NOCs and found a statistically significant association with the risk of non-cardia stomach cancer (relative risk associated with a 40 μg/day increase in endogenous NOC exposure was 1.42, 95% CI 1.14–1.78) but not with the risk of cardia cancer. Thus, the epidemiologic literature has been unable to unequivocally confirm a link between nitrite or NOC exposure and risk of gastric cancer, but the data are clearly suggestive of such a link.

MEAT INTAKE

Whilst meat consumption has been associated with increased risks of cancer of the colorectum, breast and possibly prostate, the epidemiologic evidence for a relationship with stomach cancer risk has so far been considered insufficient. However, recent cohort studies have reported substantial risk elevations among subjects in the highest intake categories, relative to those in the lowest. A meta-analysis that encompassed six prospective cohort studies and nine case-control studies [166] arrived at a summary estimate of relative risk for stomach cancer per 30 g/day increase in processed meat consumption of 1.15 (95% CI 1.04–1.27) among cohort studies and 1.38 (95% CI 1.19–1.60) among case-control studies. Thus, it appears that high intake of processed meat should be added to the list of known – but moderately strong – risk factors for stomach cancer. In the EPIC cohort, the association with processed meat was confined to non-cardia stomach cancer, with a relative risk of 2.45 for every 50 g/day increase in processed meat intake [167]. The latter study also noted positive associations with non-processed meat.

Aspirin and nonsteroidal anti-inflammatory drugs (NSAIDs)

Several epidemiologic studies have noted small reductions in risk of stomach cancer among users of aspirin and/or NSAIDs. A meta-analysis of eight case-control studies yielded a summary estimate of relative risk that indicated a statistically significant 22% risk reduction [168]. However, a randomized trial among 40 000 US women suggests

that aspirin use may not lower the risk of stomach cancer [169].

Genetic risk factors

Familial aggregation of stomach cancer has been reported in the epidemiologic literature. Typically, a 50–130% excess risk was observed among subjects with a positive family history. In an analysis of 44 788 Scandinavian twin pairs, the risk of stomach cancer among dizygotic twins with a partner who developed the same cancer was 6.6 times higher than among dizygotic twins whose partner did not have stomach cancer [170]. The corresponding excess was 10-fold in monozygotic pairs. It was estimated that inherited genes contribute 28% to the risk of stomach cancer, shared environmental effects contribute 10% and non-shared environmental factors make up the remaining 62% of the risk. Therefore, studies on twins predict the involvement of major environmental factors plus minor genetic components.

An aggregation of two or more stomach cancers in the same family is noted in about 10% of all stomach cancer cases. Among them, a number of syndromes can be identified; the most notable is the hereditary diffuse gastric cancer (HDGC – requiring two or more documented cases of diffuse stomach cancer in first/second-degree relatives, with at least one diagnosed before the age of 50; **or** three or more cases of documented diffuse stomach cancer in first/second-degree relatives, independently of age) [171]. The term "familial diffuse gastric cancer" (FDGC) is used for families with aggregation of stomach cancer and an index case with diffuse stomach cancer, but not otherwise fulfilling the criteria for HDGC, for instance due to unknown histologic type of the related cases. In a recent review of the accumulated literature [172], HDGC and FDGC accounted for 27% and 24%, respectively, of 439 screened families with familial aggregation of stomach cancer. Germline truncating mutations in the gene for the cell–cell adhesion protein E-cadherin (*CDH1*) were found in 36% of families with HDGC and in 13% of families with FDGC. In about two-thirds of HDGC families, a large proportion of FDGC families, and in the majority of families with aggregation not fulfilling criteria for HDGC or FDGC, cancer susceptibility is caused by presently unknown genetic defects.

The literature on genetic polymorphisms and stomach cancer risk is limited by a common lack of appropriate control of potential sources of bias; few studies are population-based, and the sample sizes are often insufficient even for the statistical verification of moderate main effects, let alone gene–environment interactions. Besides, information on exposure to relevant cofactors such as *H. pylori* infection, diet and smoking is often lacking. The role of functional polymorphisms in genes that code for various cytokines involved in the inflammatory response to *H. pylori* infection has attracted considerable attention in recent years. One of the key cytokines is interleukin-1 beta (IL-1β), which is an important driving force in the inflammatory responses and also a potent inhibitor of gastric acid secretion. The *IL1B* gene encoding IL-1β is highly polymorphic. Two of the polymorphisms are in the promoter region at positions –511 and –31, representing C→T and T→C transitions, respectively. The variant alleles of these loci are associated with more severe inflammation. Another cytokine that has an important influence on IL-1β levels is the endogenous interleukin-1 receptor antagonist (IL-1ra), whose gene (*IL1RN*) is also known to be polymorphic. The *IL1RN* gene has a penta-allelic 86-bp tandem repeat polymorphism (variable number of tandem repeat, VNTR) in intron 2, of which the less common allele 2 (*IL1RN*2*) – associated with enhanced IL-1β production *in vitro* – is linked to several chronic inflammatory conditions. In a landmark case-control study from Poland, El-Omar and co-workers [173] demonstrated that carriers of the C allele of *IL1B* –31 (in positive linkage disequilibrium with *IL1B* –511T) and homozygous carriers of the *2 allele of *IL1RN* had 1.6- and 2.9-fold increased risks, respectively, of stomach cancer, compared with non-carriers of these variant alleles. Carriers of the *IL1B* –31T/*IL1RN*2* haplotype had an odds ratio of 4.4. These findings have been more or less replicated in several populations, among them Portuguese, American, Mexican, Italian and Chinese. A study from Portugal with genotyping of archived gastric biopsies suggested that the combination of proinflammatory genotypes in the host with infection with high-risk *H. pylori* strains (see previous section about *H. pylori*) might involve major increases in risk, with relative risks as high as 87 [124]. However, others, including investigators from Japan, China, Taiwan, Korea, Holland, Italy, Finland and Sweden, have failed to confirm any association of the *IL1B* –31, *IL1B* –511 and/or *IL1RN* polymorphisms with stomach cancer. It appears that the relationship, if any, between polymorphisms in the *IL1* gene cluster and stomach cancer risk may be more complex than first thought.

There is a large and rapidly expanding literature on links between genetic variation in a number of potentially important carcinogenic pathways (mucin production, cytokines other than those in the *IL1* cluster, human leukocyte antigen (HLA) classes I and II, metabolic phase I and II enzymes, DNA repair systems, cyclooxygenase system, oncogenes and tumor suppressor genes) and risk of stomach cancer [174]. Unfortunately, the overall results become increasingly disappointing as the literature accumulates; notwithstanding the often apparent biological plausibility, the results are remarkably divergent. Typically, promising reports of fairly large effects are followed by null or opposite findings. Whether this diversity is mainly due to an apparent variation in epidemiologic rigor, laboratory measurement errors, or to effect modification by race, ethnicity or other external exposures cannot be determined at present. The positive findings that remain unopposed tend to be the ones that have been tested in no more than one single study. And this could, in turn, be a result of publication bias because negative studies are difficult to get published. There is an urgent need for more population-based studies with meticulous attention to epidemiologic fallacies. Carefully conducted meta-analyses of epidemiologically sound studies may also be helpful.

One notable exception is the literature on polymorphisms in the gene coding for the enzyme 5,10-methylenetetrahydrofolate reductase (MTHFR). The enzyme irreversibly converts 5,10-methylene tetrahydrofolate to 5-methyltetrahydrofolate, the predominant form of folate in the circulation. Folate is a water-soluble B vitamin that plays an important role in the maintenance of DNA integrity. Increasing evidence suggests that a low folate intake and/or an impaired folate metabolism may be implicated in the development of gastrointestinal cancers. Two common functional polymorphisms of the *MTHFR* gene, 677C/T and 1298A/C, have been identified, associated with up to 70% and 40% reductions, respectively, of MTHFR activity among individuals who are homozygous for the variant alleles. A recent meta-analysis of 11 case-control and two cohort studies that examined the association between dietary folate intake and risk of stomach cancer arrived at statistically significant 30% risk reductions for stomach cancer of both non-cardia and cardia location [175]. However, this inverse relationship was confined to studies conducted in the USA and Europe, while studies done in other populations were essentially negative. The summary estimate of relative risk for stomach among individuals with the variant TT genotype of *MTHFR* –677, relative to those with the CC genotype, was 1.68 (95% CI 1.29–2.19) and the corresponding estimate for gastric cardia cancer was 1.90 (95% CI 1.38–2.60) [175]. Available studies of the 1298A/C polymorphism did not provide any indications of a statistical relationship with stomach cancer risk.

References

1. Cover TL *et al.* Characterization of and human serologic response to proteins in *Helicobacter pylori* broth culture supernatants with vacuolizing cytotoxin activity. *Infect Immun* 1990;**58**:603.
2. Blaser MJ, Crabtree JE. CagA and the outcome of *Helicobacter pylori* infection. *Am J Clin Pathol* 1996;**106**:565.
3. Kersulyte D *et al.* Emergence of recombinant strains of *Helicobacter pylori* during human infection. *Mol Microbiol* 1999;**31**:31.
4. Odenbreit S *et al.* Translocation of *Helicobacter pylori* CagA into gastric epithelial cells by type IV secretion. *Science* 2000;**287**:1497.
5. Viala J *et al.* Nod1 responds to peptidoglycan delivered by the *Helicobacter pylori* cag pathogenicity island. *Nat Immunol* 2004;**5**:1166.
6. Occhialini A *et al.* Composition and gene expression of the cag pathogenicity island in *Helicobacter pylori* strains isolated from gastric carcinoma and gastritis patients in Costa Rica. *Infect Immun* 2001;**69**:1902.
7. Israel DA *et al. Helicobacter pylori* strain-specific differences in genetic content, identified by microarray, influence host inflammatory responses. *J Clin Invest* 2001;**107**:611.
8. Malfertheiner P *et al.* Current concepts in the management of *Helicobacter pylori* infection – the Maastricht 2–2000 Consensus Report. *Aliment Pharmacol Ther* 2002;**16**:167.
9. Schistosomes, liver flukes and Helicobacter pylori. IARC Working Group on the Evaluation of Carcinogenic Risks to Humans. Lyon, 7–14 June 1994. *IARC Monogr Eval Carcinog Risks Hum* 1994;**61**:1.
10. Wotherspoon AC *et al.* Helicobacter pylori-associated gastritis and primary B-cell gastric lymphoma. *Lancet* 1991;**338**:1175.
11. Ford AC *et al.* Eradication therapy for peptic ulcer disease in *Helicobacter pylori* positive patients. *Cochrane Database Syst Rev* 2006:CD003840.
12. Wotherspoon AC *et al.* Regression of primary low-grade B-cell gastric lymphoma of mucosa-associated lymphoid tissue type after eradication of *Helicobacter pylori*. *Lancet* 1993;**342**:575.
13. Kusters JG *et al.* Pathogenesis of *Helicobacter pylori* infection. *Clin Microbiol Rev* 2006;**19**:449.
14. DuBois S, Kearney DJ. Iron-deficiency anemia and *Helicobacter pylori* infection: a review of the evidence. *Am J Gastroenterol* 2005;**100**:453.
15. Parsonnet J. The incidence of *Helicobacter pylori* infection. *Aliment Pharmacol Ther* 1995;**9**(Suppl. 2):45.
16. Pounder RE, Ng D. The prevalence of *Helicobacter pylori* infection in different countries. *Aliment Pharmacol Ther* 1995;**9**(Suppl. 2):33.
17. Perez-Perez GI *et al.* Epidemiology of *Helicobacter pylori* infection. *Helicobacter* 2004;(Suppl. 1):1.
18. Torres J *et al.* A comprehensive review of the natural history of *Helicobacter pylori* infection in children. *Arch Med Res* 2000;**31**:431.
19. Clemens J *et al.* Sociodemographic, hygienic and nutritional correlates of *Helicobacter pylori* infection of young Bangladeshi children. *Pediatr Infect Dis J* 1996;**15**:1113.
20. Goodman KJ, Correa P. Transmission of *Helicobacter pylori* among siblings. *Lancet* 2000;**355**:358.
21. Lindkvist P *et al.* Risk factors for infection with *Helicobacter pylori* – a study of children in rural Ethiopia. *Scand J Infect Dis* 1998;**30**:371.
22. Pelser HH *et al.* Prevalence of *Helicobacter pylori* antibodies in children in Bloemfontein, South Africa. *J Pediatr Gastroenterol Nutr* 1997;**24**:135.
23. Aguemon BD *et al.* Prevalence and risk-factors for *Helicobacter pylori* infection in urban and rural Beninese populations. *Clin Microbiol Infect* 2005;**11**:611.
24. Khanna B *et al.* Use caution with serologic testing for *Helicobacter pylori* infection in children. *J Infect Dis* 1998;**178**:460.
25. Goodman KJ *et al.* Dynamics of *Helicobacter pylori* infection in a US-Mexico cohort during the first two years of life. *Int J Epidemiol* 2005;**34**:1348.
26. Genta RM. Review article: after gastritis – an imaginary journey into a *Helicobacter*-free world. *Aliment Pharmacol Ther* 2002;**16** (Suppl. 4):89.
27. Banatvala N *et al.* The cohort effect and *Helicobacter pylori*. *J Infect Dis* 1993;**168**:219.
28. Cullen DJ *et al.* When is *Helicobacter pylori* infection acquired? *Gut* 1993;**34**:1681.
29. Kumagai T *et al.* Acquisition versus loss of *Helicobacter pylori* infection in Japan: results from an 8-year birth cohort study. *J Infect Dis* 1998;**178**:717.
30. Akre K *et al.* Risk for gastric cancer after antibiotic prophylaxis in patients undergoing hip replacement. *Cancer Res* 2000;**60**:6376.
31. Melo ET *et al.* Seroprevalence of *Helicobacter pylori* antibodies in medical students and residents in Recife, Brazil. *J Clin Gastroenterol* 2003;**36**:134.
32. Triantafillidis JK *et al. Helicobacter pylori* infection in hospital workers over a 5-year period: correlation with demographic and clinical parameters. *J Gastroenterol* 2002;**37**:1005.
33. Malaty HM *et al.* Age at acquisition of *Helicobacter pylori* infection: a follow-up study from infancy to adulthood. *Lancet* 2002;**359**:931.
34. Kivi M *et al.* Concordance of *Helicobacter pylori* strains within families. *J Clin Microbiol* 2003;**41**:5604.
35. Soto G *et al. Helicobacter pylori* reinfection is common in Peruvian adults after antibiotic eradication therapy. *J Infect Dis* 2003;**188**:1263.
36. Kivi M, Tindberg Y. *Helicobacter pylori* occurrence and transmission: a family affair? *Scand J Infect Dis* 2006;**38**:407.
37. Rocha GA *et al.* Transmission of *Helicobacter pylori* infection in families of preschool-aged children from Minas Gerais, Brazil. *Trop Med Int Health* 2003;**8**:987.

38. Tindberg Y *et al. Helicobacter pylori* infection in Swedish school children: lack of evidence of child-to-child transmission outside the family. *Gastroenterology* 2001;**121**:310.

39. Rothenbacher D *et al.* Role of infected parents in transmission of *Helicobacter pylori* to their children. *Pediatr Infect Dis J* 2002;**21**:674.

40. Kivi M *et al. Helicobacter pylori* status in family members as risk factors for infection in children. *Epidemiol Infect* 2005;**133**:645.

41. Dore MP *et al.* Risk factors associated with *Helicobacter pylori* infection among children in a defined geographic area. *Clin Infect Dis* 2002;**35**:240.

42. Malaty HM *et al. Helicobacter pylori* infection: genetic and environmental influences. A study of twins. *Ann Intern Med* 1994;**120**:982.

43. Azuma T *et al.* Genetic differences between duodenal ulcer patients who were positive or negative for *Helicobacter pylori*. *J Clin Gastroenterol* 1995;**21**(Suppl. 1):S151.

44. Magnusson PKE *et al.* Gastric cancer and human leukocyte antigen: distinct DQ and DR alleles are associated with development of gastric cancer and infection by *Helicobacter pylori*. *Cancer Res* 2001;**61**:2684.

45. Zambon CF *et al.* Pro- and anti-inflammatory cytokine gene polymorphisms and *Helicobacter pylori* infection: interactions influence outcome. *Cytokine* 2005;**29**:141.

46. Hartland S *et al.* A functional polymorphism in the interleukin-1 receptor-1 gene is associated with increased risk of *Helicobacter pylori* infection but not with gastric cancer. *Dig Dis Sci* 2004;**49**:1545.

47. Aspholm-Hurtig M *et al.* Functional adaptation of BabA, the *H. pylori* ABO blood group antigen binding adhesin. *Science* 2004;**305**:519.

48. Malaty HM *et al.* Natural history of *Helicobacter pylori* infection in childhood: 12-year follow-up cohort study in a biracial community. *Clin Infect Dis* 1999;**28**:279.

49. Murray LJ *et al.* Epidemiology of *Helicobacter pylori* infection among 4742 randomly selected subjects from Northern Ireland. *Int J Epidemiol* 1997;**26**:880.

50. Everhart JE *et al.* Seroprevalence and ethnic differences in *Helicobacter pylori* infection among adults in the United States. *J Infect Dis* 2000;**181**:1359.

51. Moayyedi P *et al.* Relation of adult lifestyle and socioeconomic factors to the prevalence of *Helicobacter pylori* infection. *Int J Epidemiol* 2002;**31**:624.

52. Brenner H *et al.* Alcohol consumption and *Helicobacter pylori* infection: results from the German National Health and Nutrition Survey. *Epidemiology* 1999;**10**:214.

53. Rosenstock SJ *et al.* Association of *Helicobacter pylori* infection with lifestyle, chronic disease, body-indices, and age at menarche in Danish adults. *Scand J Public Health* 2000;**28**:32.

54. Murray LJ *et al.* Inverse relationship between alcohol consumption and active *Helicobacter pylori* infection: the Bristol Helicobacter project. *Am J Gastroenterol* 2002;**97**:2750.

55. Ogihara A *et al.* Relationship between *Helicobacter pylori* infection and smoking and drinking habits. *J Gastroenterol Hepatol* 2000;**15**:271.

56. Bazzoli F *et al.* The Loiano-Monghidoro population-based study of *Helicobacter pylori* infection: prevalence by 13C-urea breath test and associated factors. *Aliment Pharmacol Ther* 2001;**15**:1001.

57. Fontham ET *et al.* Determinants of *Helicobacter pylori* infection and chronic gastritis. *Am J Gastroenterol* 1995;**90**:1094.

58. Shinchi K *et al.* Relationship of cigarette smoking, alcohol use, and dietary habits with *Helicobacter pylori* infection in Japanese men. *Scand J Gastroenterol* 1997;**32**:651.

59. Goodman KJ *et al.* Nutritional factors and *Helicobacter pylori* infection in Colombian children. *J Pediatr Gastroenterol Nutr* 1997;**25**:507.

60. Russo A *et al.* Determinants of *Helicobacter pylori* seroprevalence among Italian blood donors. *Eur J Gastroenterol Hepatol* 1999;**11**:867.

61. Zhang HM *et al.* Vitamin C inhibits the growth of a bacterial risk factor for gastric carcinoma: *Helicobacter pylori*. *Cancer* 1997;**80**:1897.

62. Sjunnesson H *et al.* High intake of selenium, beta-carotene, and vitamins A, C, and E reduces growth of *Helicobacter pylori* in the guinea pig. *Comp Med* 2001;**51**:418.

63. McIntosh JH *et al.* Patterns of dyspepsia during the course of duodenal ulcer. *J Clin Gastroenterol* 1991;**13**:506.

64. Inadomi JM, Sonnenberg A. The impact of peptic ulcer disease and infection with *Helicobacter pylori* on life expectancy. *Am J Gastroenterol* 1998;**93**:1286.

65. Lassen A *et al.* Complicated and uncomplicated peptic ulcers in a Danish county 1993–2002: a population-based cohort study. *Am J Gastroenterol* 2006;**101**:945.

66. Aro P *et al.* Peptic ulcer disease in a general adult population: the Kalixanda study: a random population-based study. *Am J Epidemiol* 2006;**163**:1025.

67. Langman M. Population impact of strategies designed to reduce peptic ulcer risks associated with NSAID use. *Int J Clin Pract Suppl* 2003;**135**:38.

68. de Abajo FJ et al. Association between selective serotonin reuptake inhibitors and upper gastrointestinal bleeding: population based case-control study. *Br Med J* 1999;**319**:1106.

69. Higham J *et al.* Recent trends in admissions and mortality due to peptic ulcer in England: increasing frequency of haemorrhage among older subjects. *Gut* 2002;**50**:460.

70. Svanes C *et al.* Smoking and ulcer perforation. *Gut* 1997;**41**:177.

71. Kurata JH *et al.* A prospective study of risk for peptic ulcer disease in Seventh-Day Adventists. *Gastroenterology* 1992;**102**:902.

72. Everhart JE *et al.* Incidence and risk factors for self-reported peptic ulcer disease in the United States. *Am J Epidemiol* 1998;**147**:529.

73. Johnsen R *et al.* Changing incidence of peptic ulcer – facts

or artefacts? A cohort study from Tromso. *J Epidemiol Community Health* 1992;**46**:433.

74. Perez-Aisa MA *et al.* Clinical trends in ulcer diagnosis in a population with high prevalence of *Helicobacter pylori* infection. *Aliment Pharmacol Ther* 2005;**21**:65.

75. Post PN *et al.* Declining incidence of peptic ulcer but not of its complications: a nation-wide study in The Netherlands. *Aliment Pharmacol Ther* 2006;**23**:1587.

76. Rosenstock SJ, Jorgensen T. Prevalence and incidence of peptic ulcer disease in a Danish County – a prospective cohort study. *Gut* 1995;**36**:819.

77. Suadicani P *et al.* Genetic and life-style determinants of peptic ulcer. A study of 3387 men aged 54 to 74 years: The Copenhagen Male Study. *Scand J Gastroenterol* 1999;**34**:12.

78. Raiha I *et al.* Lifestyle, stress, and genes in peptic ulcer disease: a nationwide twin cohort study. *Arch Intern Med* 1998;**158**:698.

79. Sonnenberg A, Everhart JE. The prevalence of self-reported peptic ulcer in the United States. *Am J Public Health* 1996;**86**:200.

80. Kang JY *et al.* Peptic ulceration in general practice in England and Wales 1994–98: period prevalence and drug management. *Aliment Pharmacol Ther* 2002;**16**:1067.

81. Ehlin AG *et al.* Prevalence of gastrointestinal diseases in two British national birth cohorts. *Gut* 2003;**52**:1117.

82. Munnangi S, Sonnenberg A. Time trends of physician visits and treatment patterns of peptic ulcer disease in the United States. *Arch Intern Med* 1997;**157**:1489.

83. El-Serag HB, Sonnenberg A. Opposing time trends of peptic ulcer and reflux disease. *Gut* 1998;**43**:327.

84. Lewis JD *et al.* Hospitalization and mortality rates from peptic ulcer disease and GI bleeding in the 1990s: relationship to sales of nonsteroidal anti-inflammatory drugs and acid suppression medications. *Am J Gastroenterol* 2002;**97**:2540.

85. Kang JY *et al.* Recent trends in hospital admissions and mortality rates for peptic ulcer in Scotland 1982–2002. *Aliment Pharmacol Ther* 2006;**24**:65.

86. Andersen IB *et al.* Time trends for peptic ulcer disease in Denmark, 1981–1993. Analysis of hospitalization register and mortality data. *Scand J Gastroenterol* 1998;**33**:260.

87. Lam SK. Differences in peptic ulcer between East and West. *Baillieres Best Pract Res Clin Gastroenterol* 2000;**14**:41.

88. Kurata JH, Nogawa AN. Meta-analysis of risk factors for peptic ulcer. Nonsteroidal antiinflammatory drugs, *Helicobacter pylori*, and smoking. *J Clin Gastroenterol* 1997;**24**:2.

89. Meucci G *et al.* Prevalence and risk factors of *Helicobacter pylori*-negative peptic ulcer: a multicenter study. *J Clin Gastroenterol* 2000;**31**:42.

90. Gisbert JP, Pajares JM. *Helicobacter pylori* infection and perforated peptic ulcer prevalence of the infection and role of antimicrobial treatment. *Helicobacter* 2003;**8**:159.

91. Sonnenberg A, Wasserman IH. Associations of peptic ulcer and gastric cancer with other diseases in US veterans. *Am J Public Health* 1995;**85**:1252.

92. Kato I *et al.* A prospective study of gastric and duodenal ulcer and its relation to smoking, alcohol, and diet. *Am J Epidemiol* 1992;**135**:521.

93. Watanabe Y *et al.* Epidemiological study of peptic ulcer disease among Japanese and Koreans in Japan. *J Clin Gastroenterol* 1992;**15**:68.

94. Adami HO *et al.* Is duodenal ulcer really a psychosomatic disease? A population-based case-control study. *Scand J Gastroenterol* 1987;**22**:889.

95. Katschinski BD *et al.* Duodenal ulcer and refined carbohydrate intake: a case-control study assessing dietary fibre and refined sugar intake. *Gut* 1990;**31**:993.

96. Elmstahl S *et al.* Fermented milk products are associated to ulcer disease. Results from a cross-sectional population study. *Eur J Clin Nutr* 1998;**52**:668.

97. Medalie JH *et al.* The importance of biopsychosocial factors in the development of duodenal ulcer in a cohort of middle-aged men. *Am J Epidemiol* 1992;**136**:1280.

98. Tuchsen F *et al.* Employment status, non-daytime work and gastric ulcer in men. *Int J Epidemiol* 1994;**23**:365.

99. Hein HO *et al.* Genetic markers for peptic ulcer. A study of 3387 men aged 54 to 74 years: the Copenhagen Male Study. *Scand J Gastroenterol* 1997;**32**:16.

100. Sipponen P *et al.* Chronic antral gastritis, Lewis(a+) phenotype, and male sex as factors in predicting coexisting duodenal ulcer. *Scand J Gastroenterol* 1989;**24**:581.

101. Ohyauchi M *et al.* The polymorphism interleukin 8 -251 A/T influences the susceptibility of *Helicobacter pylori* related gastric diseases in the Japanese population. *Gut* 2005;**54**:330.

102. Gyulai Z *et al.* Genetic polymorphism of interleukin-8 (IL-8) is associated with *Helicobacter pylori*-induced duodenal ulcer. *Eur Cytokine Netw* 2004;**15**:353.

103. Laurén P. The two histological main types of gastric carcinoma: diffuse and so-called intestinal-type carcinoma. An attempt at a histo-clinical classification. *Acta Pathol Microbiol Scand* 1965;**64**:31.

104. Hansson LE *et al.* Survival in stomach cancer is improving: results of a nationwide population-based Swedish study. *Ann Surg* 1999;**230**:162.

105. American Cancer Society. *Cancer Facts and Figures 2006*. Atlanta: American Cancer Society, 2006.

106. Hansson LE *et al.* The decline in the incidence of stomach cancer in Sweden 1960–1984: a birth cohort phenomenon. *Int J Cancer* 1991;**47**:499.

107. Aragones N *et al.* Time trend and age-period-cohort effects on gastric cancer incidence in Zaragoza and Navarre, Spain. *J Epidemiol Community Health* 1997;**51**:412.

108. Parkin DM *et al.* Global cancer statistics, 2002. *CA Cancer J Clin* 2005;**55**:74.

109. Kamineni A *et al.* The incidence of gastric carcinoma in Asian migrants to the United States and their descendants. *Cancer Causes Control* 1999;**10**:77.

110. Cho NH *et al.* Ethnic variation in the incidence of

stomach cancer in Illinois, 1986–1988. *Am J Epidemiol* 1996;**144**:661.

111. Devesa SS *et al.* Changing patterns in the incidence of esophageal and gastric carcinoma in the United States. *Cancer* 1998;**83**:2049.

112. Ekstrom AM *et al.* Evaluating gastric cancer misclassification: a potential explanation for the rise in cardia cancer incidence. *J Natl Cancer Inst* 1999;**91**:786.

113. Ekstrom AM *et al.* Decreasing incidence of both major histologic subtypes of gastric adenocarcinoma – a population-based study in Sweden. *Br J Cancer* 2000;**83**:391.

114. Eslick GD. *Helicobacter pylori* infection causes gastric cancer? A review of the epidemiological, meta-analytic, and experimental evidence. *World J Gastroenterol* 2006;**12**:2991.

115. Maeda S *et al.* Assessment of gastric carcinoma risk associated with *Helicobacter pylori* may vary depending on the antigen used: CagA specific enzyme-linked immunoadsorbent assay (ELISA) versus commercially available *H. pylori* ELISAs. *Cancer* 2000;**88**:1530.

116. Ekstrom AM *et al. Helicobacter pylori* in gastric cancer established by CagA immunoblot as a marker of past infection. *Gastroenterology* 2001;**121**:784.

117. Hansen S *et al. Helicobacter pylori* infection and risk of cardia cancer and non-cardia gastric cancer. A nested case-control study. *Scand J Gastroenterol* 1999;**34**:353.

118. Kamangar F *et al.* Opposing risks of gastric cardia and non-cardia gastric adenocarcinomas associated with *Helicobacter pylori* seropositivity. *J Natl Cancer Inst* 2006;**98**:1445.

119. Uemura N *et al. Helicobacter pylori* infection and the development of gastric cancer. *N Engl J Med* 2001;**345**:784.

120. Brenner H *et al.* Is *Helicobacter pylori* infection a necessary condition for noncardia gastric cancer? *Am J Epidemiol* 2004;**159**:252.

121. Engel LS *et al.* Population attributable risks of esophageal and gastric cancers. *J Natl Cancer Inst* 2003;**95**:1404.

122. Hatakeyama M. Oncogenic mechanisms of the *Helicobacter pylori* CagA protein. *Nat Rev Cancer* 2004;**4**:688.

123. Held M *et al.* Is the association between *Helicobacter pylori* and gastric cancer confined to CagA-positive strains? *Helicobacter* 2004;**9**:271.

124. Figueiredo C *et al. Helicobacter pylori* and interleukin 1 genotyping: an opportunity to identify high-risk individuals for gastric carcinoma. *J Natl Cancer Inst* 2002;**94**:1680.

125. Sung JJ *et al.* Atrophy and intestinal metaplasia one year after cure of *H. pylori* infection: a prospective, randomized study. *Gastroenterology* 2000;**119**:7.

126. Correa P *et al.* Chemoprevention of gastric dysplasia: randomized trial of antioxidant supplements and anti-*Helicobacter pylori* therapy. *J Natl Cancer Inst* 2000;**92**:1881.

127. Wong BC *et al. Helicobacter pylori* eradication to prevent gastric cancer in a high-risk region of China: a randomized controlled trial. *JAMA* 2004;**291**:187.

128. Leung WK *et al.* Factors predicting progression of gastric intestinal metaplasia: results of a randomised trial on *Heli-*cobacter pylori* eradication. *Gut* 2004;**53**:1244.

129. Mera R *et al.* Long term follow up of patients treated for *Helicobacter pylori* infection. *Gut* 2005;**54**:1536.

130. You WC *et al.* Randomized double-blind factorial trial of three treatments to reduce the prevalence of precancerous gastric lesions. *J Natl Cancer Inst* 2006;**98**:974.

131. Tredaniel J *et al.* Tobacco smoking and gastric cancer: review and meta-analysis. *Int J Cancer* 1997;**72**:565.

132. Tobacco smoke and involuntary smoking. *IARC Monogr Eval Carcinog Risks Hum* 2004;**83**:1.

133. Gonzalez CA *et al.* Smoking and the risk of gastric cancer in the European Prospective Investigation Into Cancer and Nutrition (EPIC). *Int J Cancer* 2003;**107**:629.

134. Koizumi Y *et al.* Cigarette smoking and the risk of gastric cancer: a pooled analysis of two prospective studies in Japan. *Int J Cancer* 2004;**112**:1049.

135. Chow WH *et al.* Risk of stomach cancer in relation to consumption of cigarettes, alcohol, tea and coffee in Warsaw, Poland. *Int J Cancer* 1999;**81**:871.

136. Lagergren J *et al.* The role of tobacco, snuff and alcohol use in the aetiology of cancer of the oesophagus and gastric cardia. *Int J Cancer* 2000;**85**:340.

137. Mao Y *et al.* Active and passive smoking and the risk of stomach cancer, by subsite, in Canada. *Eur J Cancer Prev* 2002;**11**:27.

138. Chao A *et al.* Cigarette smoking, use of other tobacco products and stomach cancer mortality in US adults: The Cancer Prevention Study II. *Int J Cancer* 2002;**101**:380.

139. World Cancer Research Fund/American Institute of Cancer Research. *Food, Nutrition and the Prevention of Cancer: A Global Perspective.* Menasha, USA: BANTA Book Group, 1997.

140. Bagnardi V *et al.* A meta-analysis of alcohol drinking and cancer risk. *Br J Cancer* 2001;**85**:1700.

141. Larsson SC *et al.* Alcoholic beverage consumption and gastric cancer risk: A prospective population-based study in women. *Int J Cancer* 2007;**120**:373.

142. Riboli E, Norat T. Epidemiologic evidence of the protective effect of fruit and vegetables on cancer risk. *Am J Clin Nutr* 2003;**78**:559S.

143. Gonzalez CA *et al.* Fruit and vegetable intake and the risk of stomach and oesophagus adenocarcinoma in the European Prospective Investigation into Cancer and Nutrition (EPIC-EURGAST). *Int J Cancer* 2006;**118**:2559.

144. Botterweck AA *et al.* Vitamins, carotenoids, dietary fiber, and the risk of gastric carcinoma: results from a prospective study after 6.3 years of follow-up. *Cancer* 2000;**88**:737.

145. Zheng W *et al.* Retinol, antioxidant vitamins, and cancers of the upper digestive tract in a prospective cohort study of postmenopausal women. *Am J Epidemiol* 1995;**142**:955.

146. Nouraie M *et al.* Fruits, vegetables, and antioxidants and risk of gastric cancer among male smokers. *Cancer Epidemiol Biomarkers Prev* 2005;**14**:2087.

147. Jenab M *et al.* Plasma and dietary vitamin C levels and risk

of gastric cancer in the European Prospective Investigation into Cancer and Nutrition (EPIC-EURGAST). *Carcinogenesis* 2006;**27**:2250.

148. Larsson SC. Diet and gastrointestinal cancer. One carbon metabolism and other aspects. Thesis, Karolinska Institutet, Stockholm, 2006.

149. Stahelin HB *et al.* Plasma antioxidant vitamins and subsequent cancer mortality in the 12-year follow-up of the prospective Basel Study. *Am J Epidemiol* 1991;**133**:766.

150. Yuan JM *et al.* Prediagnostic levels of serum micronutrients in relation to risk of gastric cancer in Shanghai, China. *Cancer Epidemiol Biomarkers Prev* 2004;**13**:1772.

151. Jenab M *et al.* Plasma and dietary carotenoid, retinol and tocopherol levels and the risk of gastric adenocarcinomas in the European prospective investigation into cancer and nutrition. *Br J Cancer* 2006;**95**:406.

152. Taylor PR *et al.* Prospective study of serum vitamin E levels and esophageal and gastric cancers. *J Natl Cancer Inst* 2003;**95**:1414.

153. Blot WJ *et al.* Nutrition intervention trials in Linxian, China: supplementation with specific vitamin/mineral combinations, cancer incidence, and disease-specific mortality in the general population. *J Natl Cancer Inst* 1993;**85**:1483.

154. Malila N *et al.* Effects of alpha-tocopherol and beta-carotene supplementation on gastric cancer incidence in male smokers (ATBC Study, Finland*). Cancer Causes Control* 2002;**13**:617.

155. Virtamo J *et al.* Incidence of cancer and mortality following alpha-tocopherol and beta-carotene supplementation: a postintervention follow-up. *JAMA* 2003;**290**:476.

156. Hennekens CH *et al.* Lack of effect of long-term supplementation with beta carotene on the incidence of malignant neoplasms and cardiovascular disease. *N Engl J Med* 1996;**334**:1145.

157. Li JY *et al.* Nutrition intervention trials in Linxian, China: multiple vitamin/mineral supplementation, cancer incidence, and disease-specific mortality among adults with esophageal dysplasia. *J Natl Cancer Inst* 1993;**85**:1492.

158. Dawsey SM *et al.* Effects of vitamin/mineral supplementation on the prevalence of histological dysplasia and early cancer of the esophagus and stomach: results from the Dysplasia Trial in Linxian, China. *Cancer Epidemiol Biomarkers Prev* 1994;**3**:167.

159. Terry P *et al.* Inverse association between intake of cereal fiber and risk of gastric cardia cancer. *Gastroenterology* 2001;**120**:387.

160. McCullough ML *et al.* A prospective study of diet and stomach cancer mortality in United States men and women. *Cancer Epidemiol Biomarkers Prev* 2001;**10**:1201.

161. Kono S, Hirohata T. Nutrition and stomach cancer. *Cancer Causes Control* 1996;**7**:41.

162. Joossens JV *et al.* Dietary salt, nitrate and stomach cancer mortality in 24 countries. European Cancer Prevention (ECP) and the INTERSALT Cooperative Research Group. *Int J Epidemiol* 1996;**25**:494.

163. Tsugane S. Salt, salted food intake, and risk of gastric cancer: epidemiologic evidence. *Cancer Sci* 2005;**96**:1.

164. Cohen AJ, Roe FJ. Evaluation of the aetiological role of dietary salt exposure in gastric and other cancers in humans. *Food Chem Toxicol* 1997;**35**:271.

165. Jakszyn P *et al.* Endogenous versus exogenous exposure to N-nitroso compounds and gastric cancer risk in the European Prospective Investigation into Cancer and Nutrition (EPIC-EURGAST) study. *Carcinogenesis* 2006;**27**:1497.

166. Larsson SC *et al.* Processed meat consumption and stomach cancer risk: a meta-analysis. *J Natl Cancer Inst* 2006;**98**:1078.

167. Gonzalez CA *et al.* Meat intake and risk of stomach and esophageal adenocarcinoma within the European Prospective Investigation Into Cancer and Nutrition (EPIC). *J Natl Cancer Inst* 2006;**98**:345.

168. Wang WH *et al.* Non-steroidal anti-inflammatory drug use and the risk of gastric cancer: a systematic review and meta-analysis. *J Natl Cancer Inst* 2003;**95**:1784.

169. Cook NR *et al.* Low-dose aspirin in the primary prevention of cancer: the Women's Health Study: a randomized controlled trial. *JAMA* 2005;**294**:47.

170. Lichtenstein P *et al.* Environmental and heritable factors in the causation of cancer – analyses of cohorts of twins from Sweden, Denmark, and Finland. *N Engl J Med* 2000;**343**:78.

171. Caldas C *et al.* Familial gastric cancer: overview and guidelines for management. *J Med Genet* 1999;**36**:873.

172. Oliveira C *et al.* Genetics, pathology, and clinics of familial gastric cancer. *Int J Surg Pathol* 2006;**14**:21.

173. El-Omar EM *et al.* Interleukin-1 polymorphisms associated with increased risk of gastric cancer. *Nature* 2000;**404**:398.

174. Gonzalez CA *et al.* Genetic susceptibility and gastric cancer risk. *Int J Cancer* 2002;**100**:249.

175. Larsson SC *et al.* Folate intake, MTHFR polymorphisms, and risk of esophageal, gastric, and pancreatic cancer: a meta-analysis. *Gastroenterology* 2006;**131**:1271.

19 Dyspepsia

Nimish B. Vakil and Nicholas J. Talley

Key points
- Dyspepsia is a clinical syndrome defined by the presence of epigastric pain, postprandial fullness or early satiety.
- There are two major categories of dyspepsia: functional (or non-ulcer) dyspepsia, in which no cause has been established after diagnostic testing, and organic disorders, in which a cause (such as peptic ulcer disease or cancer) is demonstrated at endoscopy.
- Dyspeptic symptoms are common in population-based studies; as many as one in five patients in the population report dyspepsia.

- A small proportion of these (25–50%) seek medical attention but they still account for a large proportion of patients presenting to primary care physicians. Quality of life is impaired in patients with dyspepsia.
- The recognized risk factors include *Helicobacter pylori* infection, aspirin and non-steroidal anti-inflammatory drug (NSAID) use.
- The natural history has been studied for relatively short periods of time (less than 10 years) but appears to be generally benign.

Disease definitions

Dyspepsia has been defined by an expert consensus group as pain or discomfort centered in the upper abdomen (Rome definition of dyspepsia) [1]. Discomfort refers to a subjective negative feeling that may not be interpreted by the patient as pain and may include a variety of symptoms including fullness in the upper abdomen, early satiety (inability to finish eating a normal-sized meal), bloating or nausea. Definitions of dyspepsia, however, have been very variable. Some experts suggest dyspepsia means any upper gastrointestinal symptom (including typical symptoms of gastroesophageal reflux diseases) [2]. The Rome definition excludes patients with only reflux symptoms [1]. The rationale is that when classic heartburn or regurgitation are the only or predominant symptoms, the underlying cause is gastroesophageal reflux disease (GERD) and the patient should be managed as such. To complicate matters, patients do not use this word at all. Most recently, it has been suggested dyspepsia be restricted to mean epigastric pain, postprandial fullness or early satiety, but this remains controversial [3].

Dyspeptic symptoms may be continuous or intermittent and may be of short or long duration. Dyspeptic patients who undergo investigation and have no detectable cause for their symptoms are considered to have **non-ulcer dyspepsia** or **functional dyspepsia**. These patients should be distinguished from those who have symptoms of dys-

pepsia but have not undergone investigation (**uninvestigated dyspepsia**). To meet the criteria for the definition of this condition according to Rome III, patients must have a chronic course and have no abnormalities at endoscopy that could explain the symptoms [3]. Functional dyspepsia is therefore defined as at least 3 months of symptoms that began at least 6 months ago of:
- persistent or recurrent epigastric pain, postprandial fullness or early satiety;
- no evidence of organic disease (including at upper endoscopy) that is likely to explain the symptoms [3].

The minimum work-up for a clinical diagnosis of functional dyspepsia is a careful history, physical examination and upper endoscopy during a symptomatic period off antisecretory therapy.

Incidence and prevalence

A systematic review of population-based studies found that the prevalence of upper GI symptoms varied from 11% to 41% [4]. If heartburn was excluded, the prevalence rates ranged from 4% to 14% (Fig. 19.1) [4]. The wide range reported in different studies was not accounted for by publication bias but may be due to differences in the instruments used to measure symptoms and differences in the populations being studied [4].

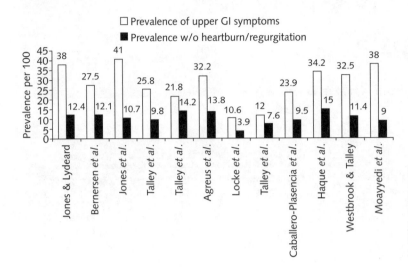

Fig. 19.1 The age-adjusted prevalence rates of uninvestigated dyspepsia reported from population-based studies that used two different definitions for dyspepsia. GI, gastrointestinal. (From El-Serag and Talley [4], with permission from Blackwell Publishing.)

Dyspepsia is the presenting complaint of approximately 4% of patients visiting primary care physicians and one of the commonest conditions encountered by primary care physicians [5,6]. In the US Householder study, the prevalence of dyspepsia was 13%, but one-third of this population had heartburn and would probably be excluded from the diagnosis by the Rome criteria [7]. In a population-based study from Norway, 2027 individuals in a community were contacted and 89% responded [8,9]. The lifetime prevalence of uninvestigated dyspepsia was 12%. The majority of patients with dyspepsia (88%) agreed to undergo endoscopy and 54% had no abnormalities at endoscopy (i.e., they had non-ulcer dyspepsia). A recent study in Olmsted County found that 34% of a random sample of the population reported symptoms of dyspepsia and that this was frequent in 17.5% of people [10]. Limited data are available in Hispanic or Black American populations. In a study from Mississippi, the prevalence of dyspeptic symptoms was similar in Black Americans (24%) and Caucasians (26%) [11].

The true incidence of dyspepsia has not been well studied but in a Scandinavian population less than 1% developed symptoms of dyspepsia over a 3-month period [12]. The number of people who develop dyspeptic symptoms is matched by those who lose their symptoms and the prevalence is therefore stable [13].

Risk factors

In a population-based study in the UK, *Helicobacter pylori* infection was a significant risk factor for dyspepsia in a

multiple logistic regression model (odds ratio = 1.21; 95% confidence interval (CI): 1.09–1.34), suggesting that 5% of dyspepsia in the population is attributable to *H. pylori* [14]. Non-steroidal anti-inflammatory drugs (NSAIDs), low educational attainment, renting accommodation, absence of central heating, sharing a bed with siblings, and being married were also significantly associated with dyspepsia in this model. Smoking, but not drinking alcohol or coffee, was marginally associated with dyspepsia, but this finding was not robust. These factors were not associated with any pattern of dyspepsia symptoms. In contrast, an Australian study of blood donors found an association between dyspeptic symptoms and smoking or the use of aspirin but no association with *H. pylori* infection measured by serology [15]. The low prevalence of *H. pylori* infection in this study (15%) probably reflects the small contribution *H. pylori* infection makes to the genesis of dyspeptic symptoms in developed countries. The most compelling data for a small but clear-cut role for *H. pylori* infection in the genesis of dyspeptic symptoms is from a population-based intervention trial performed in the UK. In a community-based trial, dyspeptic patients with *H. pylori* infection were randomized to eradication therapy or placebo and followed for 2 years [16]. Screening and eradication of *H. pylori* infection was associated with a 5% reduction in dyspeptic symptoms.

In a Danish population-based study, *H. pylori* infection was a risk factor for dyspeptic symptoms but daily NSAID or aspirin use, unemployment and cigarette smoking were associated with greater risk [17]. In a US cohort, female sex, lower education and a larger size of household were more likely to be associated with uninvestigated dyspepsia [11].

Differential diagnosis

Several studies have estimated the prevalence of endoscopic abnormalities in unselected dyspeptic patients in primary care. These studies were performed before the widespread eradication of *H. pylori* and the adoption of test-and-treat strategies in primary care. They probably overestimate the prevalence of ulcer disease in this population. These studies have found that 10–20% of dyspeptic patients in primary care have peptic ulcer disease, 5–15% have esophagitis, 10–12% have abnormalities that are less specific (gastritis, duodenitis) and approximately 50% have no visible abnormalities at endoscopy. Kagevi *et al.* [18] studied 172 patients with dyspepsia who were evaluated in a primary care center. After history-taking, physical examination, laboratory tests, upper endoscopy and flexible sigmoidoscopy, a final diagnosis was established. Six percent of patients had esophagitis, 13% had peptic ulcer disease and 64% had non-ulcer dyspepsia. In another study, Gear *et al.* [19] studied 346 patients and found that a gastric ulcer was present in 6% of cases and a duodenal ulcer in 12% of cases presenting with dyspepsia in primary care. Sixty percent of patients in that study did not have specific findings at endoscopy.

More recent studies have found a much higher prevalence of esophagitis and a lower prevalence of peptic ulcer disease than in earlier studies. A Canadian study evaluated 1040 dyspeptic patients in 49 primary care physician practices [20]. The prevalence of *H. pylori* infection was 30%, and aspirin or NSAID use was reported by 20–28% of patients. Clinically significant findings were reported in 58% of the population. Peptic ulcer disease was observed in 5% of cases. Esophagitis was found in 43%, with the largest proportion of cases having mild esophagitis (Los Angeles grade A = 51%, grade B = 37.5%, grade C = 10% and grade D = 3%).

Gastric or esophageal cancer is found infrequently (<2%) in dyspeptic patients in Western countries but in countries where gastric cancer remains common, dyspeptic symptoms may be a symptom of malignancy. In the Canadian study, only two patients were found to have a malignancy based on biopsy of nonspecific findings [20]. Chronic pancreatitis, celiac sprue and biliary disorders can occasionally be confused with dyspepsia but they are rare causes of dyspepsia. Drugs can cause dyspepsia: NSAIDS are the best studied in this regard but other drugs may also cause dyspepsia.

Clinical diagnosis

Neither the clinical impression nor computer models that evaluate symptom patterns are able to distinguish patients with functional (non-ulcer) dyspepsia from patients with an organic cause for dyspepsia [21]. A systematic review and meta-analysis found that a diagnosis reached by the clinician or computer model suggesting organic dyspepsia had a likelihood ratio (LR) of 1.6 (95% CI: 1.4–1.8), and a negative result decreased the likelihood of organic dyspepsia (LR, 0.46; 95% CI: 0.38–0.55) [21]. A diagnosis of peptic ulcer disease had a LR of 2.2 (95% CI: 1.9–2.6), but an absence of peptic ulcer disease had an LR of 0.45 (95% CI: 0.38–0.53). A clinical history suggestive of esophagitis had an LR of 2.4 (95% CI: 1.9–3.0) whereas a negative history had an LR of 0.50 (95% CI: 0.42–0.60).

Alarm features

Alarm features are symptoms and signs that suggest a more sinister underlying cause for the patient's dyspeptic symptoms (e.g., an ulcer or a malignancy). Despite the importance given to alarm features, it should be recognized that their sensitivity and specificity is low. Two UK studies found that cancer was rarely detected in patients under the age of 55 years without alarm symptoms, and when found the cancer was usually inoperable [22,23]. The rate of presentation of malignancy in patients less than 55 years without alarm symptoms was 1 per million population per year. Data from the USA and Canada have shown similar findings [24,25]. In a Danish study of 2479 patients with 13 upper GI cancers, only 1.5% of patients with dysphagia and 1.5% of those with weight loss had upper GI malignancy [26]. The rate of finding colorectal cancer was similar to the rate of finding upper GI cancer in patients with dyspepsia and weight loss. A systematic review and meta-analysis evaluated 15 prospective studies that included a total of 57 363 patients, of whom 458 (0.8%) had cancer [27]. The sensitivity of alarm symptoms varied from 0% to 83%, with considerable heterogeneity between studies. The specificity also varied significantly from 40% to 98%. The study concluded that alarm features have limited predictive value for an underlying malignancy. Their use in dyspepsia management strategies needs further refinement and study.

Natural history and mortality

In a population-based study in Osthammer, Sweden, a postal questionnaire on symptoms was mailed to a random sample and repeated at 1 year and 7 years [28]. The prevalence of dyspeptic symptoms decreased with time from 11.7% to 8.1%.

Of the 99 patients with dyspepsia in the original sample, 32% had upper abdominal pain at the original assessment, and this proportion decreased slightly to 30% at 7 years; the proportion of patients with minor symptoms decreased from 33% to 23%. There was a concomitant increase in predominant reflux symptoms in the dyspeptic cohort from 6% to 11%, and in irritable bowel syndrome (IBS) symptoms from 15% to 18%. These data suggest that dyspeptic symptoms tend to persist over long periods of time. While the proportion of patients with dyspeptic symptoms remained relatively stable over time there was a shift in symptom patterns in individual patients. Some dyspeptic patients developed symptoms of irritable bowel syndrome and vice versa, suggesting that these disorders may overlap when patients are followed for long periods of time.

There is little information on how dyspeptic symptoms affect survival. As this is a symptom complex, a number of underlying conditions will need to be accounted for in such an analysis. The most important factor in determining mortality is likely to be infection with *H. pylori*, which can cause peptic ulcer disease and gastric cancer, both of which are associated with an increased risk of death.

Disability, quality of life and healthcare seeking

A systematic review found no data on quality of life in functional dyspepsia in a population-based setting (Fig. 19.2) [29]. All the studies that met the authors' inclusion criteria were carried out among patients with functional dyspepsia who presented with symptoms in a referral setting. In uninvestigated dyspepsia, quality of life has been shown to be impaired compared with the general population and to improve after *H. pylori* eradication in some studies. In other studies no significant benefit in quality of life was observed [30]. In a recent US study, quality of life was impaired in both Caucasian and Black American subjects with dyspepsia and remained statistically significant after adjusting for income, education and other factors that affect quality of life [11]. Only a minority with dyspepsia consult; US data suggest just one in four seek

medical care for the symptom complex [31,32]. What drives healthcare seeking for dyspepsia remains poorly defined [31,32].

Prevention

Eradication of *H. pylori* has a modest effect in preventing the development of dyspeptic symptoms and this has been demonstrated in large randomized controlled trials [30,33]. The benefit is small but has been shown to reduce dyspepsia-related costs [33,34]. To a substantial degree, this depends on the prevalence of *H. pylori* infection in a community and the potential benefit of eradication in preventing gastric cancer. The latter may be a more important factor in economic models than relief of dyspeptic symptoms [35,36]. Discontinuation or avoidance of aspirin and NSAIDs is a simple strategy to prevent drug-related dyspeptic symptoms.

Areas for further study

Our knowledge of dyspepsia is limited by the definitions that have been used in various studies to identify the condition. Many of the criteria are artificial and not applicable to clinical practice or to epidemiologic studies. A clinically meaningful definition and classification of dyspepsia would be an important addition. Several aspects of the epidemiology of dyspepsia remain unclear. For example, drivers of healthcare seeking and the economic burden in consulters and non-consulters is poorly documented. The disease burden in the elderly is also little studied. In North America, little information is available for Black Americans and Hispanic people, and the natural history of the disease in these populations is unknown. Long-term data on *H. pylori*-negative dyspeptic patients are lacking, particularly in the group of patients who fail to show any response to acid inhibition.

Conclusions

Dyspeptic symptoms are common in population-based studies and as many as one in five patients in the population report dyspepsia. A small proportion of these seek medical attention but they still account for a large proportion of patients presenting to primary care physicians. The differential diagnosis is complicated by the lack of reliability of symptoms and physical examination. Dys-

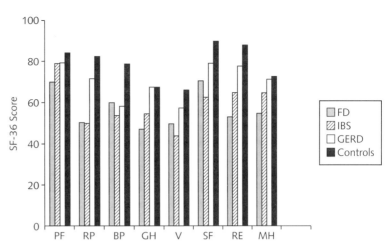

Fig. 19.2 SF-36 scores for patients with functional dyspepsia (FD), controls from the general population, patients with irritable bowel syndrome (IBS) and patients with gastroesophageal reflux disease (GERD): PF, physical functioning; RP, physical role ; BP, bodily pain; GH, general health; V, vitality; SF, social functioning; RE, emotional role; MH, mental health. (From El-Serag and Talley [29], with permission from Blackwell Publishing.)

peptic symptoms change over time, with some individuals evolving to a symptom complex more suggestive of the irritable bowel syndrome. The recognized risk factors include *H. pylori* infection, aspirin and NSAID use. Smoking, alcohol use and educational status have been variably reported to be associated with dyspeptic symptoms. Although the data are limited, they suggest that quality of life is impaired in patients with dyspepsia. Eradication of *H. pylori* can prevent the development of dyspeptic symptoms and may be cost-effective. The natural history has been studied for relatively short periods of time (less than 10 years) and appears to be generally benign, but long-term data are needed as some causes of dyspepsia (e.g., *H. pylori* infection) can result in serious morbidity and death (e.g., by causing gastric cancer).

References

1. Talley NJ *et al.* Functional gastroduodenal disorders. In: Drossman DA (ed.) *Rome II: the Functional Gastrointestinal Disorders*. McLean, VA: Degnon Associates, 2000:299.
2. Veldhuyzen van Zanten S *et al.* An evidence-based approach to the management of uninvestigated dyspepsia in the era of *Helicobacter pylori*. *Can Med Assoc J* 2000;**162**(12 Suppl.):S3.
3. Tack J, Talley NJ. Functional gastrointestinal disorders. *Gastroenterology* 2006;**131**:390.
4. El-Serag H, Talley N. Systematic review: the prevalence and clinical course of functional dyspepsia. *Aliment Pharmacol Ther* 2004;**19**:643.
5. Jones R, Lydeard S. Prevalence of symptoms of dyspepsia in the community. *Br Med J* 1989;**298**:30.
6. Marsland DW *et al.* Content of family practice. Part I. Rank order of diagnoses by frequency. Part II. Diagnosis by disease category and age/sex distribution. *J Fam Pract* 1976;**3**:37.
7. Drossman D *et al.* U.S. householder survey of functional gastrointestinal disorders. Prevalence, sociodemography, and health impact. *Dig Dis Sci* 1993;**38**:1569.
8. Bernersen B *et al.* Towards a true prevalence of peptic ulcer: the Sorreisa gastrointestinal disorder study. *Gut* 1990;**31**:989.
9. Bernersen B *et al.* Non-ulcer dyspepsia and peptic ulcer: the distribution in a population and their relation to risk factors. *Gut* 1996;**38**:822.
10. Castillo EJ *et al.* A community-based, controlled study of the epidemiology and pathophysiology of dyspepsia. *Clin Gastroenterol Hepatol* 2004;**2**:985.
11. Minocha A *et al.* Detailed characterization of epidemiology of uninvestigated dyspepsia and its impact on quality of life among African Americans as compared to Caucasians. *Am J Gastroenterol* 2006;**101**:336.
12. Agreus L *et al.* Irritable bowel syndrome and dyspepsia in the general population: Overlap and lack of stability over time. *Gastroenterology* 1995;**109**:671.
13. Talley N *et al.* Onset and disappearance of gastrointestinal symptoms and functional gastrointestinal disorders. *Am J Epidemiol* 1992;**136**:165.
14. Moayyedi P *et al.* The proportion of upper gastrointestinal symptoms in the community associated with *Helicobacter pylori*, lifestyle factors, and nonsteroidal anti-inflammatory drugs. Leeds HELP Study Group. *Am J Gastroenterol* 2000;**95**:1448.
15. Nandurkar S *et al.* Dyspepsia in the community is linked to smoking and aspirin use but not to *Helicobacter pylori* infection. *Arch Intern Med* 1998;**158**:1427.
16. Moayyedi P *et al.* Effect of population screening and treatment for *Helicobacter pylori* on dyspepsia and quality of life in the community: a randomised controlled trial. Leeds HELP Study Group. *Lancet* 2000;**355**:1665.
17. Wildner-Christensen M *et al.* Risk factors for dyspepsia in a general population: non-steroidal anti-inflammatory drugs,

cigarette smoking and unemployment are more important than *Helicobacter pylori* infection *Scand J Gastroenterol* 2006;**41**:149.

18. Kagevi I *et al.* Endoscopic findings and diagnoses in unselected dyspeptic patients at a primary health care center. *Scand J Gastroenterol* 1989;**24**:145.

19. Gear MWL, Barnes RJ. Endoscopic studies of dyspepsia in general practice. *Br Med J* 1980;**1**:1136.

20. Thomson A *et al.* The prevalence of clinically significant endoscopic findings in primary care patients with uninvestigated dyspepsia: the Canadian Adult Dyspepsia Empiric treatment-prompt endoscopy (CADET-PE) study. *Aliment Pharmacol Ther* 2003;**17**:1481.

21. Moayyedi P *et al.* Can the clinical history distinguish between organic and functional dyspepsia? *JAMA* 2006;**295**:1566.

22. Christie J *et al.* Gastric cancer below the age of 55: implications for screening patients with uncomplicated dyspepsia. *Gut* 1997;**41**:513.

23. Gillen D, McColl KE. Does concern about missing malignancy justify endoscopy in uncomplicated dyspepsia in patients aged less than 55? *Am J Gastroenterol* 1999;**94**:2329.

24. Canga C 3rd, Vakil N. Upper GI malignancy, uncomplicated dyspepsia, and the age threshold for early endoscopy. *Am J Gastroenterol* 2002;**97**:600.

25. Breslin NP *et al.* Gastric cancer and other endoscopic diagnoses in patients with benign dyspepsia. *Gut* 2000; **46**:93.

26. Meineche-Schmidt V, Jorgensen T. 'Alarm symptoms' in patients with dyspepsia: A three-year prospective study from general practice. *Scand J Gastroenterol* 2002;**37**:999.

27. Vakil N *et al.* Limited value of alarm features in the diagnosis of upper gastrointestinal malignancy: systematic review and meta-analysis. *Gastroenterology* 2006;**131**:390; quiz 659.

28. Agréus L *et al.* Natural history of gastroesophageal reflux disease and functional abdominal disorders: a population-based study. *Am J Gastroenterol* 2001;**96**:2905.

29. El-Serag HB, Talley NJ. Health-related quality of life in functional dyspepsia. *Aliment Pharmacol Ther* 2003;**18**:387.

30. Wildner-Christensen M *et al.* Rates of dyspepsia one year after *Helicobacter pylori* screening and eradication in a Danish population. *Gastroenterology* 2003;**125**:372.

31. Ahlawat SK *et al.* Dyspepsia consulters and patterns of management: a population-based study. *Aliment Pharmacol Ther* 2005;**22**:251.

32. Koloski NA *et al.* Predictors of conventional and alternative health care seeking for irritable bowel syndrome and functional dyspepsia. *Aliment Pharmacol Ther* 2003;**17**:841.

33. Ford AC *et al.* A community screening program for *Helicobacter pylori* saves money: 10-year follow-up of a randomized controlled trial. *Gastroenterology* 2005;**129**:1910.

34. Chiba N *et al.* Economic evaluation of *Helicobacter pylori* eradication in the CADET – *Helicobacter pylori* randomized controlled trial of *H. pylori*-positive primary care patients with uninvestigated dyspepsia. *Aliment Pharmacol Ther* 2004;**19**:349.

35. Mason J *et al.* The cost-effectiveness of population *Helicobacter pylori* screening and treatment: a Markov model using economic data from a randomized controlled trial. *Aliment Pharmacol Ther* 2002;**16**:559.

36. Lane JA *et al.* Impact of *Helicobacter pylori* eradication on dyspepsia, health resource use, and quality of life in the Bristol helicobacter project: randomised controlled trial. *Br Med J* 2006;**332**:199.

20 Upper Gastrointestinal Bleeding

James Lau and Joseph Sung

Key points
- Upper gastrointestinal bleeding has become a disease of the elderly with comorbid illnesses. This trend keeps the mortality of the condition relatively high despite advances in endoscopic and pharmacologic therapies.
- Although *Helicobacter pylori*-related peptic ulcer is declining, usage of NSAIDs and aspirin has become an increasingly important cause of upper gastrointestinal bleeding.
- There is also an increase in non-*Helicobacter*, non-NSAID-related ulcer reported in both the East and the West. These ulcers are likely to recur.
- The most important risk factors predicting death in upper gastrointestinal bleeding are old age, comorbidities, severe bleeding as manifested by shock at presentation or fresh hematemesis, continued or recurrent bleeding, onset of bleeding while hospitalized for other causes and major stigmata of bleeding.

Clinical summary

Upper gastrointestinal bleeding is among the commonest gastrointestinal emergencies. The condition accounts for 1–2% of all hospital admissions, representing substantial hospital resource utilization [1]. Owing to an aging population with comorbid illnesses, mortality from upper gastrointestinal bleeding has remained at around 10% for several decades. Hematemesis and melena are signs that indicate bleeding from an upper gastrointestinal source (proximal to the ligament of Treitz). In about 5% of patients, exigent bleeding leads to hematochezia.

Population-based studies: incidence and prevalence

Epidemiological studies of upper gastrointestinal bleeding have varied in their designs and sample populations. The reported incidence ranges widely and is approximately 100 per 100 000 population [2–7]. The American Society of Gastrointestinal Endoscopy conducted a national survey in 1990 among its members [2]. Subsequently, data from members belonging to a large HMO from a defined population in southern California indicated an annual incidence of 102 per 100 000 [3]. Two large UK audits became available in the 1990s. The National United Kingdom audit was a population-based, prospective collection of data over a 4-month period in 74 acute hospitals totaling 4185 cases [4]. The West of Scotland study was a case ascertainment study with prospective case identification over a 6-month period in a defined region [5]. In both audits, it is noteworthy that at least 20% of patients admitted had no documented source of bleeding. A prospective cohort study in The Netherlands reported a lower incidence of 45 per 100 000 [6]. The Canadian Registry on Nonvariceal Upper Gastrointestinal Bleeding and Endoscopy (RUGBE) represented a registry of randomly selected patients endoscoped for upper gastrointestinal bleeding [7]. Findings of major population-based studies are summarized in Table 20.1.

Acute upper gastrointestinal bleeding is a disease primarily affecting older age groups. From the National United Kingdom Audit [4], 68% and 27% of the cohort were older than 60 and 80 years, respectively. When compared with historic British series, a steady rise in the incidence was noticed over the last few decades. The crude mortality rate increased from 9.9% in the 1940s to 11% in the 1990s. When age standardized, a slight decrease in mortality could be observed. It is often argued that advances in the care of patients with upper gastrointestinal bleeding have been offset by an aging population (Table 20.2).

There has also been a trend towards increasing admissions among older subjects and a corresponding decline for younger patients resulting in little change in the overall admissions. Higham and colleagues [8] reviewed hospital

Table 20.1 Population-based epidemiology studies on acute upper gastrointestinal hemorrhage in the last decade

Author and year	Region	No. of population	Median age in years	Incidence per 100 000	Crude mortality (%)
Longstreth, 1994 [3]	California	258	61	102	5
Rockall et al., 1995 [4]	England	4183	71	103	14
Blatchford et al., 1997 [5]	Scotland	1882	NA	172	14
Vreeburg et al., 1997 [6]	The Netherlands	951	71	45	13.9

episode statistics for admissions obtained from the Office of National Statistics in the UK. From 1989 to 1999, admission rates for peptic ulcer hemorrhage increased among older subjects. Over the period, admissions increased by 33% among women aged more than 74 years and by 49% among elderly men. Much of the rise related to admissions for hemorrhage.

Causes of acute upper gastrointestinal bleeding

Traditionally, upper gastrointestinal bleeding (GIB) is categorized as variceal or nonvariceal in etiology. Among the nonvariceal causes, peptic ulcer is the commonest in most series. In large population-based studies, variceal bleeding constitutes only 5–10% of all patients with upper GIB. Variceal bleeding is associated with a poorer prognosis. Mortality during the first bleed approaches 30%. In over 50% of patients with variceal bleeding, the bleeding is likely to be more severe and will continue or recur. The causes of acute upper GIB and their occurrences are listed in Table 20.3. This chapter focuses on the condition of peptic ulcer bleeding.

Risk factors: *Helicobacter pylori*, NSAIDs and aspirin

Helicobacter pylori, non-steroidal anti-inflammatory drugs (NSAIDs) and aspirin are risk factors for bleeding peptic ulcers. They seem to act independently although some studies suggest synergistic roles among these factors.

H. pylori is strongly associated with peptic ulcer disease. Its pathogenic role in peptic ulcer bleeding has been less clear. The reported prevalence of *H. pylori* in patients with bleeding ulcers varies from 46% to 99%, and these figures may be 15–20% lower than in patients with non-bleeding ulcers [9]. Eradication of *H. pylori* prevents ulcer relapse and decreases recurrent bleeding among those infected. This fact suggests a strong etiologic role for *H. pylori* and bleeding in peptic ulcers. In a Cochrane database systematic review [10], *H. pylori* eradication therapy was compared with non-eradication therapy with or without long-term antisecretory therapy. *H. pylori* eradication led to fewer rebleeds (2.9% vs 20% among 578 patients; odds ratio (OR) 0.17; 95% confidence interval (CI) 0.1–0.32) in seven trials that did not use long-term maintenance antisecretory therapy. Even compared with long-term main-

Table 20.2 Previous British studies showing age structure and age-standardized mortality ratio. (Adapted from Rockall et al. [4], with permission from the British Medical Group)

Series	Year	No. of cases	Age >60	Age >80	Mortality emergency admissions	Age-standardized mortality ratio (95% CI)
Jones	1940–47	687	33	2	9.9	147 (109–195)
Schiller	1953–67	2149	48	8	8.9	110 (95–126)
Johnston	1967–68	817	49	9	10.6	122 (100–146)
Mayberry	1972–78	583	NA	NA	10.3	–
Katchinski	1984–86	1017	63	18	11.8	91 (73–112)
Rockall	1993	4185	68	27	11.0	100 (reference)

Table 20.3 Diagnoses based on data from the National UK Audit. (Adapted from Rockall *et al.* [4], with permission from the British Medical Group)

Diagnosis	Percent
Peptic ulcer	35
Malignancy	4
Varices	4
Mallory–Weiss syndrome	5
Erosive disease	11
Esophagitis	10
Other diagnosis	6
None	25

tenance antisecretory therapy, *H. pylori* eradication was better in preventing rebleeding (1.6 vs 5.6%; OR 0.25; 95% CI 0.08–0.76) in three trials consisting of 470 patients. All patients with peptic ulcer bleeding should therefore be tested for *H. pylori* infection and eradication therapy prescribed to those who test positive.

The use of non-steroidal anti-inflammatory drugs is an important risk factor for bleeding ulcers. Prospective data collected in the Arthritis, Rheumatism, and Aging Medical Information System (ARAMIS) in the USA showed a conservative estimate of 16 500 deaths related to NSAIDs in the year 1997 [11]. The figure was similar to that from acquired immunodeficiency syndrome (AIDS) in the country and was ranked 15th most common cause of death in the USA. From prospective observational cohort studies, GI complications occur in 7.3–13 of every 1000 patients taking NSAIDs for 12 months. During the same time, only 4–8% of patients will present with symptomatic gastroduodenal ulcers. As a whole, NSAID use increases the risk of gastrointestinal bleeding by a factor of 4–5. In a case control study, 46.3% and 10.7% of patients had used an NSAID or low-dose aspirin, respectively, prior to their admissions, compared with 10.3% and 9.2% among controls (OR 7.4 and 2.4, respectively) [12]. The use of nitrates or antisecretory drugs, by contrast, confers some protection against upper gastrointestinal bleeding (Table 20.4). Elderly patients with a history of ulcer disease, especially with a complication, are at increased risk of developing gastroduodenal complications. Factors that predict development of NSAID-associated peptic ulcers among patients are listed in Table 20.5 [13]. Certain NSAIDs are more toxic than others. For instance, piroxicam is associated with a substantially higher risk (relative risk (RR) 3.8) when compared with ibuprofen [14].

It is conjectural whether *H. pylori* infection potentiates or mitigates ulcer bleeding among NSAID or aspirin users. In a pooled analysis of observational studies on the prevalence of *H. pylori* infection and NSAID use in patients with peptic ulcer bleeding, *H. pylori* infection and NSAID use increased risk of ulcer bleeding 1.79-fold and 4.85-fold, respectively. The relative risk increased to 6.13 when both factors were present [15]. In a randomized trial, the role of *H. pylori* eradication in patients with bleeding peptic ulcers using NSAIDs was evaluated. Healing in NSAID-associated bleeding ulcers given a proton pump inhibitor was similar with or without *H. pylori* eradication (86 vs 83% at 8 weeks, ITT analysis) [16]. In another trial, patients on naproxen or low-dose aspirin were randomized to receive maintenance proton pump inhibitor therapy or *H. pylori* eradication. The rate of recurrent bleeding at 6 months was higher in naproxen users who received *H. pylori* therapy without a maintenance proton pump inhibitor (19% vs 4%). The rate of rebleeding in aspirin users was low and similar between groups [17]. Current evidence suggests that NSAIDs, aspirin and *H. pylori* infection are independent risk factors with little synergism among factors.

The management of patients with peptic ulcer bleeding on NSAIDs is complex. The issues include careful selection of anti-inflammatory drugs – NSAIDs or selective cyclooxygenase 2 (COX-2) inhibitors (coxibs) – based upon patients' ulcer history and a review over use of as-

Table 20.4 Frequency of drug use and risk of upper gastrointestinal bleeding (adjusted odds ratios) in patients and controls. (Adapted from Lanas *et al.* [12], with permission from the British Medical Group)

Type of drug	No. of patients affected (%) (total = 1122)	No. of controls affected (%) (total = 2231)	Adjusted odds ratio (95% CI)
NSAIDs	520 (46.3)	229 (10.3)	7.4 (4.5–12)
Low-dose aspirin use	120 (10.7)	206 (9.2)	2.4 (1.8–3.3)
Nitrovasodilator use	60 (5.3)	137 (6.1)	0.6 (0.4–0.9)
Antisecretory therapy	135 (12)	206 (9.2)	0.6 (0.44--00.8)

Table 20.5 Risk factors for the development of NSAID-associated gastroduodenal ulcers. (Adapted from Wolfe *et al.* [13], with permission from the Massachusetts Medical Society)

Established risk factors
Advanced age (linear increase in risk)
History of ulcer
Concomitant use of corticosteroids
Higher doses of NSAIDs, including the use of more than one NSAID
Concomitant administration of anticoagulants
Comorbid illnesses

Possible risk factors
Concomitant *Helicobactor pylori* infection
Cigarette smoking
Alcohol consumption

pirin therapy. The withdrawal of certain COX-2 inhibitors due to their associated adverse cardiovascular events has simplified choices. Testing and cure of *H. pylori*, if present, is indicated. For patients who present with peptic ulcer bleeding but require NSAIDs long term, long-term proton pump inhibitor or misoprostol in prophylaxis against recurrent bleeding is recommended. The management of patients taking low-dose aspirin is complex,

but eradication of *H. pylori* infection alone in those with a past history of bleeding does not guarantee complete protection and therefore a proton pump inhibitor should also be given.

Do *H. pylori* and NSAID/aspirin account for all the peptic ulcer bleeding? Pooled data from the USA showed that some 27% of duodenal ulcers lack evidence of *H. pylori* infection or probable NSAID usage (Table 20.6) [19].

As one might expect, the recurrence of ulcer after eradication of *H. pylori* (Hp) in these so-called "non-Hp, non-NSAID ulcers" is appreciable. Laine *et al.* summarized seven double-blinded randomized controlled studies in the USA that attempted to eradicate *H. pylori*, and found ulcer recurrence in 20% even after successful eradication of the infection (Fig. 20.1) [19].

Non-*H. pylori*, non-NSAID ulcer leading to bleeding may not be as common, at least in the last decade. In a study surveying over 1000 cases of peptic ulcer from Hong Kong, only 4% of cases could not be explained by *H. pylori* infection or NSAID usage (Fig. 20.2) [20]. However, when the same investigators repeated the study more recently, 18.8% of the bleeding ulcers were non-Hp and non-NSAID related [21]. These ulcers were found in older patients with more comorbid illnesses. They are also more likely to recur despite initial treatment success. The etiol-

Reference	Year of study	N	Percent confirmed *H. pylori* negative
Unpublished data	1991	1225	28 (280/1010)
Unpublished data	1991	1130	26 (237/896)
Graham	1993	139	33 (40/122)
Graham	1993	132	21 (23/112)
Peterson	1993	128	27 (30/112)
Lanza	1993	156	33 (47/142)
Total		2910	27 (657/2394)

Table 20.6 Published studies on the rate of *H. pylori* negative duodenal ulcers in the USA. (Adapted from Ciociola *et al.* [18], with permission from Blackwell Publishing)

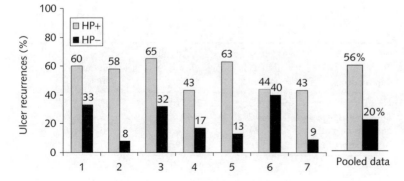

Fig. 20.1 Recurrence of duodenal ulcer after eradication of *H. pylori* infection.

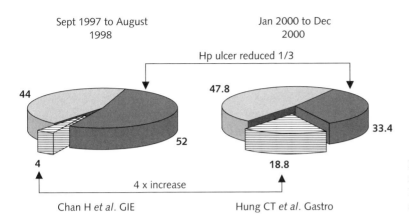

Sept 1997 to August 1998

Jan 2000 to Dec 2000

Hp ulcer reduced 1/3

44

47.8

52

33.4

4

18.8

4 x increase

Chan H *et al.* GIE

Hung CT *et al.* Gastro

Fig. 20.2 Proportion of peptic ulcers resulting from *H. pylori* infection and NSAID usage. (Based on Chan *et al.* [20] and Hung *et al.* [21].)

Table 20.7 Summary of statistically significant predictors of persistent or recurrent bleeding as assessed by multivariate analyses in studies over the past decade (modified from Barkun [26], with permission from the American College of Physicians)

Risk factor	Odds ratio for increased risk
Clinical factors	
Age	
>65 years	1.3
≥70 years	2.3
Shock (systolic BP <100 mmHg)	1.2–3.65
Health status (ASA class 1 vs 2–5)	1.94–7.63
Comorbid illness	1.6–7.63
Erratic mental status	3.21
Ongoing bleeding	3.14
Laboratory factors	
Initial hemoglobin ≤100 g/L or hematocrit <0.3	0.8–2.99
Prolonged partial thromboplastin time	1.96
Presentation of bleeding	
Melena	1.6
Red blood on rectal examination	3.76
Blood in gastric aspirate or stomach	1.1–11.5
Hematemesis	1.2–5.7
Endoscopic factors	
Active bleeding on endoscopy	2.5–6.48
Endoscopic high-risk stigmata	1.91–4.81
Clot	1.72–1.9
Ulcer size ≥2 cm	2.29–3.54
Diagnosis of gastric or duodenal ulcer	2.7 (1.2–4.9)
Ulcer location:	
High on lesser curvature	2.79
Superior wall	13.9
Posterior wall	9.2

ogy of these ulcers has not been thoroughly established. Surreptitious use of NSAIDs, undiagnosed Crohn's disease and stress-related ulcer may account for some of these cases. Over the last decade, prescription of selective serotonin reuptake inhibitors (SSRIs) has increased 15-fold [8]. Evidence from case-control studies suggests that SSRIs may increase the risk of upper gastrointestinal bleeding 2–3-fold [22,23].

Natural history and risk stratification

Upper gastrointestinal bleeding is usually a self-limiting condition; 80% of bleeding stops spontaneously and recovery in this group of patients is uneventful. The remaining 20% of patients account for the majority of morbidity and mortality from the condition. It is therefore logical to stratify risks and provide the appropriate level of care. Several risk scores, such as those of Rockall *et al.* or Blatchford *et al.*, have been devised [24,25]. The Blatchford score is a pre-endoscopy scoring system based on simple clinical parameters such as admission hemoglobin level, blood urea, pulse rate, blood pressure and evidence of hepatic or cardiac diseases. Other scores such as the Rockall score incorporate findings at endoscopy. However, none of them is in common use (Table 20.5) [26]. Major risk factors predicting death include old age, comorbidities, severe bleeding as manifested by shock at presentation or fresh hematemesis, continued or recurrent bleeding, onset of bleeding while hospitalized for other causes, and major stigmata of bleeding. Large ulcers (often defined by size >2 cm) in proximity to and eroding into large artery complexes, such as those at the lesser curve or posterior bulbar duodenum, are predicted to rebleed.

Early endoscopy (often defined by endoscopy performed within 24 hours of admission) identifies the source of bleeding in most instances. The approach allows risk stratification and triages patients. Actively bleeding ulcers mandate endoscopic hemostasis. The technique has been shown to reduce recurrent bleeding, the need for surgery and, in pooled analyses [27], death. Ulcers with stigmata of recent bleeding such as a nonbleeding visible vessel (a protuberant discoloration) or an adherent clot also warrant therapy. These ulcers constitute the high-risk group. Patients with ulcers harboring flat dots or a clean base can be discharged early. Laine and Peterson [28] summarized studies that did not use endoscopic treatment of ulcers and found that rate of further bleeding correlated with stigmata of bleeding seen at endoscopy: <5% in clean ulcer base; 10% with a flat spot; 22% with an adherent clot; 43% with a nonbleeding visible vessel; and 55% in those with active bleeding. In patients with ongoing bleeding or at risk of recurrent bleeding, endoscopic therapy reduces bleeding-associated morbidity and mortality. Low-risk patients can be discharged early, as the approach of early endoscopy reduces hospital resource utilization [29].

It is becoming clear that the use of a proton pump inhibitor is beneficial in the management of bleeding peptic ulcer. In a pooled analysis [30], the use of a proton pump inhibitor was associated with reductions in both recurrent bleeding and surgery. A proton pump inhibitor is used as an adjunctive therapy to endoscopic treatment in high-risk ulcers. The optimal dose remains controversial. In theory, a high dose given as a continuous infusion over 3 days is required to maintain intragastric pH at 6 or above. With gastric neutrality, platelet function is optimized thereby facilitating clot formation over ulcers. The adjunctive use of a high-dose proton pump inhibitor after endoscopic control of a bleeding peptic ulcer has been shown to be cheaper in preventing an episode of recurrent bleeding [31]. This is implicit with savings on reintervention during an episode of recurrent bleeding and hospitalization.

Healthcare utilization

Upper gastrointestinal hemorrhage is a common disorder resulting in 250 000–300 000 hospitalizations per year in the USA, and costs associated with upper gastrointestinal hemorrhage have been estimated to exceed $2.5 billion annually. Data from ARAMIS suggested that at least 100 000 hospitalizations were due to NSAID-related GI complications. Cost reduction will have to come from two sources: management of the acute condition and prevention of gastrointestinal bleeding. The emphasis on outcomes research and development of practice guide-

lines aims to identify management guidelines that are cost-efficient. It is generally believed that inconsistency in practices leads to inappropriate and wasteful utilization of resources without improving patients' outcomes. As mentioned above, in the acute management of an episode of upper gastrointestinal bleeding, early endoscopy in selected low-risk patients enables their early discharge and reduces hospitalization.

Prevention

Prevention is certainly preferable to treatment. Effective strategies in both primary and secondary prevention are well established. Physicians should clearly identify patients at risk for gastrointestinal complications (e.g., old age and previous ulcer bleeding) before prescribing NSAIDs. Good practices include avoidance of concomitant aspirin, anticoagulants or corticosteroids, the use of lowest possible doses, and use of a single or safer NSAID, such as diclofenac. In patients with risk factors, the use of misoprostol, proton pump inhibitors, selective COX-2 inhibitors or a combination of these is effective. The choice will depend on the assessment of gastrointestinal risk as well as the cardiovascular risk in individual patients. In patients tested positive for *H. pylori* infection, eradication therapy should be prescribed. *H. pylori* eradication is especially important in secondary prophylaxis.

Gaps in epidemiology knowledge

Although endoscopy and proton pump inhibitors (PPI) currently have central roles in treating gastrointestinal bleeding, questions remain concerning what is the best form of therapy. Would clipping be superior to thermal coagulation? How about oral PPI compared with intravenous PPI? What is the best protection for high-risk patients who require antiplatelet agents such as clopidogrel [32]? What about the risk of double antiplatelet agents? What about the risk of COX-2 specific inhibitors in combination with antiplatelet agents? Many questions remain to be answered, for which carefully designed clinical trials are much needed.

Summary

Upper gastrointestinal bleeding continues to be a challenge to clinicians. In an aging population, bleeding is often an agonal event in many patients with severe comorbid illnesses. Advances in medical care of such patients are unlikely to impact on mortality. The best strategy may lie with prevention of ulcer bleeding among elderly patients. Further studies are required to determine if upper gastrointestinal bleeding is becoming less or more prevalent. Widespread *H. pylori* eradication may see a decline in the cohort of infected patients. But as the population ages, the proportion of old people presenting with upper gastrointestinal bleeding, along with NSAID-associated ulcers, will probably grow. Preventive strategies, such as the use of co-therapy or safer NSAIDs, need to be better studied in terms of their clinical efficacies and cost-effectiveness.

References

1. Dulai GS *et al.* Utilization of healthcare resources for low-risk patients with acute, non-variceal upper GI hemorrhage (UGIH). *Gastrointest Endosc* 2002;**55**:321.
2. Silverstein FE *et al.* The national ASGE survey on upper gastrointestinal bleeding. II. Clinical prognostic factors. *Gastrointest Endosc* 1981;**27**:80.
3. Longstreth GF. Epidemiology of hospitalization for acute upper gastrointestinal hemorrhage: a population-based study. *Am J Gastroenterol* 1995;**90**:206.
4. Rockall TA *et al.* Incidence of and mortality from acute upper gastrointestinal haemorrhage in the United Kingdom. *Br Med J* 1995;**311**:222.
5. Blatchford O *et al.* Acute upper gastrointestinal haemorrhage in west of Scotland: Case ascertainment study. Br Med J 1997;**315**:510.
6. Vreeburg EM *et al.* Acute upper gastrointestinal bleeding in the Amsterdam area: Incidence, diagnosis and clinical outcome. *Am J Gastroenterol* 1997;**92**:236.
7. Barkun A *et al.* The Canadian Registry on Nonvariceal Upper Gastrointestinal Bleeding and Endoscopy (RUGBE): Endoscopic hemostasis and proton pump inhibition are associated with improved outcomes in a real-life setting. *Am J Gastroenterol* 2004;**99**:1238.
8. Higham J *et al.* Recent trends in admissions and mortality due to peptic ulcer in England: Increasing frequency of haemorrhage among older subjects. *Gut* 2002;**50**;460.
9. Gisbert JP, Pajares JM. *Helicobacter pylori* and bleeding peptic ulcer: what is the prevalence of the infection in patients with this complication? *Scand J Gastroenterol* 2003;**38**:2.
10. Gisbert JP *et al. H. pylori* eradication therapy vs. antisecretory non-eradication therapy (with or without long-term maintenance antisecretory therapy) for the prevention of recurrent bleeding from peptic ulcer. *Cochrane Database Syst Rev* 2003;**4**:CD004062.
11. Singh G, Triadafilopoulos G. Epidemiology of NSAID induced gastrointestinal complications. *J Rheumatol* 1999;**26**(Suppl. 26):18.
12. Lanas A *et al.* Nitrovasodilators, low-dose aspirin, other nonsteroidal antiinflammatory drugs, and the risk of upper gastrointestinal bleeding. *N Engl J Med* 2000;**343**:834.
13. Wolfe MM *et al.* Medical progress: gastrointestinal toxicity of nonsteroidal antiinflammatory drugs. *N Engl J Med* 1999;**340**:1888.
14. Hernandez-Diaz S, García Rodríguez LA. Epidemiologic assessment of the safety of conventional nonsteroidal antiinflamatory drugs. *Am J Med* 2001;**110**:20S.
15. Huang JQ *et al.* Role of *Helicobacter pylori* infection and non-steroidal anti-inflammatory drugs in peptic-ulcer disease: A meta-analysis. *Lancet* 2002;**359**:14.
16. Chan FK *et al.* Preventing recurrent upper gastrointestinal bleeding in patients with *Helicobacter pylori* infection who are taking low-dose aspirin or naproxen. *N Engl J Med* 2001;**344**:967.
17. Chan FK *et al.* Eradication of *Helicobacter pylori* and risk of peptic ulcers in patients starting long-term treatment with non-steroidal anti-inflammatory drugs: A randomized trial. *Lancet* 2002;**359**:9.
18. Ciociola AA *et al. Helicobacter pylori* infection rates in duodenal ulcer patients in the United States may be lower than previously estimated. *Am J Gastroenterol* 1999;**94**:1834.
19. Laine L *et al.* Has the impact of *Helicobacter pylori* therapy on ulcer recurrence in the United States been overstated? *Am J Gastroenterol* 1998;**93**:1409.
20. Chan HL *et al.* Long-term outcome of *Helicobacter pylori*-negative idiopathic bleeding ulcers: a prospective cohort study. *Gastrointest Endosc* 2001;**53**:438.
21. Hung LC *et al.* Long-term outcome of *Helicobacter pylori*-negative idiopathic bleeding ulcers: a prospective cohort study. *Gastroenterology* 2005;**128**:1845.
22. de Abajo FJ *et al.* Association between selective serotonin reuptake inhibitors and upper gastrointestinal bleeding: population based case-control study. *Br Med J* 1999;**319**:1106.
23. Dalton SO *et al.* Use of selective serotonin reuptake inhibitors and risk of upper gastrointestinal tract bleeding: a population-based cohort study. *Arch Intern Med* 2003;**163**:59.
24. Rockall TA *et al.* Risk assessment after acute upper gastrointestinal haemorrhage. *Gut* 1996;**38**:316.
25. Blatchford O *et al.* A risk score to predict need for treatment for upper gastrointestinal haemorrhage. *Lancet* 2000;**356**:1318.
26. Barkun A *et al.* Consensus recommendations for managing patients with non-variceal upper gastrointestinal bleeding. *Ann Intern Med* 2003;**139**:843.
27. Cook DJ *et al.* Endoscopic therapy for acute nonvariceal upper gastrointestinal hemorrhage: a meta-analysis. *Gastroenterology* 1992;**102**:139.
28. Laine L, Peterson WL. Bleeding peptic ulcer. *N Engl J Med* 1994;**331**:717.
29. Spiegel BM *et al.* Endoscopy for acute nonvariceal upper gas-

trointestinal tract hemorrhage: is sooner better? *Arch Intern Med* 2001;**161**:1393.

30. Leontiadis GI *et al.* Proton pump inhibitor treatment for acute peptic ulcer bleeding. *Cochrane Database Syst Rev* 2006;**1**:CD002094.

31. Barkun AN *et al.* High-dose intravenous proton pump in-hibition following endoscopic therapy in the acute management of patients with bleeding peptic ulcers in the USA and Canada: a cost-effectiveness analysis. *Aliment Pharmacol Ther* 2004;**19**:591.

32. Sung JJY. Combining aspirin with antithrombotic agents. *Br Med J* 2006;**333**:712.

21 Celiac Disease

Alberto Rubio-Tapia and Joseph A. Murray

Key points
- Celiac disease is a global health problem.
- At present, "atypical" or screen-detected cases of celiac disease are the most frequent clinical presentations of the disease.
- Health-related quality of life can be worsened by delayed detection and improved by treatment of celiac disease.
- Greater knowledge of celiac disease epidemiology may aid in the early diagnosis of celiac disease and lead to decreased morbidity and mortality.

Clinical summary

Celiac disease (CD), also known as gluten-sensitive enteropathy, is defined as a permanent intolerance to ingested gluten (the storage protein components of wheat, barley and rye) that damages the small intestine by inducing crypt hyperplasia and villous atrophy; and that resolves with removal of gluten from the diet [1]. CD results from the interaction between the environment (gluten intake) and genetic susceptibility (HLA haplotypes DQ2 or DQ8) that leads to an aberrant immune response in the gut. The inflammation and perpetuation of the autoimmune process is induced in part by tissue transglutaminase-mediated gliadin deamidation (resulting in enhanced antigen presentation) and interactions between cytokines and inflammatory cells (principally T cell lymphocytes).

Clinical features vary by type of presentation (classical vs atypical), severity (mild vs severe) and patient age at diagnosis (children vs adult). The constellation of symptoms and signs includes steatorrhea, weight loss or failure to thrive, as well as less-specific gastrointestinal complaints – such as bloating, abdominal pain, diarrhea, constipation, flatulence, secondary lactose intolerance and dyspepsia – and non-gastrointestinal complaints – such as fatigue, depression, arthralgias, osteomalacia or osteoporosis, and iron-deficiency anemia. Furthermore, CD can be "silent" without any symptoms. Thus, a high index of suspicion is necessary to establish the diagnosis in a wide variety of conditions and settings [2].

The detection of celiac disease most often begins with serologic testing. Confirmation of the disease requires histological examination of intestinal biopsies and ultimately a positive objective response to a gluten-free diet. In selected cases, HLA typing may provide adjunctive information, especially in patients who do not respond to a gluten-free diet or in patients where histologic or serologic determination has been rendered insensitive by prior treatment with a gluten-free diet.

The absence of the susceptibility-associated genotype has a high negative predictive value. Empiric treatment with a gluten-free diet is not recommended and renders most of the other tests inaccurate [3]. In most cases, a presumptive diagnosis can be made when serology and histology are both consistent with the ultimate proof occurring with the measurable objective response to a gluten-free diet.

Disease definition

CD is defined according to the clinical presentation and has been likened to an iceberg (Fig. 21.1). The tip of the iceberg represents the most obvious part of the clinical spectrum (classic malabsorption). If the patient's symptoms are characteristic of the malabsorption syndrome (diarrhea, steatorrhea, weight loss, fatigue) then the adjective "classical" is used. There is also "atypical" or "nonclassical" CD, these adjectives being applied when patients have nonspecific symptoms such as abdominal discomfort, bloating, indigestion or non-gastrointestinal symptoms.

157

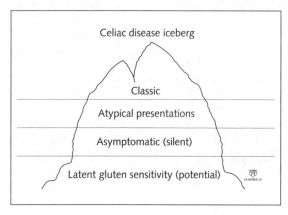

Fig. 21.1 Concept of the celiac disease "iceberg."

Finally, the submerged portion of the iceberg consists of "silent" patients who are clinically asymptomatic (but have histological evidence of CD if biopsied); thus most cases remain undiagnosed. Furthermore, there is an additional group – "latent" disease refers to genetically susceptible persons, without symptoms or histologic evidence of CD, who will ultimately go on to develop celiac disease [4]. These individuals are typically identified by repeat testing those with persistently positive autoantibodies, patients with dermatitis herpetiformis who initially have a normal small intestine biopsy, or asymptomatic family members of individuals with CD.

Prevalence and incidence

CD is common in Western countries including North America. Population-based data from the USA demonstrate an estimated prevalence of just over 1% based on confirmed diagnosis [5]. However, this figure may underestimate the true prevalence of CD due to lack of testing in all those with atypical, silent or latent CD. Furthermore, other reported prevalence studies (mainly based on serologic testing) indicate that CD could be a common disease around the world, suggesting that CD might be a global health problem (Table 21.1).

The incidence of CD varies internationally. In most countries, there has been a significant increase in the overall incidence and, hence, prevalence of celiac disease. However, this change has not been uniform across the age spectra. In the UK and Republic of Ireland, although childhood celiac disease reached epidemic proportions in the late 1960s and early 1970s, a substantial decrease in childhood celiac disease was observed in the latter half of the 1970s. This decrease was ascribed to a public health campaign to delay the introduction of solids and to encourage breastfeeding in newborns. Sweden also had a dramatic increase in celiac disease incidence in childhood through the 1980s (200–240 cases per 100 000 person years) and into the 1990s followed by an equally abrupt decline in incidence of symptomatic celiac disease (50–60 cases per 100 000 person years) after 1995 [16]. This decrease was attributed to a change in public policy whereby the quantity of gluten in infant foodstuffs was reduced and a national recommendation was made to encourage breastfeeding during the period when gluten-containing foods are introduced into the diet [17]. In contrast, the overall annual incidence of CD in North America has shown a gradual increase. A study from Olmsted County showed that the incidence was 0.9 per 100 000 in 1950–1989, 3.3 per 100 000 in the 1990s, and 9.1 per 100 000 in

Table 21.1 Prevalence of CD in different countries based on selected serologic studies

Country [ref.]	Type of study	Antibodies tested	Intestinal biopsy	Positive/tested	Prevalence/1000
Tunisia [6]	BD	EMA, tTG	Yes	2/1418	1.4
USA [7]	BD	AGA, EMA	No	8/2000	4
England [8]	PB	EMA, tTG	No	87/7527	10
Brazil [9]	BD	AGA, EMA	Yes	3/2045	1.4
Italy [10]	PB	EMA	Yes	17/3483	5
Israel [11]	BD	AGA, tTG, EMA	Yes	10/1571	6.3
Argentina [12]	PB	AGA, EMA	Yes	12/2000	6
Finland [13]	PB	tTG, EMA	Yes	27/3654	7.3
The Netherlands [14]	BD	EMA	Yes	3/1000	3
Mexico [15]	BD	tTG	No	27/1009	27

BD, blood donors; PB, population-based study; EMA, anti-endomysium antibodies; AGA, antigliadin antibodies; tTG, anti-tissue transglutaminase antibodies.

2000 and 2001. Serology prompted biopsy in a substantial proportion of recently diagnosed subjects suggesting that the increase in this population was due in part to an increased detection rate arising from increased physician awareness of the disorder and thus higher rates of screening for CD, although a true increase in incidence may have also occurred [18]. This phenomenon could be present in other countries; for example, a national prospective study in The Netherlands showed a significant continual increase in reported incidence of CD (0.1–0.4/1000 live births from 1975 to 1990, to 0.81/1000 live births for 1993 to 2000) [19]. This increase in prevalence could be explained by an increase in wheat consumption globally, but especially in North America over the last 20 years, with a 70% increase in per capita wheat consumption. Thus it remains to be determined whether the higher incidence of CD is due to a true increase or simply reflects increased testing for CD. If other studies suggest this rise is a real phenomenon, more research is needed to explain fully the possible factor(s) that have contributed to the increase in CD incidence.

Risk factors for disease

Gender

Cases predominate in females (by about 2:1) [20]. Interestingly, a high male preponderance (3:1) was found among the new cases of CD in members of nuclear families with two affected children [21]. Additionally, in a US cohort of biopsy-proven adult patients with CD, men show indirect evidence of greater malabsorption than females and have female-predominant associated autoimmune diseases [22].

Geography

As was described above, CD is recognized in every continent. The extent of celiac disease mirrors the coincidence of consumption of wheat and a high frequency of the genetic susceptibility genotype DQ2. Ironically, wheat cultivation started in the fertile crescent (a historical region in the Middle East related to the origins of agriculture) wherein Caucasians also originated, and the areas of the world that have the highest prevalence of the celiac disease susceptibility genotype have relied on wheat and similar grains as major staples to enable population growth and civilization. The world's "celiac icebergs" are shown in Fig. 21.2.

Socioeconomic factors

There appears to be little association between CD and specific socioeconomic factors. However, the presentation of CD may be associated with more severe nutritional consequences in developing countries, as exemplified by lower height-for-age and hemoglobin levels among CD-affected Saharawi children [23].

Familial aggregation/genetics

CD occurs commonly in families. The inheritance pat-

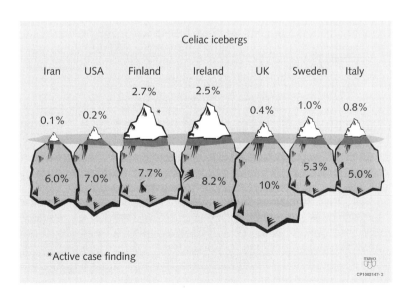

Fig. 21.2 "Celiac icebergs:" the tips represent the prevalence of diagnosed CD; the submerged portions represent undiagnosed CD.

tern is complex and determined by the effects of several genes and the environment. CD is strongly associated with the HLA class II genes *DQA1*05, DQB1*02* that encode the molecule DQ2, and less frequently *DQAI*0301, DQB1*0302* that encode DQ8. Such is the strength of the association that these HLA haplotypes are virtually essential for the disease to occur and they are a valuable tool for diagnosis in selected cases [24]. Furthermore, homozygosity for the *DQB1*0201* allele has been associated with a more severe form of CD characterized by total villous atrophy on small bowel biopsy, younger age of disease onset, more severe diarrhea and a lower level of blood hemoglobin at the time of diagnosis. This allele has also been associated with a slower recovery of villous atrophy after commencing a gluten-free diet (GFD) [25].

However, despite the fact that the majority of family members will carry the at-risk HLA haplotype, far fewer of these will actually develop the disease. This indicates that genes other than HLA, or environmental factors have a major effect on causation of the disease in family members.

Other diseases

Several other diseases are associated with a high prevalence of CD (Table 21.2).

CD is strongly associated with type 1 diabetes mellitus, thyroid disease, Addison's disease, osteopenic bone disease and Down syndrome; but also with less common conditions such as autoimmune myocarditis [26]. The prevalence of CD among osteoporotic individuals (3.4%) is higher than that among non-osteoporotic individuals (0.2%) [27]. Furthermore, female patients >50 years with CD demonstrated a higher risk of fracture, and also for more multiple fractures [28]. Thus, osteopenia and osteoporosis are serious consequences of CD.

Natural history and mortality

The natural history of CD recognizes that, at certain points in time, the disease is not associated with clinical manifestations. There may be a long latent phase followed by a "silent" phase. At some point, intestinal and/or extraintestinal symptoms develop and the diagnosis is made by demonstrating the villous atrophy and strongly positive anti-tissue transglutaminase (tTG) and anti-endomysial IgA autoantibodies [29]. Celiac disease is a chronic disease and one that will persist unless treated. Many patients may remain undiagnosed and the ultimate outcome in these individuals remains unknown.

The Denver studies have followed a birth cohort of individuals who had HLA typing performed at birth. Using tTG antibodies, this cohort was followed on a yearly basis up to the age of 7 years. One percent of these children, most of whom had the at-risk HLA haplotype, developed CD [30], but most of these had minimal or no symptoms. This suggests that CD probably starts in the first decade, although the majority of patients are not diagnosed until later (Fig. 21.3).

Patients with untreated or partially treated symptomatic CD are at high risk of complications and mortality associated with the disease. Enteropathy-associated T-cell lymphoma (EATL) is a rare form of high-grade, T-cell non-Hodgkin lymphoma of the upper small intestine that is specifically associated with CD [31,32]. EATL is the most common malignant cause of death in poorly treated CD patients, with an estimated odds ratio (OR) of 28 [33].

Associated conditions	Consequences
Isolated hypertransaminasemia	Infertility
Autoimmune thyroiditis	Hyposplenism
Microscopic colitides	Arthralgia or arthropathy
Autoimmune hepatitis	Ataxia
IgA deficiency	Dental enamel hypoplasia
Psoriasis	Epilepsy
Primary biliary cirrhosis	Folate or iron deficiency anemia
Dermatitis herpetiformis	Recurrent pancreatitis
Down syndrome	Oral aphthous ulcers
Type 1 diabetes mellitus	Lymphoma
Turner syndrome	Osteoporosis

Table 21.2 Associated conditions and consequences of celiac disease (partial list)

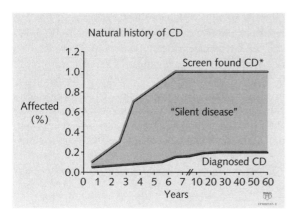

Fig. 21.3 Natural history of CD.

A significant excess of mortality is evident during the first 3 years after diagnosis and in patients with malabsorption syndromes, but not in those diagnosed because of minor symptoms or through antibody screening [34].

A population-based cohort study in the UK demonstrates that the increased risk of malignancy (other than lymphoproliferative disease) is primarily in the first year after diagnosis. Interestingly, people with CD also have a reduced risk of breast cancer [35]. Adenocarcinoma of the small intestine, nasopharyngeal, melanoma and esophageal cancer are also more common in patients with CD than the general population [36].

Infections as a consequence of immunodeficiency associated with malnutrition could be a major cause of death. Also, in the setting of severe malnutrition and/or functional intestinal failure, complications from total parenteral nutrition or central venous catheter-related sepsis could be major issues. Fatal pneumococcal septicemia has been reported in celiacs with hyposplenism, and prophylactic vaccination may be appropriate in this clinical scenario [37].

Disability and quality of life

As a chronic condition, symptomatic CD impairs health-related quality of life. Before treatment onset, 66% of patients report that their perceived quality of life is either moderate bad to poor [38]. Several studies have shown that quality of life improves after treatment with a gluten-free diet (GFD). Longstanding clinical experience reports that a GFD will generally result in a dramatic improvement in what are often severe GI symptoms, including symptoms

other than the typical ones of diarrhea, steatorrhea and weight loss [39]. It would be expected that such improvement in symptoms could result in improved quality of life. However, because (i) the disease is chronic and (ii) the treatment is lifelong, the rather restrictive GFD may have negative effects on quality of life. Careful studies, incorporating patients who have minimal or no GI symptoms at the onset of treatment, need to be performed to identify the degree of ultimate benefit for overall quality of life of the early detection and treatment of nonsymptomatic celiac disease.

Adherence to a GFD for at least 1 year causes 82% of classic CD patients to consider that they reached a "well" or "very well" feeling of well-being as assessed by a modified version of the Zung Self-Related Depression Scale [40]. A Finnish study demonstrated that after 1 year of following a GFD, quality of life for patients with screen-detected CD significantly improved as measured by a generic quality of life questionnaire (Psychological General Well-Being Questionnaire) [41]. In a Spanish population, it was found that CD impaired the perceived health of affected individuals, and that their health improved when on a GFD reaching levels comparable with the general population, as assessed by administering two generic health-related quality of life questionnaires: EuroQol-5D and Gastrointestinal Quality of Life [42]. Another study found that, using the SF-36, adherence to a GFD causes patients to perceive a health-related quality of life comparable to that of the general population [43].

It must be noted that no CD-specific quality-of-life measure exists to date, and that this remains an open area for development and research.

Prevention

Protective factors, such as breastfeeding and delayed introduction of large amounts of gluten into the infant diet, seem to reduce the likelihood of developing CD at an early age. In Sweden, the prevalence of symptomatic CD (clinically detected) declined after a national change in infant feeding recommendations was proposed in 1996: a slow introduction to gluten during weaning was stressed, and the recommendation was to maintain breast-feeding during the period when smaller quantities of gluten are introduced into the diet, beginning at the age of 4 months instead of the introduction of larger amounts of gluten at the age of 6 months. However, no difference was found in undiagnosed CD between the screened children born before and after 1996. Thus, a slow introduction of gluten in infancy could protect some children against developing symptomatic CD, but it might not protect them from subclinical or silent forms of this disease in childhood [44]. Serologic testing in high-risk populations, such as type 1 diabetics, could be a good approach for early detection of the disease. However, the utility of that approach to prevent complications or cancer-related mortality remains to be proved. Finally, the issue of mass population screening and the benefit or harm of treatment in asymptomatic patients remains unclear. Massive population screening would need to be carefully evaluated in terms of risk and its cost-benefit analysis before its introduction.

Issues and gaps in epidemiology

There are several notable issues and unresolved questions in the epidemiology of celiac disease. These include:
• What are the benefits and drawbacks of screening high-risk populations for CD?
• What is the clinical significance of CD detected by mass screening?
• What is the prevalence of undiagnosed CD?
• What are the most appropriate CD-specific quality-of-life measures?
• What is the true cost of healthcare utilization for the diagnosis and treatment of CD and its complications?

Recommendations for future studies

Much remains unknown about the natural history of undiagnosed and, hence, untreated celiac disease. Studies that could address this topic, possibly examining historical cohorts from patients with silent celiac disease that were not treated or patients in whom the diagnosis could be established retrospectively in stored sera, may give some helpful insights into the natural history of untreated celiac disease. Inherent in this evaluation of outcome of untreated disease is the possibility that in some circumstances, such as societies where excess calories are a major cause of morbidity, it may be reasonable to consider the potential positive effects of subtle malabsorption on cardiovascular risk.

Conclusions

Over the last decade, the epidemiology of CD has changed because of the emergence of a new generation of serologi-

cal tools, permitting a better understanding of the true incidence and prevalence of CD around the world. It has also become apparent that CD can have many faces on presentation, so clinicians must be familiar with all of them in order to obtain an early diagnosis of the disease before complications appear or become irreversible. As a global health problem, CD warrants additional study to allow better detection of disease, as well as better prevention of the development of disease and its complications.

The Mayo Foundation retains copyright on all original artwork.

References

1. Farrell RJ *et al.* Celiac sprue – current concepts. *N Engl J Med* 2002;**346**:180.
2. Green PHR *et al.* Celiac disease. *Annu Rev Med* 2006;**57**:207..
3. Abdulkarim AS *et al.* Review article: the diagnosis of celiac disease. *Aliment Pharmacol Ther* 2003;**17**:987.
4. American Gastroenterology Association. Medical position statement: celiac sprue. *Gastroenterology* 2001;**120**:1526.
5. Fasano A *et al.* Prevalence of celiac disease in at-risk and not-at-risk groups in the United States: a large multicenter study. *Arch Intern Med* 2003;**163**:269.
6. Bdioui F *et al.* Prevalence of celiac disease in Tunisian blood donors. *Gastroenterol Clin Biol* 2006;**30**:33.
7. Not T *et al.* Celiac disease risk in the USA: high prevalence of antiendomysium antibodies in healthy blood donors. *Scand J Gastroenterol* 1998;**33**:494.
8. West J *et al.* Seroprevalence, correlates, and characteristics of undetected celiac disease in England. *Gut* 2003;**52**:960.
9. Gandolfi L *et al.* Prevalence of celiac disease among blood donors in Brazil. *Am J Gastroenterol* 2000;**95**:689.
10. Volta U *et al.* High prevalence of celiac disease in Italian general population. *Dig Dis Sci* 2001;**46**:1500.
11. Shaaminr R *et al.* The use of a single serological marker underestimates the prevalence of celiac disease in Israel: a study of blood donors. *Am J Gastroenterol* 2002;**97**:2589.
12. Gomez JC *et al.* Prevalence of celiac disease in Argentina: screening of an adult population in the La Plata area. *Am J Gastroenterol* 2001;**96**:2700.
13. Mäki M *et al.* Prevalence of celiac disease among children in Finland. *N Engl J Med* 2003;**348**:2517.
14. Rostami K *et al.* High prevalence of celiac disease in apparently healthy blood donors suggests a high prevalence of undiagnosed celiac disease in the Dutch population. *Scand J Gastroenterol* 1999;**34**:276.
15. Remes-Troche JM *et al.* Celiac disease could be a frequent disease in Mexico: prevalence of tissue transglutaminase antibody in healthy blood donors. *J Clin Gastroenterol* 2006;**40**:697.

16. Cavell B *et al.* Increasing incidence of childhood celiac disease in Sweden. Results of a national study. *Acta Paediatr* 1992;**81**: 589.

17. Ivarsson A *et al.* Epidemic of coeliac disease in Swedish children. *Acta Pediatr* 2000;**89**:165.

18. Murray JA *et al.* Trends in the identification and clinical features of celiac disease in a North America community, 1950–2001. *Clin Gastroenterol Hepatol* 2003;**1**:19.

19. Steens RF *et al.* A national prospective study on childhood celiac disease in the Netherlands 1993–2000: an increasing recognition and a changing clinical picture. *J Pediatr* 2005;**147**:239.

20. Ciacci C *et al.* Gender and clinical presentation in adult celiac disease. *Scand J Gastroenterol* 1995;**30**:1077.

21. Gufjondfottir AH *et al.* The risk of celiac disease in 107 families with at least two affected siblings. *JPGN* 2004;**38**:338.

22. Bai D *et al.* Effect of gender on the manifestations of celiac disease: evidence for greater malabsorption in men. *Scand J Gastroenterol* 2005;**40**:183.

23. Ratsch IM *et al.* Celiac disease: a potentially treatable health problem of Saharawi refugee children. *Bull World Health Organ* 2001;**79**:541.

24. Van Heel DA *et al.* Genetics in celiac disease. *Best Pract Res Clin Gastroenterol* 2005;**19**:323.

25. Karinen H *et al.* Gene dose effect of the DQB1*0201 allele contributes to severity of celiac disease. *Scand J Gastroenterol* 2006;**41**:191.

26. Frustaci A *et al.* Celiac disease associated with autoimmune myocarditis. *Circulation* 2002;**105**:2611.

27. Stenson WF. Increased prevalence of celiac disease and need for routine screening among patients with osteoporosis. *Arch Intern Med* 2005;**165**:393.

28. Davie MW *et al.* Excess non-spine fractures in women over 50 years with celiac disease: a cross-sectional, questionnaire-based study. *Osteoporos Int* 2005;**16**:1150.

29. Rewers M. Epidemiology of celiac disease: What are the prevalence, incidence and progression of celiac disease? *Gastroenterology* 2005;**128**:S47.

30. Hoffenberg EJ *et al.* A prospective study of the incidence of childhood celiac disease. *J Pediatr* 2003;**143**:308.

31. Viljamaa M. Malignancies and mortality in patients with celiac disease and dermatitis herpetiformis: 30-year population-based study. *Digest Liver Dis* 2006;**38**:374.

32. Catassi C *et al.* Association of celiac disease and intestinal lymphomas and other cancers. *Gastroenterology* 2005;**128**: S79.

33. Mearin ML *et al.* European multi-centre study on celiac disease and non-Hodgkin lymphoma. *Eur J Gastroenterol Hepatol* 2006;**18**:187.

34. Corrao G *et al.* Mortality in patients with celiac disease and their relatives: a cohort study. *Lancet* 2001;**358**:356.

35. West J *et al.* Malignancy and mortality in people with celiac disease: population based cohort study. *Br Med J* 2004;**329**:716.

36. Green PHR *et al.* Risk of malignancy in patients with celiac disease. *Am J Med* 2003;**115**:191.

37. Johnston SD *et al.* Fatal pneumococcal septicemia in a celiac patient. *Eur J Gastroenterol Hepatol* 1998;**10**:353.

38. Green PHR *et al.* Characteristics of adult celiac disease in the USA: results of a national survey. *Am J Gastroenterol* 2001;**96**:126.

39. Murray JA *et al.* Effect of a gluten-free diet on gastrointestinal symptoms in celiac disease. *Am J Clin Nutr* 2004;**79**:669.

40. Ciacci C *et al.* Self-related quality of life in celiac disease. *Dig Dis Sci* 2003;**48**:2216.

41. Mustalahti K *et al.* Gluten-free diet and quality of life in patients with screen-detected celiac disease. *Eff Clin Pract* 2002;**5**:105.

42. Casellas F *et al.* Perceived health status in celiac disease. *Rev Esp Enferm Dig* 2005;**97**:794.

43. O'Leary C *et al.* Celiac disease and the transition from childhood to adulthood: a 28-year follow-up. *Am J Gastroenterol* 2004;**99**:2437.

44. Carlsson A *et al.* Prevalence of celiac disease: Before and after a national change in feeding recommendations. *Scand J Gastroenterol* 2006;**41**:553.

22 Measuring Utilization of Colonoscopy in Clinical Practice

David Lieberman

Key points

- The utilization of endoscopy in the USA is uncertain. The Clinical Outcome Research Initiative (CORI) was created to capture endoscopic data from diverse clinical practices.
- Colonoscopy is the most commonly used endoscopic procedure in the USA. Understanding the utilization of colonoscopy can help improve appropriate use and outcomes.

- Endoscopic databases can be used to track practice trends and monitor quality.
- CORI provides a model for capturing key clinical data within the flow of clinical practice, with the goal of improving patient outcomes.

Introduction

Endoscopy plays a major role in the diagnosis and management of gastrointestinal (GI) diseases. Although many clinical research studies have demonstrated the benefit of endoscopic diagnosis and therapy, few studies have examined the "effectiveness" of endoscopy as it is actually used in general clinical practice. Previously, administrative databases have been studied to describe variation in practice patterns [1–3]. These databases often lack key information about patients and medical decision-making, such as patient symptoms, comorbidities and details of exam findings [4].

Practice-based networks and clinical registries provide models for collecting more detailed clinical data. The work of the Northern New England Cardiovascular Disease Study Group, a regional network of cardiovascular surgeons, cardiologists and other health professionals, illustrates the potential for practice-based networks to explore practice variation and improve quality of care [5]. Other successful practice networks in internal medicine include the ARAMIS project in rheumatology [6].

Tools that can collect data in the flow of clinical practice offer an opportunity for effectiveness research [7]. Attempts to use computerized databases to collect endoscopic data date back to the early 1980s with the American Society for Gastrointestinal Endoscopy (ASGE) database and development of an endoscopic report generator in the late 1980s by Cotton *et al.* [8]. However, efforts to collect community-based data in gastroenterology have been regional [8–10] – a potentially significant limitation in a large country such as the USA.

The Clinical Outcomes Research Initiative (CORI) evolved from a strategic planning session of the ASGE, which identified the evaluation of the effectiveness of endoscopy in broad clinical practice settings as a high priority. The CORI database was developed as a uniform, computerized endoscopic report generator to capture endoscopic data from many practicing sites. To date, CORI is the largest endoscopic research database in the USA, receiving more than 220 000 endoscopic reports each year from 73 clinical practice sites since 2000. This chapter will describe utilization of colonoscopy in the CORI consortium in the USA, focusing on patient demographics, procedure indications and key endoscopic findings. Data specifically regarding other endoscopic procedures such as esophagogastroduodenoscopy, endoscopic retrograde cholangiopancreatography and endoscopic ultrasound will not be reviewed in this chapter. These are the first descriptive data of colonoscopy practice in the USA in diverse settings and populations, illustrating that the CORI database provides a model that can be utilized in epidemiologic research in GI and other specialties.

Methods

Principles of CORI

CORI was developed to study utilization and outcomes of endoscopic procedures in diverse practice settings.

Box 22.1. Research goals of CORI

- Describe patients undergoing endoscopy in diverse practice settings: patient demographics and procedure indications.
- Describe endoscopic use patterns, and observe changes in practice patterns over time.
- Evaluate the frequency of specific endoscopic findings and their relationship with reasons for performing the procedure, with the goal of improving risk stratification of patients.
- Observe the natural history of chronic GI diseases for which endoscopic surveillance is used.
- Determine the success and effectiveness of endoscopic therapies.
- Determine the impact of endoscopic diagnoses and therapies on patient outcomes, including disease-specific quality of life, functional status and healthcare utilization.
- Determine the impact of medical therapies following endoscopic diagnoses.
- Evaluate the frequency of endoscopic complications, and risk factors for complications.
- Prospectively monitor the utilization and findings of new endoscopic innovations.
- Measure quality improvement.
- Create patient registries for clinical trials.
- Develop parallel systems to study outcomes in pediatric endoscopy.

Research goals included analyses of patterns of practice, trends over time, prospective follow-up of patients receiving endoscopy, and analyses of rare events such as procedure complications (Box 22.1). Analysis of de-identified data can provide "snapshots" of endoscopic practice and outcomes. Prospective studies with patient follow-up require informed consent.

CORI: participants and methods

Participating sites were selected based on geographic and practice-type diversity. The CORI consortium includes 73 practice sites in 24 states with more than 400 physicians (Fig. 22.1). Participating physicians use a structured, computerized endoscopic report generator to produce their endoscopic reports. The report generator includes key descriptive elements of the endoscopy report, based on guidelines from the ASGE [11]. When possible, terms from the international Minimum Standard Terminology (MST) are used [12]. Mandatory fields are included to ensure collection of key information including procedure indication, endoscopic findings, patient demographics and adverse events.

The data file from the report is transmitted electronically to a central data repository, after removal of patient and physician identifiers. This "de-identified" data is reviewed for missing fields, duplicative reports and data points outside normal ranges. Practice sites are contacted if reports are incomplete. The data are transmitted to a Data Warehouse where data from multiple sites are merged. Specific data are extracted for analyses. These analyses are limited to adult practices, and exclude patients less than 20 years old. This discussion will focus on utilization of colonoscopy and will focus on 146 457 unique patients who had colonoscopy from 2000 to 2002. Reports were received from private practice settings (68%), academic universities (20%) and Veterans Affairs (VA) medical centers (12%).

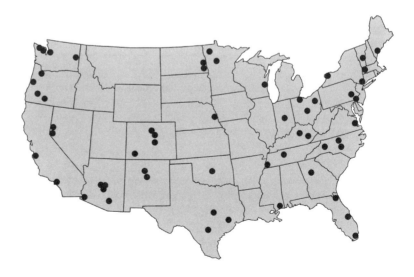

Fig. 22.1 Map of CORI sites in the USA.

Colonoscopy

Who receives colonoscopy?

Among adults receiving colonoscopy for any reason, 55% are women (excluding VA sites). Twenty percent are less than 50 years old and 6.5% are over 80 years [13]. That women are more likely to receive colonoscopy than men is an interesting observation. Because women have lower age-adjusted rates of colorectal cancer (CRC) compared with men [14], one might expect higher rates of colonoscopy utilization in men. Our observation may reflect a generally higher level of health awareness in women, and possibly increased physician interactions as a result of routine cervical and breast cancer screening.

Eighty-four percent of the cohort comprised White (non-Hispanic) people, a proportion that differs from the US population as a whole (69.1% in the 2000 census). This racial difference from the general population may be due to systematic bias in the CORI sampling – participating sites may have higher numbers of Whites compared with non-participating sites. Nonetheless, the racial data may be a true reflection of the patients who receive colonoscopy in the USA. In the same participating practices, we find that the proportion of White (non-Hispanic) people receiving upper endoscopy for dyspepsia is 76.7% [15]. This is a subject for further study because of implications in colon cancer screening in minorities. Research is needed to determine if patients from minority groups are even offered colonoscopy or are declining to have colonoscopy when offered.

Why do they receive colonoscopy?

Among patients less than 50 years old (Table 22.1), we find

that irritable bowel syndrome (IBS: defined by indications such as abdominal pain, bloating, change in bowel habits, nonbloody diarrhea and constipation, excluding all other indications) and rectal bleeding account for more than 50% of procedures. The severity of hematochezia is unknown, but it is likely that in many cases it may represent relatively trivial outlet bleeding. The role of colonoscopy for hematochezia in patients aged under 50 years is controversial [16]. The benefit of colonoscopy for evaluation of IBS symptoms in young patients is unknown. Although the rate of serious pathology is low (see below), there may be unmeasured benefits such as reduction in anxiety and healthcare utilization that cannot be assessed with this database alone.

Among patients aged 50–74 years, the most common indications for colonoscopy are asymptomatic screening (average-risk, family history, positive FOBT) in 40% of colonoscopies, surveillance of adenomatous polyps in 17%, evaluation of rectal bleeding in 20% and evaluation of IBS symptoms in 17%. In patients older than 74 years, screening (28%), adenoma surveillance (24%), rectal bleeding 16%, anemia (13%) and IBS symptom evaluation (17%) are the most common indications. Women over 50 years are far more likely than men to have colonoscopy to evaluate IBS symptoms (23% vs 12%; $P < 0.001$). Summarizing the age data, the database demonstrates that, perhaps unsurprisingly, individuals under 50 years of age undergo colonoscopy for active symptoms, those aged 50–74 years are predominantly asymptomatic prior to testing, and many aged over 74 are still undergoing diagnostic testing while asymptomatic, but with a greater proportion undergoing adenoma surveillance as well as testing for anemia.

Table 22.1 Most common indications for colonoscopy by age and gender (adapted from Lieberman *et al.* [13])

Age	<50 years		50–74 years		>74 years	
Gender	Women	Men	Women	Men	Women	Men
Number of patients	16 257	13 510	45 142	48 989	11 296	11 263
Family history of CRC (%)	20	18	16	12	8	5
Screening colonoscopy (%) (average-risk)	–	–	12	13	8	7
Positive FOBT (%)	8	10	10	13	13	14
Surveillance of adenoma (%)	–	–	14	21	21	28
Surveillance of cancer (%)	–	–	–	–	7	8
Hematochezia (%)	31	37	19	21	16	16
IBS cluster (%)	29	18	23	12	22	13

> 5% of indications for the group.
CRC, colorectal cancer; FOBT, fecal occult blood test; IBS, irritable bowel syndrome.

The CORI database can also be used to analyze the proportion of indications by race and ethnicity. Non-White patients were more likely to have colonoscopy to evaluate symptoms such as anemia, hematochezia and weight loss than Whites (36.4% vs 27.1%; $P < 0.001$). This statistic may suggest that non-White patients do not receive colonoscopy until they may be more likely to have serious advanced pathology. Further study is needed to corroborate these trends and to determine the reasons for this observation (e.g., lack of awareness suggesting need for greater health education, insufficient access to healthcare).

Rate of key findings

Based on the indications cited, most colonoscopies are performed to detect and/or remove neoplastic lesions. Some, but not all CORI sites add pathology data after the procedure. In the absence of definitive pathology, a surrogate endpoint of importance, polyp(s) >9 mm, was evaluated [17]. This endpoint was chosen because (i) most polyps >9 mm will be adenomas and (ii) adenomas of this size are considered "advanced" and hence clinically important. Multivariate analysis of prevalence rates of polyp(s) >9 mm demonstrated that risk increased with age, male gender and Black race. In patients undergoing asymptomatic screening, the number needed to endoscope (NNE) to detect one patient with a polyp >9 mm declined from 42 (age <50 years) to 14 (age >79 years) in

women, and from 28 (age <50 years) to 10 (age >79 years) in men (Table 22.2). Men had lower age-adjusted NNE than women across all indications. In addition, procedure indications associated with a higher risk than screening (lower NNE) included hematochezia, iron deficiency anemia and weight loss. Patients with IBS symptoms actually had higher NNE compared with patients undergoing screening colonoscopy. These data can be used to aid clinical and perhaps healthcare policy decisions of diagnostic yield for malignant or premalignant lesions based on procedural indication.

Trends in practice

Since 1998, we have analyzed the proportion of procedures performed in each GI practice, comparing the relative proportions of EGD, colonoscopy and flexible sigmoidoscopy within the practice. From 1998 to 2004, the rate of colonoscopy increased from 41% of all endoscopic procedures to 62%. These data parallel trends in the USA, which show an increased utilization of colonoscopy. Among the indications, screening colonoscopy and adenoma surveillance have steadily increased as a proportion of colonoscopy procedures [18]. Rates of screening colonoscopy (as a proportion of all colonoscopies) increased from less than 4% in 1999 to 14.2% by 2002 [19]. The rate of colorectal cancer per 1000 colonoscopies declined from 110 to 72 from 2000 to 2003, which may reflect increased use of screening exams and sur-

Table 22.2 Number needed to endoscope (NNE) to identify one patient with polyp/mass >9 mm (adapted from Lieberman *et al.* [17])

Gender	Female				Male			
Age (years)	<50	50–59	60–69	70–79	<50	50–59	60–69	70–79
Screening								
Average risk	42	28	20	18	28	18	13	12
Positive family history CRC	34	22	16	14	22	15	11	10
Positive FOBT	24	15	9	8	16	10	7	6
Surveillance								
Prior adenoma	17	17	14	13	15	15	13	12
Prior cancer	35	23	17	15	23	15	11	10
Evaluation of symptoms								
Hematochezia	27	18	13	12	18	12	9	8
Anemia	27	18	13	12	18	12	9	8
IBS[a]	47	31	22	20	30	20	15	13

CRC, colorectal cancer; FOBT, fecal occult blood test.
[a]IBS = irritable bowel syndrome, defined as one or more of the following symptoms: diarrhea, constipation, abdominal pain/bloating and change in bowel habits and excluding all patients with weight loss, bleeding and anemia.

veillance, with lower rates of cancer detection than in symptomatic patients [20]. The result may also possibly reflect the effectiveness of prevention of progression to cancer with the use of therapeutic polypectomy. Overall, these trends indicate increased public and physician awareness of colorectal cancer screening over a short period of time.

Limitations of CORI

The collection of endoscopic data in the flow of clinical practice is an important function of CORI, but there are several important limitations. Although the consortium was designed to mirror endoscopic practice in the USA, we cannot exclude the possibility of "site selection" bias. Practice sites that participate in CORI are comfortable using computers for endoscopic reporting and sharing data from their practice. Such practices may differ in important ways from those that will not share data or do not use electronic records to monitor quality in their practice. Some of the practices participating in CORI use the computerized report generator for procedures performed in an ambulatory surgical center, but not in the hospital, due to hospital policies regarding information technologies. Therefore, these data may not reflect the full spectrum of inpatient hospital procedures performed by the participants. Because most colonoscopy procedures are performed in the outpatient setting, the current data should provide a valid reflection of outpatient colonoscopy.

Some data may be incomplete or inaccurate. Race and ethnicity data are not self-reported, but are provided by the physician or nurse, and therefore may not be as accurate as self-report. Indications for colonoscopy are provided by the physician by checking an item on a computer screen. Physicians may be parsimonious, and enter some, but not all, reported symptoms or problems. The endoscopy report also lacks clinical perspective; for example, we do not know what diagnostic tests or treatments were performed prior to colonoscopy. We used mass or polyp >9 mm as a surrogate endpoint for serious pathology, and assumed that more than 90% of such lesions would be adenomatous. Although this analysis has focused on one key endpoint, we recognize that other findings at colonoscopy may be clinically important. Despite these important limitations, the CORI repository is a valuable hypothesis-generating tool. Observational snapshots of clinical practice identify important research questions, which will require more precise data collection in prospective studies.

Summary and future directions

CORI provides a model for collecting detailed epidemiologic data within the flow of clinical practice while protecting patient privacy [21,22]. This chapter provides some examples of how such a database can be used to improve understanding of the utilization of endoscopic procedures. The proliferation of endoscopic databases throughout the world offers opportunities for new epidemiologic research in endoscopy. In Europe, a consortium of members from the European Union have developed the Networked European Endoscopy Database (NEED), which is modeled after CORI. In Asia, investigators of the Asia Pacific Working Group on Colorectal Cancer have utilized CORI as a prototype for a colonoscopy reporting system in 10 Asian countries (Joseph Sung, personal communication).

Until recently, there was little information about who received endoscopy and why. CORI provides an important tool for understanding the utilization of endoscopic procedures in clinical practice. Future studies will measure key patient outcomes in specific disease states or clinical syndromes.

References

1. Chassin MR *et al.* Variations in the use of medical and surgical services by the Medicare population. *N Engl J Med* 1986;**314**:285.
2. Wennberg JE *et al.* An assessment of prostatectomy for benign urinary tract obstruction: geographic variations and the evaluation of medical care outcomes. *JAMA* 1988;**259**:3027.
3. Kahn KL *et al.* The use and misuse of upper gastrointestinal endoscopy. *Ann Intern Med* 1988;**109**:664.
4. Palmer RH. Process-based measures of quality: the need for detailed clinical data in large health care databases. *Ann Intern Med* 1997;**127**:733.
5. Malenka DJ, O'Connor GT. The Northern New England Cardiovascular Disease Study Group: a regional collaborative effort for continuous quality improvement in cardiovascular disease. *Jt Comm J Qual Improv* 1998;**10**:594.
6. Fries JF, McShane DJ. ARAMIS (the American Rheumatism Association Medical Information System). A prototypical national chronic-disease data bank. *Western J Med* 1986;**145**:798.
7. Nelson EC *et al.* Building measurement and data collection into medical practice. *Ann Intern Med* 1998;**128**:460.
8. Brazer SR *et al.* Studies of gastric ulcer disease by community-based gastroenterologists. *Am J Gastroenterol* 1990;**85**:824.
9. Lieberman DA *et al.* Risk factors for Barrett's esophagus in community-based practice. GORGE consortium. *Gastro-*

enterology Outcomes Research Group in Endoscopy. *Am J Gastoenterol* 1997;**92**:1293.

10. Ellis KK *et al.* Management of symptoms of gastroesophageal reflux disease: does endoscopy influence medical management? *Am J Gastroenterol* 1997;**92**:1472.

11. Computer Committee. *Standard Format and Content of the Endoscopic Procedure Report.* American Society for Gastrointestinal Endoscopy, 1992.

12. Delvaux M (ed.) *Digestive Endoscopy: Minimal Standard Terminology,* V 1.0. European Society of Gastrointestinal Endoscopy, 1995.

13. Lieberman DA *et al.* Utilization of colonoscopy in the United States: results from a national consortium. *Gastrointest Endosc* 2005;**62**: 875.

14. Jemal A *et al.* Cancer statistics 2005. *CA Cancer J Clin* 2005;**55**:10.

15. Lieberman DA *et al.* Endoscopic evaluation of patients with dyspepsia: Results from the national endoscopic data repository. *Gastroenterology* 2004;**127**:1067.

16. Lieberman D. Rectal bleeding and dimunitive colon polyps. *Gastroenterology* 2004;**126**:1167.

17. Lieberman DA *et al.* Prevalence of polyps greater than 9 mm in a consortium of diverse clinical practice settings in the United States. *Clin Gastroenterol Hepatol* 2005;**3**:798.

18. Cram P *et al.* The impact of a celebrity promotional campaign on the use of colon cancer screening: the Katie Couric effect. *Arch Intern Med* 2003;**163**:1601.

19. Harewood GC, Lieberman DA. Colonoscopy practice patterns since introduction of Medicare coverage for average-risk screening. *Clin Gastroenterol Hepatol* 2004;**2**:72.

20. Auslander JN *et al.* Endoscopic procedures and diagnoses are not influenced by seasonal variations. *Gastrointest Endosc* 2006;**63**:267.

21. Nelson EC *et al.* Building measurement and data collection into medical practice. *Ann Intern Med* 1998;**128**:460.

22. Gostin L. Health care information and the protection of personal privacy: ethical and legal considerations. *Ann Intern Med* 1997;**127**:683.

23 Colorectal Carcinoma

Steven B. Ingle and Paul Limburg

Key points
- Colorectal cancer affects about 1 in every 18 persons in the USA.
- Environmental factors likely influence colorectal cancer risk, but the key exposures remain incompletely defined.
- Nearly all colorectal cancers are preceded by premalignant, adenomatous polyps.
- Regular screening evaluations can reduce the number of incident colorectal cancer cases by approximately 76–90%.

Clinical summary

The symptoms of colorectal cancer (CRC) are nonspecific and can vary by anatomic subsite. Cecal, ascending colon and transverse colon cancers are often associated with abdominal pain, weight loss or occult bleeding, while descending colon, sigmoid colon and rectal cancers can cause narrowed stools, obstipation or hematochezia. Diagnostic colonoscopy is the test of choice for patients who present with symptoms or signs that are suggestive of CRC, because visual inspection and mucosal sampling can be performed during the same procedure.

Preoperative staging of newly diagnosed CRC cases typically includes an abdominopelvic CT (computed tomography) scan and a chest X-ray to look for distant metastases. For rectal cancer cases, endoscopic ultrasound is also routinely obtained to assess tumor depth and regional lymph node status. Final determination of CRC stage incorporates pathology review of surgically resected tissue specimens. The TNM system (Box 23.1) is used to formulate treatment recommendations (Table 23.1). Five-year survival rates decline progressively across TNM stages: stage I = 93%, stage II = 72–83%, stage III = 44–83% and stage IV = 8%. However, the recent development of molecularly targeted chemotherapy agents appears to extend both disease-free and overall survival rates for patients with stage IV CRC [1,2].

Disease definition

CRC represents a histologically diverse group of ma-

lignant tumors, including adenocarcinoma, carcinoid, lymphoma, leiomyosarcoma, melanoma and squamous cell carcinoma. However, adenocarcinomas comprise the large majority (~95%) of invasive colorectal lesions.

Incidence and prevalence

Global statistics indicate that 1 023 256 incident CRC cases are recognized each year [3], which is nearly 10% of the world total for all cancers [4]. In the USA, CRC is the third

---

Box 23.1 TNM staging classification for colorectal cancer

Primary tumor (T)

T0	No evidence of primary tumor
T1	Tumor invades submucosa
T2	Tumor invades muscularis propria
T3	Tumor invades through the muscularis propria
T4	Tumor invades surrounding organs or structures

Regional lymph nodes (N)

N0	No regional lymph node metastases
N1	Metastases in 1–3 regional lymph nodes
N2	Metastases in ≥ 4 regional lymph nodes

Distant metastasis (M)

M0	No distant metastasis
M1	Distant metastasis

(Used with the permission of the American Joint Committee on Cancer (AJCC), Chicago, Illinois. The original source for this material is the *AJCC Cancer Staging Manual*, Sixth Edition (2002) published by Springer – New York, www.springeronline.com.)

Table 23.1 Standard treatment recommendations for colorectal cancer, by presenting stage

Presenting stage	TNM grouping(s)	Treatment recommendations	
		Colon cancer	Rectal cancer
Stage I	T1 N0 M0 T2 N0 M0	Surgical resection	Surgical resection
Stage II	T3 N0 M0 T4 N0 M0	Surgical resection; consider adjuvant chemotherapy if pathologic features suggest high recurrence risk	Neoadjuvant chemo/radiation therapy + surgical resection + adjuvant chemo/radiation therapy
Stage III	Any T N1 M0 Any T N2 M0	Surgical resection + adjuvant chemotherapy	Neoadjuvant chemo/radiation therapy + surgical resection + adjuvant chemo/radiation therapy
Stage IV	Any T Any N M1	Chemotherapy and/or symptomatic care; consider potentially curative treatment for isolated liver or lung metastases	Chemotherapy and/or symptomatic care; consider potentially curative treatment for isolated liver or lung metastases

most common cancer type among both women and men, with age-adjusted annual incidence rates of 47.9 and 65.9 per 100000 persons, respectively [5]. Approximately 1 in 18 US residents will develop CRC over the course of a lifetime. Encouragingly, data from 1998–2002 suggest that overall CRC incidence rates are gradually declining [5]. However, not all race/ethnicity subgroups exhibit the same favorable trend, with African Americans having higher CRC incidence rates than Caucasians [6]. Two large average-risk screening studies conducted within the US Veterans' Affairs health system reported CRC prevalence rates of 1% among men and 0.1% among women [7,8]. A retrospective, population-based study from Israel found a 1.1% CRC prevalence rate among average-risk colonoscopy patients [9].

Risk factors for disease

Age and gender

Like many cancers, CRC risk increases with advancing age (Table 23.2). The median age at diagnosis is 71 years. Fewer than 9% of all CRC cases occur among persons younger than age 50 years [10]. Premalignant colorectal adenomas are also more common among older patients [7,8]. As noted above, CRC incidence rates are higher for men than women. Tumor distribution patterns also differ by gender, with male:female incident CRC rate ratios increasing progressively across the proximal colon (1.17), descending colon (1.35) and distal colorectum (1.39) [11].

Geography

CRC incidence rates vary considerably across global regions, with a 5-fold or greater difference in high- (~50 per 100000 population) versus low-incidence (~10 per 100000 population) areas [4]. International migrant studies have shown that CRC incidence rates can change within a single generation, emphasizing the role of environmental factors in CRC causation. Significant geographic variation also exists within the USA, for reasons that remain incompletely defined [12].

Family history

Familial clustering is observed in 15–25% of CRC patients, with heritable cancer syndromes accounting for approximately 6% of all cases. Familial adenomatous polyposis (FAP), an autosomal dominant condition caused by germline mutation in the *APC* gene, is characterized by hundreds of colorectal adenomas distributed throughout the colorectum. The lifetime CRC risk for FAP patients approaches 100% unless total proctocolectomy is performed. Hereditary non-polyposis colorectal cancer (HNPCC), another autosomal dominant condition caused by germline mutation in one of at least five DNA mismatch repair protein genes, is typified by relatively few, proximally located colorectal adenomas. HNPCC-associated CRCs exhibit microsatellite instability, which is a laboratory finding that results from abnormal insertion or deletion of short nucleotide repeat sequences. Without

Age	Cumulative risk				Table 23.2 Cumulative risk of developing colorectal cancer across 10-year age categories, by gender
	Men (%)	1 in…	Women (%)	1 in…	
10 years	0.0001	10 000 000	0.0001	10 000 000	
20 years	0.0018	55 556	0.0020	50 000	
30 years	0.0153	6 536	0.0144	6 944	
40 years	0.0745	1 342	0.0681	1 468	
50 years	0.2857	350	0.2615	382	
60 years	0.9597	104	0.7747	129	
70 years	2.3686	42	1.8247	55	
80 years	4.2552	24	3.4459	29	
90 years	5.5015	18	4.9387	20	

Data obtained using DevCan 6.1.1 software, available from the National Cancer Institute website (http://srab.cancer.gov/devcan).

prophylactic surgery, the lifetime CRC risk for HNPCC patients is approximately 60–80%. In the absence of a defined heritable syndrome, patients with one or more first-degree relatives with CRC have a 2–4-fold increase in CRC risk compared with the general population, whereas family history confined to second-degree relatives appears to confer a more modest increase in CRC risk [13].

Diet and lifestyle

Dietary modifications and lifestyle alterations could theoretically prevent at least 70% of all CRC cases [14]. However, at present, the most relevant, potentially modifiable exposures remain unknown. Dietary fats induce the excretion of primary bile acids, which are converted to procarcinogenic secondary bile acids by colonic bacteria. Certain fatty acid subtypes, such as *trans*-fatty acids, may directly affect colonocyte growth. Red meat, particularly when consumed with a heavily browned surface, may be an independent risk factor for both benign and malignant colorectal neoplasia. Excess carbohydrate consumption induces hyperinsulinemia, which appears to stimulate colorectal carcinogenesis. Tobacco smoke contains several putative carcinogens, and data from several large prospective studies suggest that cigarette smoking increases CRC risk after a prolonged latency period of 20 or more years. Conversely, fruit and vegetable intake has consistently been shown to reduce CRC risk (while affording benefits with respect to other chronic health conditions as well).

Prior colorectal neoplasia

Patients who have a personal history of colorectal adenoma(s) are at 3–6-fold increased risk for metachronous neoplasia [15]. Patients who have undergone CRC resection are also prone to develop recurrent CRC, second primary CRC and metachronous adenomas. Overall, about 2–4% of colon cancer patients develop recurrent disease at the site of their surgical anastomosis; for rectal cancer patients, the local recurrence rate may be 10 or more times higher [16], due to differences in surgical technique and/or tumor biology.

Inflammatory bowel disease (IBD)

Chronic ulcerative colitis, one of the two major subtypes of IBD, is associated with a substantially increased risk for CRC, which continues to rise over time: cumulative CRC incidence rates range from 2% after 10 years of ulcerative colitis, 8% after 20 years, and 18% after 30 years of disease [17]. Extensive colitis, early age at onset and primary sclerosing cholangitis have been proposed as additional risk factors for IBD-associated CRC. Fewer studies have examined CRC risk among Crohn's disease patients, but recent recommendations suggest that involvement of at least one-third of the colonic mucosa should be considered a CRC risk factor [18]. Current data do not support increased CRC risk in the setting of either lymphocytic colitis or collagenous colitis.

Other conditions

In a recent meta-analysis of 15 observational studies, type 2 diabetes mellitus was found to be associated with a 30% increase in CRC risk [19], perhaps due to chronic hyperinsulinemia. Patients with acromegaly may also be at increased CRC risk because of excess circulating growth hormone and/or insulin-like growth factor concentrations. However, the relative rarity of this condition has hindered the precision of CRC risk estimates reported from most prior observational studies.

Natural history and mortality

Premalignant adenomas are thought to precede nearly all CRCs. When dysplastic cells invade across the basement membrane, the requisite criterion for transformation from a benign adenoma to a malignant adenocarcinoma is achieved. Advanced adenomas are typically defined as size ≥1 cm, any component of villous morphology, or high-grade dysplasia [15], and are thought to be the near-term precursor to most CRCs, although flat adenomas (height less than half the diameter) may contribute to a small minority of cases. Aberrant crypt foci appear to represent an earlier stage in colorectal carcinogenesis [20], but further study is needed to understand the true biology of these microscopic lesions. Small, distally located hyperplastic polyps do not appear to have malignant potential, whereas the risk of CRC associated with large, diffusely distributed hyperplastic polyps remains controversial.

Quality of life

Because the majority of CRC patients survive for 5 years or longer after completing therapy, quality of life (QOL) is an important outcome measure. The spectrum of CRC treatment options, including multiple surgical, chemotherapy and radiation therapy approaches (alone and in combination), further highlights the need to evaluate post-treatment QOL, in addition to prolongation of life. However, most randomized controlled trials have focused primarily on the latter outcome measure [21]. Both first-line and palliative chemotherapies can improve or stabilize QOL, especially in symptomatic patients who respond favorably to treatment. Yet, CRC survivors are prone to depression and anxiety. Rectal cancer patients who require colostomy may experience greater changes in QOL compared with

other rectal cancer survivors, although existing data remain inconsistent [22].

Costs and expenditures

CRC imposes a substantial economic burden, with an estimated annual cost of $5.3 billion in the USA alone [23]. Hospital facility fees and office visits contribute most heavily to the direct costs. CRC screening could have a considerable impact on current expenditures, with an estimated cost-effectiveness of $11900 per year of life gained [24].

Prevention

Early detection

Regular screening programs have been shown to reduce CRC incidence and CRC mortality. For average-risk patients, multiple screening options have been endorsed by national organizations (Table 23.3) [15]. In general, onset of CRC screening is recommended at age 50 years for asymptomatic adults who have no identifiable risk factors. Selection of a particular screening option should be based on an informed discussion between patient and provider, with consideration given to the effectiveness, risks and costs associated with various tests. Positive CRC screening exams should be followed up with diagnostic colonoscopy. For high-risk patients, colonoscopy is the preferred test for both the initial screening and subsequent surveillance examinations.

Chemoprevention

Chemoprevention refers to the use of chemical compounds to prevent, inhibit or reverse carcinogenesis at a preinvasive stage. In its broadest sense, chemoprevention includes both nutritional and pharmaceutical interventions. Leading candidate agents include selective and nonselective cyclooxygenase-2 inhibitors, estrogen compounds, calcium, folate and selenium [25].

Future studies

Opportunities exist to favorably affect the natural history of colorectal carcinogenesis at multiple levels. Additional well-designed cohort studies are needed to clarify the role

Table 23.3 Colorectal cancer screening guidelines for average-risk patients	Screening option	Screening interval[a]
	Fecal occult blood test (FOBT)	Annually
	Flexible sigmoidoscopy (FS)	Every 5 years
	FOBT and flexible sigmoidoscopy	FOBT annually with FS every 5 years
	Double-contrast barium enema (DCBE)	Every 5 years
	Colonoscopy	Every 10 years

[a]Assuming no findings on current screening test(s).

of specific environmental factors associated with CRC risk. Further laboratory investigation of the molecular signatures expressed by benign and malignant neoplasia might also afford greater predictive and prognostic capabilities, respectively. Lastly, clinical trials of novel anticancer agents should lead to more effective, less toxic intervention strategies.

Conclusions

CRC is a common disease with a well-defined natural history. Colorectal carcinogenesis is influenced by personal, familial and environmental risk factors. Non-modifiable risk factors can be used to define early detection algorithms, whereas modifiable risk factors represent potential targets for dietary, lifestyle or behavioral interventions. At present, early detection remains the cornerstone of CRC prevention. Recently introduced chemotherapy drugs contribute to prolonged survival for CRC patients, and emerging chemoprevention agents show promise for interrupting the disease process at a preinvasive stage.

References

1. Cunningham D *et al.* Cetuximab monotherapy and cetuximab plus irinotecan in irinotecan-refractory metastatic colorectal cancer. *N Engl J Med* 2004;**351**:337.
2. Hurwitz H *et al.* Bevacizumab plus irinotecan, fluorouracil, and leucovorin for metastatic colorectal cancer. *N Engl J Med* 2004;**350**:2335.
3. Kamangar F *et al.* Patterns of cancer incidence, mortality, and prevalence across five continents: defining priorities to reduce cancer disparities in different geographic regions of the world. *J Clin Oncol* 2006;**24**:2137.
4. Parkin DM. International variation. *Oncogene* 2004;**23**:6329.
5. Jemal A *et al.* Cancer statistics, 2006. *CA Cancer J Clin* 2006;**56**:106.
6. Irby K *et al.* Emerging and widening colorectal carcinoma disparities between Blacks and Whites in the United States (1975–2002). *Cancer Epidemiol Biomarkers Prev* 2006;**15**:792.
7. Lieberman DA *et al.* Use of colonoscopy to screen asymptomatic adults for colorectal cancer. Veterans Affairs Cooperative Study Group 380. *N Engl J Med* 2000;**343**:162.
8. Schoenfeld P *et al.* Colonoscopic screening of average-risk women for colorectal neoplasia. *N Engl J Med* 2005;**352**:2061.
9. Strul H *et al.* The prevalence rate and anatomic location of colorectal adenoma and cancer detected by colonoscopy in average-risk individuals aged 40–80 years. *Am J Gastroenterol* 2006;**101**:255.
10. Fairley TL *et al.* Colorectal cancer in U.S. adults younger than 50 years of age, 1998–2001. *Cancer* 2006;**107**(5 Suppl): 1153.
11. Cheng X *et al.* Subsite-specific incidence rate and stage of disease in colorectal cancer by race, gender, and age group in the United States, 1992–1997. *Cancer* 2001;**92**:2547.
12. Lai SM *et al.* Geographic variation in the incidence of colorectal cancer in the United States, 1998–2001. *Cancer* 2006;**107**(5 Suppl): 1172.
13. Butterworth AS *et al.* Relative and absolute risk of colorectal cancer for individuals with a family history: a meta-analysis. *Eur J Cancer* 2006;**42**:216.
14. Giovannucci E. Modifiable risk factors for colon cancer. *Gastroenterol Clin North Am* 2002;**31**:925.
15. Winawer SJ *et al.* Guidelines for colonoscopy surveillance after polypectomy: a consensus update by the US Multi-Society Task Force on Colorectal Cancer and the American Cancer Society. *Gastroenterology* 2006;**130**:1872.
16. Rex DK *et al.* Guidelines for colonoscopy surveillance after cancer resection: a consensus update by the American Cancer Society and the US Multi-Society Task Force on Colorectal Cancer. *Gastroenterology* 2006;**130**:1865.
17. Eaden J. Review article: colorectal carcinoma and inflammatory bowel disease. *Aliment Pharmacol Ther* 2004;**20** (Suppl. 4):24.
18. Itzkowitz SH, Present DH. Consensus conference: Colorectal cancer screening and surveillance in inflammatory bowel disease. *Inflamm Bowel Dis* 2005;**11**:314.
19. Larsson SC *et al.* Diabetes mellitus and risk of colorectal cancer: a meta-analysis. *J Natl Cancer Inst* 2005;**97**:1679.
20. Alrawi SJ *et al.* Aberrant crypt foci. *Anticancer Res* 2006;**26**:107.

21. de Kort SJ *et al*. Quality of life versus prolongation of life in patients treated with chemotherapy in advanced colorectal cancer: A review of randomized controlled clinical trials. *Eur J Cancer* 2006;**42**:835.

22. Pachler J, Wille-Jorgensen P. Quality of life after rectal resection for cancer, with or without permanent colostomy. *Cochrane Database Syst Rev* 2005:CD004323.

23. Sandler RS *et al*. The burden of selected digestive diseases in the United States. *Gastroenterology* 2002;**122**:1500.

24. Maciosek MV *et al*. Colorectal cancer screening: health impact and cost effectiveness. *Am J Prev Med* 2006;**31**:80.

25. Hawk ET *et al*. Colorectal cancer chemoprevention – an overview of the science. *Gastroenterology* 2004;**126**:1423.

24 Irritable Bowel Syndrome

Yuri A. Saito, Nicholas J. Talley and G. Richard Locke III

Key points
- Irritable bowel syndrome (IBS) is an extremely common disorder, affecting about 1 in every 5–10 persons.
- Environmental factors – such as diet, stress, abuse and infections – have clear links to IBS development or exacerbation, yet the pathophysiology of IBS remains poorly understood.
- IBS results in significant work absenteeism, decreased productivity, and impaired health-related quality of life, and results in high direct and indirect healthcare costs.

Clinical summary

Irritable bowel syndrome (IBS) is a chronic disorder characterized by recurrent abdominal pain or discomfort associated with altered bowel habits. Disturbed bowel habits may include symptoms of diarrhea, constipation or both. Typically, the abdominal pain or discomfort is associated with a change in stool consistency (harder or looser) or stool frequency (increased or decreased), and is often relieved by passage of stool. Other symptoms may include abdominal bloating or distension, straining, sensation of incomplete evacuation, or passage of mucus. Subtypes of IBS exist, based on the predominant symptom: constipation-predominant IBS (C-IBS), diarrhea-predominant IBS (D-IBS) and mixed IBS (M-IBS) [1].

The exact pathophysiology of IBS remains unknown, although various mechanisms including gastrointestinal dysmotility and visceral hypersensitivity have been well-studied in IBS. No diagnostic tests are presently available to diagnose IBS. Individuals presenting with typical symptoms of IBS may not require additional laboratory, radiologic or endoscopic evaluation, but those with severe symptoms may warrant additional testing to rule out other disease. Treatment is selected based on the predominant symptom. For example, antispasmodics or visceral neuromodulators may be used for those with significant pain; antidiarrheals may be used in those with diarrhea; and laxatives (fiber, osmotic, stimulant) or other prokinetic agents may be used in those with constipation.

Disease definition

IBS is typically defined by symptom-based diagnostic criteria known as the "Rome criteria." These consensus-derived criteria have been assembled by an international panel of experts in the field of functional gastrointestinal disorders. The most recent criteria are referred to as the "Rome III" criteria. By these criteria, IBS is defined as "recurrent abdominal pain or discomfort, at least 3 days per month in the last 3 months associated with two or more of the following: (i) improvement with defecation, (ii) onset associated with a change in frequency of stool and (iii) onset associated with a change in form (appearance) of stool." [2]

Two special points should be made about the disease definition in IBS. First, various diagnostic criteria for IBS have been employed over the last three decades including the Manning criteria [3], Rome 1989 [4], Rome 1990 [5], Rome I (1992) criteria [6] and Rome II (1999) criteria [7]. The Rome III criteria are the most recently published, so the majority of epidemiologic studies are based on the older criteria rather than the Rome III criteria. Second, although formal diagnostic criteria are increasingly recognized and utilized in clinical practice, there are several studies documenting less than optimal or even suboptimal knowledge of formal diagnostic criteria among gastroenterologists and general practitioners [8–10], as well as poor agreement between diagnostic criteria and physicians [11], suggesting that many providers make the diagnosis based on clinical impression alone. Which disease definition was utilized may dramatically impact conclusions [12], thus, any review of epidemiology literature related to IBS must be cognizant of the disease definition utilized.

Prevalence and incidence

In the USA, IBS is a common disorder. Community-based prevalence estimates in the USA have varied from 3% to 20%, and the study details and results are summarized in Table 24.1. The variation in prevalence may reflect true regional differences, but likely reflects differences in study methodology – particularly with respect to the definition of IBS selected for each study. Several studies suggest that there is a female preponderance for IBS [13,14], although at least two studies found a slight female predominance but with confidence intervals of prevalence estimates

overlapping between men and women [12,15], and at least one study observed that the gender predilection may vary with study definition of IBS used.

In the USA, the only data regarding incidence estimates have come from Olmsted County, Minnesota. Two serial surveys were sent to a random age- and gender-stratified sample of 1120 residents 12–20 months apart [16]. Among the residents who did not meet Manning or Rome criteria for IBS at baseline and responded to both surveys, 9% developed symptoms over the 795 person-years of follow-up. In a separate study involving medical record review of county residents without a diagnosis of IBS in the previous 10 years for a new clinical diagnosis of IBS over a 3-year period, the age- and sex-adjusted incidence rate was 2 per 1000 person-years, which significantly increased with age [17]. The age-adjusted incidence was higher in women than men – 2.4 vs 1.4 per 1000 (P =

Table 24.1 US population-based studies estimating the prevalence of IBS

Study	Sample[a]	Survey method	Study definition	Prevalence estimate (%)
US government national health surveys Sandler [13]	122 859 Adults NHIS 1987	Face-to-face interview with	Self-report "spastic colitis" during previous year	4–10
US government national health surveys Sandler [13]	18 447 12–74-year-olds NHANES II 1976–1980	Face-to-face interview	Self-report physician diagnosis of "spastic colon or mucous colitis" ever	3
Olmsted County, MN Talley et al. [15]	835 30–64-year-old County residents 1987	Mailed questionnaire	1. Pain and ≥2 Manning 2. Pain and ≥3 Manning 3. Pain and ≥4 Manning	17 13 9
Olmsted County, MN Talley et al. [68]	328 65–93-year-olds County residents	Mailed questionnaire	1. Pain and ≥3 Manning 2. Pain and ≥4 Manning	11 5
US householder Drossman et al. [14]	5430 households Marketing database 1990	Mailed questionnaire	Rome 1990	9
US government national health survey Hahn et al. [69]	42 392 Adults NHIS 1989	Face-to-face interview	1. Self-report "IBS," "spastic colon," "irritable colon within 12 months" 2. ≥2 or Manning 3. Rome 1990	~3.6% ~8% ~3%
Olmsted County, MN Saito et al. [12,70]	643 30–69-year-olds Country residents 1992	Mailed questionnaire	1. Pain and ≥2 Manning 2. Pain and ≥3 Manning 3. Pain and ≥4 Manning 4. Rome 1989 5. Rome 1990	20 16 9 12 9

[a]NHIS, National Health Interview Survey; NHANES, National Health and Nutrition Examination Survey.

0.0004). Another population-based study conducted in England and Wales, using first-diagnosis of IBS by a general practitioner, found an estimated incidence of 2.6 per 1000 person-years [18]. The different estimates between the three studies likely reflect the difference in symptom presence (with or without seeking medical attention in the first study) and seeking medical attention (in the second and third study).

Risk factors for disease

Age and gender

As summarized above, based on prevalence data, IBS appears to be more common in women than men, with up to a 2:1 ratio. The ratio may increase further when outpatient studies are examined; however, it is unclear if the increased ratio in outpatients may reflect greater healthcare seeking by women than men with comparable symptoms.

No real data exist regarding the age-of-onset of IBS. Without objective data, it remains unclear whether increasing age is associated with increased risk of developing IBS. However, clinical experience suggests this situation is not the case, and is supported by the stable prevalence of IBS across various adult age groups [13–15].

Geography

IBS is a common disorder around the world, with studies reporting prevalence rates of 6% to 22% in Western countries and 2% to 17% in Asian countries [19,20]. Although IBS has been studied in other continents, such as Africa and South America, population-based studies from these regions are lacking. A recent systematic review evaluating geographic and ethnic differences in IBS did not find real differences between countries in the East and countries in the West with respect to overall prevalence rate [20]. Rates of IBS subtypes varied considerably from study to study – some showed equal distribution, others showed one subtype predominating; however, definitions of IBS used varied considerably.

Race and ethnicity

Studies evaluating race within the same country suggest that IBS may affect Caucasians more than other ethnic groups. For example, studies of the 1987 National Health Interview Survey (NHIS), the 1976–1980 Second National Health and Nutrition Examination Survey (NHANES II), and the 1985 National Ambulatory Medical Care Survey (NAMCS) show that the rate of self-reported spastic colon or mucous colitis was consistently greater in Caucasians than in Black people or African-Americans [13]. Data from other ethnic groups were not reported. However, these figures were based on "being told" of these diagnoses, and thus may reflect reduced access to healthcare rather than true differences in prevalence between racial/ethnic groups. Another study comparing the prevalence of IBS among US African-Americans and Caucasians also found that Caucasians were over twofold more likely to report IBS, after adjusting for age, education and household income [21]. Of note, the study sample was a convenience sample (rather than population-based), raising the question of participation and selection bias affecting the final estimates; but, recognizing the paucity of data regarding race, the finding suggests that even after taking into account education level and socioeconomic status, Caucasians may be at higher risk than African-Americans for IBS. Another non-population-based study comparing Hispanic people with non-Hispanic people showed that IBS-type symptoms were less common in Hispanics compared with non-Hispanic White people, although no significant ethnic difference was found after controlling for covariates [22]. The authors also reported that Hispanic people were less likely to see a physician for their bowel symptoms [23]. In summary, studies suggest that IBS is more common among Caucasians than non-Caucasians, but further investigation is warranted.

Diet

Many patients report dietary triggers for their symptoms, various food substances have been reported to be associated with exacerbating IBS symptoms, and some dietary elimination studies show positive symptom benefit. And yet, the role of diet and specific dietary components in causing IBS is perplexing as there is considerable heterogeneity in response to foods [24]. The only population-based study comparing diet among cases and controls demonstrated little difference in the diet and nutrient intakes of those reporting IBS-like symptoms and those not reporting symptoms, suggesting that food sensitivity rather than dietary excess is associated with IBS [25]. To date, food allergy has not clearly been shown to be a cause of IBS [26]. In summary, there may be certain food substances that worsen or trigger symptoms, but in themselves they do not cause IBS.

Psychological factors

Psychological and psychiatric comorbidity has been frequently linked with IBS, and several treatments for IBS either treat the psychological disorders directly or act as nerve-modulating agents [27,28]. Some have suggested that the high level of comorbidity observed in IBS patients may be a reflection of factors that drive healthcare seeking. However, there are other data arguing that consulters with IBS are not different psychologically from non-consulters with IBS [29,30], and that neuroticism, psychological morbidity and abuse history are not predictors of healthcare seeking [31].

Abuse

Many clinic-based studies have reported a higher prevalence of abuse history in IBS patients compared with controls [32–34], although it should be noted that there are also several clinic-based studies that have not found an association between abuse and IBS [35,36]. One community-based study in Olmsted County affirmed the association between IBS and sexual, emotional or verbal abuse in childhood or adulthood [37]. However, a similar study in Penrith, Australia, conducted by the same investigator, although finding an association between childhood abuse and IBS, observed that the association disappeared after controlling for age, gender and psychological factors [38]. This study suggested that abuse may lead to increased neuroticism, and consequently, greater healthcare seeking. Other studies have shown that patients with past abuse demonstrate higher levels of current psychological distress [35], and that the abuse history, although not linked with IBS specifically, may result in an increased number of gastrointestinal and extragastrointestinal symptoms, irrespective of the presence of an underlying functional or organic disorder [36]. In summary, although abuse has been linked to IBS, abuse may not lie in the causal pathway to IBS, but this association remains an area of relative controversy.

Infection

Several patient-based or outbreak studies have shown that a subset of individuals with acute gastroenteritis go on to develop persistent IBS [39–44]. One population-based study utilized a database of clinical diagnoses in the UK and observed that the cohort with bacteriologically confirmed gastroenteritis was 12-fold more likely to develop IBS within the next year [45]. Another population-based study of patients presenting with bacterial gastroenteritis at a primary care practice in the UK observed that after excluding those with IBS at baseline [46], IBS was 10-fold more common in cases than controls [47]. Another study conducted in Walkerton, Canada, following a large outbreak of acute *Escherichia coli* O157:H7 and *Campylobacter jejuni* gastroenteritis, yielded a threefold risk for the development of postinfectious IBS after clinically suspected gastroenteritis [48]. Thus, postinfectious IBS appears to be a real clinical entity. However, it is unlikely that infection is the underlying etiology for all IBS cases, and may represent the major risk factor in only a small subset of patients. Furthermore, psychological characteristics appear to be independent risk factors for the development of postinfectious IBS [39,40], and the role and interaction of inflammatory mediators with IBS remain to be determined.

Family history

Various clinical studies confirm that IBS appears to aggregate in families [49–51]. However, only one population-based study has been performed to date [52]. This small study did find that reporting a first-degree relative with abdominal pain or bowel problems was associated with self-report of IBS, with an estimated odds ratio of 2.3 (95% confidence interval: 1.3–3.9). In contrast, reporting a spouse with pain or bowel problems was not associated with IBS. These studies do suggest that a positive family history of IBS remains a relevant risk factor for a diagnosis of IBS; however, whether this is due to genetics or shared environment (including learned illness behavior) remains to be determined.

Natural history

Reviews of studies evaluating the natural history of IBS demonstrate that it is indeed a chronic disorder in clinic-based patients [53]. With long-term follow-up, 20–50% of patients have unchanged symptoms, 2–18% of patients have worsening symptoms, and for the remainder, symptoms improve. For example, in a large 1-year prospective, observational study of 400 primary care and gastroenterology clinic patients in Spain, half of the patients and half of the physicians considered their symptoms to have improved, although objective review of diary data showed that the improvement was small and that the major predictor of improvement was severe baseline symptoms [54].

Population-based studies that include patients as well as non-consulters show considerable fluctuation of IBS and non-IBS symptoms. For example, a random sample survey in Sweden in 1988, 1989 and 1995 showed that among those with IBS at baseline, 55% continued to report IBS at both follow-up surveys [55]; 3% were symptom-free at year 1, and 13% were symptom-free at year 7, thus implying that among a small subset, there is perhaps complete resolution of symptoms. A change from IBS symptoms to dyspepsia symptoms at years 1 and 7, was reported by 15% and 8% respectively, suggesting that other GI symptoms may develop or predominate in the natural history of IBS. Another study in Olmsted County observed that only 38% of those with IBS at baseline no longer met criteria for IBS after 146 person-years of follow-up [16], whereas a 5-year follow-up study in Denmark showed that only 5% of those with IBS at baseline were symptom-free years later [28].

The diagnosis of IBS also appears to be durable, with only an estimated 2–5% of IBS patients being given an initial misdiagnosis that is subsequently changed [53].

Disability and quality of life

A number of studies have been conducted to quantitate the disability that results from IBS. A recent systematic review of the available literature found that the average number of days off work per year because of IBS was between 8.5 and 21.6 [56]. Patients also report being late for work or leaving work early, and having to make other work–life adjustments including working shorter hours, refraining from applying for promotions or a new job [57], and/or selecting work based on settings for reasons such as restroom access (including working from home or being self-employed). IBS also impacts the personal and social lives of affected individuals, resulting in avoidance or reduction of activities, inhibited personal relationships, interference with sex life and embarrassment at using public toilets [57–59].

Not surprisingly, health-related quality of life (HRQoL) is lower in patients with IBS compared with the general population. A number of studies have evaluated HRQoL in patients with IBS, some of which were evaluated and summarized in a recent well-conducted systematic review [60]. This review found:
1 HRQoL is lower in patients with moderate to severe IBS compared with healthy controls;
2 patients with IBS have impaired HRQoL comparable with diseases such as moderate to severe gastroesophageal

reflux disease (GERD), end-stage renal disease, peptic ulcer disease, inflammatory bowel disease and liver disease;
3 patients with a response to therapy have a correlative improvement in HRQoL;
4 the subtype of IBS does not affect the degree of impact of IBS on HRQoL;
5 the degree of impairment of HRQoL is directly related to severity of bowel symptoms.

Healthcare utilization and costs

In 2002, the American Gastroenterological Association (AGA) published findings of their study to determine the burden of selected gastrointestinal diseases [61]. Using publicly available and proprietary databases to assess inpatient hospital stays, physician office visits, emergency room visits and hospital outpatient visits, the study found that IBS was second only to GERD as the most prevalent chronic gastrointestinal disorder. In a separate study using the National Ambulatory Medical Care Survey (NAMCS) and comparing IBS with non-GI diseases, IBS-related outpatient physician visits occurred at the same rate as for asthma and 2.6 times the rate of visits for migraine headaches [62]. Thus, visits directly related to IBS care appear to be extremely common in the USA.

Besides visits directly related to IBS, patients with IBS utilize more healthcare resources overall. Studies of managed care administrative databases [63–65], administrative claims data from a national Fortune 100 manufacturer collecting information on medical, pharmaceutical and disability claims for employees, spouses and retirees [66], and Medicaid administrative databases [67] have demonstrated that overall healthcare utilization was greater in patients with IBS compared with controls without the syndrome.

Estimates for the direct and indirect costs attributed to IBS have been evaluated in many settings. The AGA figures estimated that the direct costs for inpatient and outpatient visits and prescription medications for IBS exceeded $1.6 billion in 1998, or $1.7 billion in year 2000 dollars. The costs arose from 3.65 million physician visits, 500 000 hospital inpatient stays, 150 000 hospital outpatient visits and 87 000 emergency room visits. Estimated indirect costs, based exclusively on lost work days due to consumption of healthcare, were estimated at $205 million, but using different methodology applying wage figures to age, work loss was estimated at $19.2 billion in 1998, or $20.2 billion in 2000 dollars.

Prevention

Because the cause of IBS remains unknown, measures to prevent the development of IBS are nonexistent.

Issues/gaps in epidemiology knowledge

Until the pathophysiology of IBS is better understood, there remain many lines of further study. Several gaps in our understanding of the epidemiology of IBS remain:
• The accuracy of symptom-based diagnostic criteria, such as the Rome criteria.
• The determination of whether IBS is one disorder, or an etiologically heterogeneous collection of multiple disorders.
• The identification of environmental and genetic risk factors that lead to the clustering of IBS in families, including the role of learned illness behavior in IBS.
• The determination of the long-term natural history of IBS, including better description of its onset (e.g., incidence, age-of-onset), its evolution from childhood through adulthood, and its long-term consequences (mortality, morbidity).

Conclusions

IBS is a common disorder that exists in individuals of all ages and various ethnic and cultural backgrounds. It is one of the most prevalent gastrointestinal disorders, and results in disability, decreased productivity and absenteeism in working-age individuals, and costs the healthcare system considerable dollars. Hence, a better understanding of the pathophysiology is needed. Several environmental risk factors – such as diet and stress – have been well studied, but clearly are not the sole determinants of disease development and exacerbation. Further epidemiologic studies are warranted to identify the environmental, psychosocial and genetic risk factors for IBS occurrence and prognosis so that better diagnostic tests and treatments may be developed.

References

1. Talley NJ, Spiller R. Irritable bowel syndrome: a little understood organic bowel disease. *Lancet* 2002;**360**:555.
2. Longstreth GF *et al*. Functional bowel disorders. *Gastroenterology* 2006;**130**:1480.
3. Manning AP *et al*. Towards positive diagnosis of the irritable bowel. *Br Med J* 1978;**ii**:653.
4. Thompson WG *et al*. Irritable bowel syndrome: guidelines for the diagnosis. *Gastroenterology International* 1989;**2**:92.
5. Drossman DA *et al*. Identification of sub-groups of functional gastrointestinal disorders. *Gastroenterology International* 1990;**3**:159.
6. Thompson WG *et al*. Functional bowel disease and functional abdominal pain. *Gastroenterology International* 1992;**5**:75.
7. Thompson WG *et al*. Functional bowel disorders and functional abdominal pain. *Gut* 1999;**45**(Suppl. 2):II43.
8. Lea R *et al*. Diagnostic criteria for irritable bowel syndrome: utility and applicability in clinical practice. *Digestion* 2004;**70**:210.
9. Charapata C, Mertz H. Physician knowledge of Rome symptom criteria for irritable bowel syndrome is poor among non-gastroenterologists. *Neurogastroenterol Motil* 2006;**18**:211.
10. Longstreth GF, Burchette RJ. Family practitioners' attitudes and knowledge about irritable bowel syndrome: effect of a trial of physician education. *Fam Pract* 2003;**20**:670.
11. Vandvik PO *et al*. Diagnosing irritable bowel syndrome: poor agreement between general practitioners and the Rome II criteria. *Scand J Gastroenterol* 2004;**39**:448.
12. Saito YA *et al*. A comparison of the Rome and Manning criteria for case identification in epidemiological investigations of irritable bowel syndrome. *Am J Gastroenterol* 2000;**95**:2816.
13. Sandler RS. Epidemiology of irritable bowel syndrome in the United States. *Gastroenterology* 1990;**99**:409.
14. Drossman DA *et al*. U.S. householder survey of functional gastrointestinal disorders. Prevalence, sociodemography, and health impact. *Dig Dis Sci* 1993;**38**:1569.
15. Talley NJ *et al*. Epidemiology of colonic symptoms and the irritable bowel syndrome. *Gastroenterology* 1991;**101**:927.
16. Talley NJ *et al*. Onset and disappearance of gastrointestinal symptoms and functional gastrointestinal disorders. *Am J Epidemiol* 1992;**136**:165.
17. Locke GR 3rd *et al*. Incidence of a clinical diagnosis of the irritable bowel syndrome in a United States population. *Aliment Pharmacol Ther* 2004;**19**:1025.
18. Garcia Rodriguez LA *et al*. Detection of colorectal tumor and inflammatory bowel disease during follow-up of patients with initial diagnosis of irritable bowel syndrome. *Scand J Gastroenterol* 2000;**35**:306.
19. Cremonini F, Talley NJ. Irritable bowel syndrome: epidemiology, natural history, health care seeking and emerging risk factors. *Gastroenterol Clin North Am* 2005;**34**:189.
20. Kang JY. Systematic review: the influence of geography and ethnicity in irritable bowel syndrome. *Aliment Pharmacol Ther* 2005;**21**:663.
21. Wigington WC *et al*. Epidemiology of irritable bowel syndrome among African Americans as compared with whites: a population-based study. *Clin Gastroenterol Hepatol* 2005;**3**:647.
22. Zuckerman MJ *et al*. Comparison of bowel patterns in His-

panics and non-Hispanic whites. *Dig Dis Sci* 1995;**40**:1763.

23. Zuckerman MJ *et al.* Health-care-seeking behaviors related to bowel complaints. Hispanics versus non-Hispanic whites. *Dig Dis Sci* 1996;**41**:77.

24. Lea R, Whorwell PJ. The role of food intolerance in irritable bowel syndrome. *Gastroenterol Clin North Am* 2005;**34**:247.

25. Saito YA *et al.* Diet and functional gastrointestinal disorders: a population based case-control study. *Am J Gastroenterol* 2003;**98**:S275.

26. Bischoff S, Crowe SE. Gastrointestinal food allergy: new insights into pathophysiology and clinical perspectives. *Gastroenterology* 2005;**128**:1089.

27. Palsson OS, Drossman DA. Psychiatric and psychological dysfunction in irritable bowel syndrome and the role of psychological treatments. *Gastroenterol Clin North Am* 2005;**34**:281.

28. Kay L *et al.* The epidemiology of irritable bowel syndrome in a random population: prevalence, incidence, natural history and risk factors. *J Intern Med* 1994;**236**:23.

29. Weinryb RM *et al.* Psychological factors in irritable bowel syndrome: a population-based study of patients, non-patients and controls. *Scand J Gastroenterol* 2003;**38**:503.

30. Kanazawa M *et al.* Patients and nonconsulters with irritable bowel syndrome reporting a parental history of bowel problems have more impaired psychological distress. *Dig Dis Sci* 2004;**49**:1046.

31. Talley NJ *et al.* Predictors of health care seeking for irritable bowel syndrome: a population based study. *Gut* 1997;**41**:394.

32. Walker EA *et al.* Histories of sexual victimization in patients with irritable bowel syndrome or inflammatory bowel disease. *Am J Psychiatry* 1993;**150**:1502.

33. Delvaux, M *et al.* Sexual abuse is more frequently reported by IBS patients than by patients with organic digestive diseases or controls. Results of a multicentre inquiry. French Club of Digestive Motility. *Eur J Gastroenterol Hepatol* 1997;**9**:345.

34. Talley NJ *et al.* Self-reported abuse and gastrointestinal disease in outpatients: association with irritable bowel-type symptoms. *Am J Gastroenterol* 1995;**90**:366.

35. Hobbis IC *et al.* A re-examination of the relationship between abuse experience and functional bowel disorders. *Scand J Gastroenterol* 2002;**37**:423.

36. Baccini F *et al.* Prevalence of sexual and physical abuse and its relationship with symptom manifestations in patients with chronic organic and functional gastrointestinal disorders. *Dig Liver Dis* 2003;**35**:256.

37. Talley NJ *et al.* Gastrointestinal tract symptoms and self-reported abuse: a population-based study. *Gastroenterology* 1994;**107**:1040.

38. Talley NJ *et al.* Is the association between irritable bowel syndrome and abuse explained by neuroticism? A population based study. *Gut* 1998;**42**:47.

39. Gwee KA *et al.* Psychometric scores and persistence of irritable bowel after infectious diarrhoea. *Lancet* 1996;**347**:150.

40. Gwee KA *et al.* The role of psychological and biological factors in postinfective gut dysfunction. *Gut* 1999;**44**:400.

41. Neal KR *et al.* Prevalence of gastrointestinal symptoms six months after bacterial gastroenteritis and risk factors for development of the irritable bowel syndrome: postal survey of patients. *Br Med J* 1997;**314**:779.

42. Urfer E *et al.* Outbreak of *Salmonella braenderup* gastroenteritis due to contaminated meat pies: clinical and molecular epidemiology. *Clin Microbiol Infect* 2000;**6**:536.

43. Thornley JP *et al.* Relationship of *Campylobacter* toxigenicity in vitro to the development of postinfectious irritable bowel syndrome. *J Infect Dis* 2001;**184**:606.

44. Cumberland P *et al.* The infectious intestinal disease study of England: a prospective evaluation of symptoms and health care use after an acute episode. *Epidemiol Infect* 2003;**130**:453.

45. Rodriguez LA, Ruigomez A. Increased risk of irritable bowel syndrome after bacterial gastroenteritis: cohort study. *Br Med J* 1999;**318**:565.

46. Parry SD *et al.* Is irritable bowel syndrome more common in patients presenting with bacterial gastroenteritis? A community-based, case-control study. *Am J Gastroenterol* 2003;**98**:327.

47. Parry SD *et al.* Does bacterial gastroenteritis predispose people to functional gastrointestinal disorders? A prospective, community-based, case-control study. *Am J Gastroenterol* 2003;**98**:1970.

48. Marshall JK *et al.* Incidence and epidemiology of irritable bowel syndrome after a large waterborne outbreak of bacterial dysentery. *Gastroenterology* 2006;**131**:445; quiz 660.

49. Whorwell PJ *et al.* Non-colonic features of irritable bowel syndrome. *Gut* 1986;**27**:37.

50. Bellentani S *et al.* A simple score for the identification of patients at high risk of organic diseases of the colon in the family doctor consulting room. The Local IBS Study Group. *Fam Pract* 1990;**7**:307.

51. Levy RL *et al.* Intergenerational transmission of gastrointestinal illness behavior. *Am J Gastroenterol* 2000;**95**:451.

52. Locke GR 3rd *et al.* Familial association in adults with functional gastrointestinal disorders. *Mayo Clin Proc* 2000;**75**:907.

53. El-Serag HB *et al.* Systemic review: Natural history of irritable bowel syndrome. *Aliment Pharmacol Ther* 2004;**19**:861.

54. Mearin F *et al.* Predictive factors of irritable bowel syndrome improvement: 1-year prospective evaluation in 400 patients. *Aliment Pharmacol Ther* 2006;**23**:815.

55. Agreus L *et al.* Natural history of gastroesophageal reflux disease and functional abdominal disorders: a population-based study. *Am J Gastroenterol* 2001;**96**:2905.

56. Maxion-Bergemann S *et al.* Costs of irritable bowel syndrome in the UK and US. *Pharmacoeconomics* 2006;**24**:21.

57. Silk DB. Impact of irritable bowel syndrome on personal relationships and working practices. *Eur J Gastroenterol Hepatol* 2001;**13**:1327.

58. Dapoigny M *et al.* Irritable bowel syndrome in France: a common, debilitating and costly disorder. *Eur J Gastroenterol Hepatol* 2004;**16**:995.

59. Hungin AP *et al.* Irritable bowel syndrome in the United States: prevalence, symptom patterns and impact. *Aliment Pharmacol Ther* 2005;**21**:1365.

60. El-Serag HB *et al.* Health-related quality of life among persons with irritable bowel syndrome: a systematic review. *Aliment Pharmacol Ther* 2002;**16**:1171.

61. Sandler RS *et al.* The burden of selected digestive diseases in the United States. *Gastroenterology* 2002;**122**:1500.

62. Kozma CM *et al.* A comparison of office-based physician visits for irritable bowel syndrome and for migraine and asthma. *Manag Care Interface* 2002;**15**:40,49.

63. Levy RL *et al.* Costs of care for irritable bowel syndrome patients in a health maintenance organization. *Am J Gastroenterol* 2001;**96**:3122.

64. Patel RP *et al.* The economic impact of irritable bowel syndrome in a managed care setting. *J Clin Gastroenterol* 2002;**35**:14.

65. Longstreth GF *et al.* Irritable bowel syndrome, health care use, and costs: a U.S. managed care perspective. *Am J Gastroenterol* 2003;**98**:600.

66. Leong SA *et al.* The economic consequences of irritable bowel syndrome: a US employer perspective. *Arch Intern Med* 2003;**163**:929.

67. Martin BC *et al.* Utilization patterns and net direct medical cost to Medicaid of irritable bowel syndrome. *Curr Med Res Opin* 2003;**19**:771.

68. Talley NJ *et al.* Prevalence of gastrointestinal symptoms in the elderly: a population-based study. *Gastroenterology* 1992;**102**:895.

69. Hahn *et al.* Differences between individuals with self-reported irritable bowel syndrome (IBS) and IBS-like symptoms. *Dig Dis Sci* 1997;**42**:2585.

70. Saito YA *et al.* The effect of new diagnostic criteria for irritable bowel syndrome on community prevalence estimates. *Neurogastroenterol Motil* 2003;**15**:687.

25 Constipation

John F. Johanson

Key points
- Constipation is among the most common gastrointestinal disorders, affecting nearly 15% of the US population.
- Constipation is more common in women, the elderly and those in lower socioeconomic classes.
- Constipation is associated with decreased productivity and results in diminished quality of life.
- The unique epidemiologic distribution of constipation suggests the influence of environmental factors that have yet to be identified.

Clinical summary

Constipation is among the most common gastrointestinal disorders. It is so prevalent that it has been considered endemic in the elderly population. In the USA alone, more than 3 million prescriptions are written and more than $800 million is spent for over-the-counter laxatives [1].

Despite its significant impact, the pathophysiology of constipation remains largely unknown. A number of different constipation subtypes have been described including slow transit, defecatory dysfunction, normal transit or functional constipation, and irritable bowel syndrome with constipation. It is not clear, however, whether these conditions represent distinct pathophysiologic entities or whether they represent a spectrum of the same underlying process.

The onset of constipation is generally slow and unrelated to any specific event. Symptoms of constipation may begin at any time. Early in its course, infrequent or difficult defecation may be the only symptom. Specific constipation symptoms may vary according to the type of constipation. Slow transit constipation, for example, is often associated with very infrequent defecation and bloating in young women. By contrast, disordered defecation commonly presents with hard stools, straining, a feeling of rectal blockage or pressure, manual attempts at disimpaction, or feelings of incomplete evacuation. However, constipation is a slowly progressive disorder. As it increases in severity, patients frequently develop bloating and abdominal discomfort. Individuals who have suffered with constipation for many years may also note fatigue, malaise, anorexia or other constitutional symptoms. Despite its slowly progressive course, constipation rarely leads to severe morbidity or mortality.

Disease definition

Any description of the epidemiology of constipation is dependent upon how the disorder is defined. Attempts to provide an objective definition of constipation date back to the early 1960s. At that time, Connell and colleagues surveyed the bowel habits of factory workers in England and found that more than 99% had bowel frequencies ranging between three per day and three per week [2]. Based on this one study, constipation has, for the past 30 years, been defined as less than three bowel movements per week. However, the symptom of "infrequent bowel movements" captures a relatively small percentage of individuals with constipation. A population-based survey done by Paré and colleagues in Canada [3] revealed that patients consider other symptoms to more commonly represent constipation; 81% believed that constipation meant straining, while 72% believed that constipation was present if stools were hard. Other definitions included an inability to defecate when desired (54%) and abdominal bloating (37%). Infrequent bowel movements were considered constipation by only 36% of respondents.

The recognition of these varied symptoms led to development of the Rome criteria for defining constipation. The initial intention was to provide a consistent method of identifying individuals with constipation to facilitate enrollment of comparable patients into clinical trials. However, the Rome criteria are increasingly being employed in clinical practice. The Rome III criteria for functional constipation [4] comprise two or more of the following abnormalities:

- hard or lumpy stools;
- straining;
- a sensation of incomplete evacuation;
- a feeling of anorectal obstruction or the need for manual maneuvers (digital disimpaction);
more than 25% of the time, and
- less than three bowel movements per week.

Additionally, criteria for IBS must not be present, and loose stools must occur only rarely without the use of laxatives.

Even if the Rome criteria are used in epidemiologic studies, many patients with constipation may not be captured. Defining constipation as hard stools, straining with defecation or even infrequent defecation may be inadequate because individuals often complain of being constipated even though they may not have any of these specific symptoms. Many individuals feel constipated based solely on the perception that their bowel habits are not normal. Even if they do not meet an accepted definition of constipation, they are likely to seek treatment.

Although this may appear to be a question of semantics, it is important to understand the various definitions of constipation when studying its epidemiology. Population-based data sources, particularly large databases, rely on ICD-9 (International Classification of Diseases 9) diagnosis codes, which are ultimately based on physician coding. If a physician's belief is that constipation is present only when defecation frequency is less than three per week, prevalence rates based on these data may underestimate the true prevalence of constipation. Moreover, coding (or miscoding) practices may be influenced by other issues such as reimbursement. Even when epidemiologic studies employ the Rome criteria, they may underestimate the prevalence of constipation [5]. However, relying solely on an individual's perception that their bowel habits are not normal may lead to overestimating the true prevalence of constipation.

Nevertheless, objective criteria are necessary to define constipation in order to examine its epidemiology in a consistent manner. The various definitions of constipation have their own strengths and limitations. For purposes of interpretation and application of the findings of epidemiologic studies, however, it is important to know the definition upon which the results were based.

Incidence and prevalence

Incidence

It is difficult to estimate the incidence of constipation because of the widespread availability of over-the-counter (OTC) therapies. Many patients self-medicate when they first develop symptoms, and onset is often insidious, both of which make it difficult to determine the exact incidence of constipation.

There have been two studies that provide estimates of the incidence of constipation. Talley and colleagues observed rates of 40/1000 person-years when resurveying residents of Olmsted County 15 months after an initial survey of the same population [6]. A study by Everhart *et al.* identified a 27.3% increase in the number of patients self-reporting constipation over a 10-year period [7].

A third study examined the incidence of constipation among nursing home patients. In this retrospective study of 21 000 Medicare recipients, the incidence of constipation after admission to a nursing home facility was estimated to be 7% in the first 3 months [8]. This corresponds to an incidence rate of 280/1000 person years, sevenfold greater than that seen in ambulatory Olmsted County residents.

Prevalence

The prevalence of constipation ranges between 2% and 27% depending on which definition of constipation is utilized. A systematic review of all population-based epidemiologic studies of constipation in North America identified 10 studies [5]. In these studies, a number of different case definitions of constipation were employed. One of the studies actually compared three definitions of constipation among the same individuals, finding that self-report led to the highest prevalence of constipation (27.2%), whereas Rome I (14.9%) and Rome II criteria (16.7%) provided similar prevalence rates. The average prevalence of constipation among the various studies was 14.8% (Fig. 25.1), similar to that identified by both Rome criteria [5].

Although national population-based surveys tend to be the most reliable, case ascertainment is based on ICD-9 coding, which allows for significant variability in the definition of constipation. Smaller, regional population-based studies benefit from the ability to define constipation more precisely. These studies also permit analysis of the epidemiology of different subsets of constipation, such as normal transit constipation or disordered defecation.

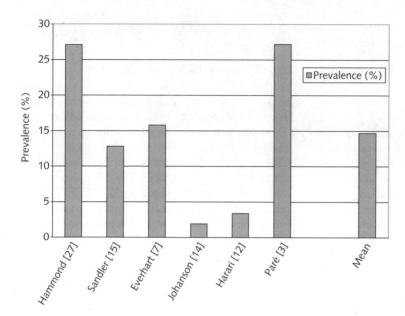

Fig. 25.1 The prevalence of self-reported constipation.

Talley performed two mail surveys of White adults between the ages of 30 and 64 years residing in Olmsted County [9,10], documenting prevalence rates of between 11% (for cases defined by Rome I outlet obstruction) to 19% (for cases defined by Rome I functional constipation). In the same manner, a meta-analysis of 30 regional epidemiologic studies revealed a broad range of prevalence rates depending upon the specific definition of constipation employed. Prevalence rates ranged from 1.4% for infrequent defecation to 16.9% for straining [11].

Given the uniformity of prevalence rates among the various studies, the overall prevalence of constipation is approximately 15%.

Risk factors for disease

Age

The relationship between age and constipation has been examined in numerous studies. Unfortunately, most of these studies divided age groups differently. In general, constipation demonstrates a progressive increase with increasing age. Harari [12], Johanson [13,14] and Sandler [15], for example, observed trends toward increased constipation with increasing age in various national databases.

Gender

The majority of epidemiologic studies report a higher prevalence of constipation in females, with female-to-male ratios ranging from 1.0 to 3.8 (Fig. 25.2). This is true across a range of case definitions, although higher ratios were typically observed in the studies that utilized self-reported constipation (average 2.65), compared with Rome criteria (average 1.75) [5,14].

Race/ethnicity

The prevalence of constipation is higher among non-Caucasian populations, with non White to White ratios ranging from 1.13 to 2.89. Self-reported constipation again generated the highest ratio and Rome II criteria the smallest [5]. The prevalence of constipation among individual racial or ethnic groups is more difficult to determine. Non-White racial groups are not typically stratified because of small numbers of non-White participants even in population-based studies. Moreover, it is difficult to compare prevalence rates of constipation among different countries to examine the influence of race or ethnicity, because the definition of constipation can vary significantly.

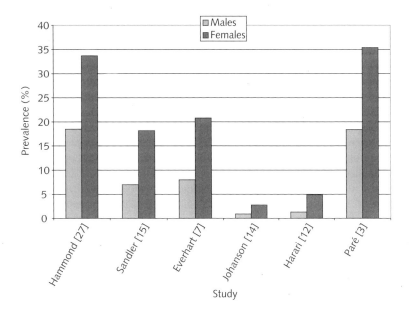

Fig. 25.2 The prevalence of constipation by gender.

Geography

Analysis of the prevalence of self-reported constipation indicates that constipation is more common in the South and Midwest of the USA [13]. A more refined geographic analysis of Medicare data demonstrated that constipation is more common in rural, northern, mountainous and poorer states [16]. This distribution suggests the influence of three environmental factors: rural living, colder temperatures and lower socioeconomic status. How these factors influence the development of constipation remains speculative.

Socioeconomic factors

The influence of socioeconomic status on the prevalence of constipation also appears to be consistent among published studies. Although specific income groups varied across studies, subjects with lower incomes consistently demonstrated significantly greater rates of constipation than those in higher income groups [14]. This effect was not as obvious in studies defining constipation by the Rome criteria [5].

An inverse correlation of education with prevalence of constipation has also been reported. There appears to be a trend toward increased prevalence with less education in the NHANES I data [15]. A similar trend toward increasing self-reported constipation with less education

was seen by Johanson [14]. An association of constipation with a lower level of education is less consistent in several other studies, particularly among those defining constipation using the Rome criteria [5]. This finding, therefore, may simply represent a surrogate marker for socioeconomic status.

Other diseases

Constipation occurs commonly among patients with other diseases. In many instances, these conditions are the actual cause of an individual's constipation. For example, hypothyroidism is well known to cause constipation. In other cases the associations may be coincidence or may be the result of shared risk factors. Using the Medicare database, Johanson studied the association of constipation with other diseases [17]. Not surprisingly, a number of known causes of constipation were found to be strongly associated with constipation, including laxative abuse (odds ratio, OR, 18.8), Hirschsprung's disease (OR 6.5), intestinal obstruction (OR 6.3) and hypothyroidism (OR 1.6).

Further analysis demonstrated a number of associations between constipation and neuropsychiatric disorders, including herpes zoster (OR 5.1), depression (OR 6.5), multiple sclerosis (OR 3.9), Parkinson's disease (OR 3.2) and vertebral column fracture (OR 10.1). These associations suggest a potential link between central nervous system dysfunction and constipation.

The prevalence of constipation among patients with specific neurologic diseases has also been studied. Hinds *et al.* [18] found that 43% of outpatients with multiple sclerosis complained of constipation regardless of the severity of their multiple sclerosis. Similarly, 31% of patients with spinal cord injuries suffered from severe constipation, while 24% had difficulty evacuating their stool [19]. Finally, in a study of developmentally delayed individuals with IQs less than 50, 70% were constipated. When compared with controls, the constipated individuals were more likely to have cerebral palsy, be nonambulatory, use anticonvulsants and have an IQ less than 35 [20].

Natural history and mortality

There has been little study of the natural history of constipation. It would appear that constipation represents a slowly progressive disorder that rarely if ever resolves. This is in part supported by Talley's data from Olmsted County, where 89% of respondents had no change in their symptoms of constipation during a 15-month interval between surveys [6].

Despite its unrelenting course, constipation rarely leads to severe morbidity. Hospitalization for constipation is uncommon, and mortality from constipation is quite rare [14]. Potential complications of chronic constipation include fecal impaction, fecal incontinence, sigmoid volvulus and stercoral ulcerations of the sigmoid colon or rectum. An association between constipation and colon cancer remains to be established.

Disability and quality of life

Constipation is associated with considerable disability. On an annual basis, patients with constipation experience nearly 14 million days of restricted activity, meaning they are not able to participate in desired activities because of their constipation. This corresponds to 3.6 days per patient per year [21]. Furthermore, constipation affects work productivity. Patients with constipation miss 2–3 days of work per month directly as a result of their constipation. Even while at work, 60% of patients with constipation have difficulty performing necessary job functions, leading to a 21% decrease in productivity [22].

Available data indicate that constipation likewise diminishes health-related quality of life. Irvine and colleagues found decreased mental and physical SF-36 subscores in a population-based sample of Canadians with constipa-

tion [23]. The decrease was statistically significant when compared with the Canadian norm, but was less than five points, thus the clinical relevance of this decrease is unclear. A more recent study by Damon and colleagues examined quality of life among patients with constipation and fecal incontinence who presented to their laboratory for anorectal manometry [24]. In this obviously selected referral population, quality of life was profoundly altered among their patients with constipation. Quality of life was considered to be significantly decreased if the GIQLI was less than 105. Total scores averaged 92.3 (±24.8) and 126 (±18) for patients with chronic constipation and normals, respectively. Other studies by O'Keefe in Olmsted County and Cheng in Hong Kong have demonstrated similar findings [25,26].

Given these findings, the true impact of constipation on quality of life may be hidden in the heterogeneity of constipation inherent among population-based studies. Although studies such as Irvine's provide a good estimate of its general effects on quality of life, a more homogeneous population may demonstrate more striking affects of constipation on quality of life.

Healthcare utilization

The majority of population-based data on healthcare utilization among patients with constipation date back 10 years or more. Despite their age, these data probably remain valid.

Although many individuals with constipation self-medicate, constipation leads to 2.9 million physician visits for constipation, which corresponds to 1.2 visits per 100 population (1.2%). During these visits, a prescription for laxatives is given between 85% and 100% of the time depending on the specific database examined [14]. Hospitalization for constipation is significantly less common, with approximately 20 000 discharges annually for a primary diagnosis of constipation. Mortality from constipation is exceedingly rare, with an annual average of 29 deaths per year directly attributable to constipation. However, when other complications of constipation such as volvulus or megacolon are considered, the annual mortality rate increases to 841 per year [14].

Prevention

The variety of symptoms and potential risk factors associated with constipation suggest that its etiology is multifactorial. Despite extensive investigation, clearly defined risk factors remain elusive, making it difficult to identify strategies for preventing constipation. Although advancing age, female gender, low socioeconomic status, and rural living appear to be important factors, they cannot be easily altered. Despite evidence to suggest that enteric nerve damage is closely associated with the development of constipation, environmental factors contributing to degeneration of enteric nerves have not been identified.

Based on the weight of evidence, increased dietary fiber intake does not seem to normalize transit or ease defecation in the majority of constipated individuals. Although speculative, endogenous neurotoxins may play a pathogenic role. Whether a diet rich in fresh fruits and vegetables containing antioxidants may ultimately prove to be an effective primary preventive measure is unknown.

The goal of secondary prevention is to inhibit the development of complications. Although chronic constipation is rarely associated with severe morbidity or mortality, potential complications include stercoral ulcers, fecal impaction and volvulus. Regular emptying of the rectum induced by oral laxatives or suppositories may prevent the development of fecal impaction, reducing the occurrence of overflow incontinence. Treatment of constipation may also prevent the formation of sigmoid volvulus, a potentially fatal disorder.

Issues/gaps in epidemiology knowledge

The basic epidemiologic distributions of constipation have been well described. However, a number of epidemiologic issues remain. First, a better understanding of the incidence of constipation is needed. Second, the natural history of constipation remains poorly understood. Elucidating both of these would provide better data upon which to base strategies for treatment and/or prevention of constipation. Finally, newer and better data are needed to define the impact of constipation on healthcare utilization, particularly as it relates to its effects on indirect costs, as well as the effects of constipation on disability and health-related quality of life.

Conclusions

Constipation is among the most common gastrointestinal disorders, affecting nearly 15% of the US population. It is clearly more common in women, the elderly and those in lower socioeconomic classes. Constipation is associated with decreased productivity and results in diminished quality of life.

Despite its significant impact, the etiology of constipation remains largely unknown. The variety of symptoms and risk factors associated with constipation suggests that its etiology is multifactorial. Although epidemiologic studies cannot establish cause and effect relationships, consistent epidemiologic distributions suggest potential etiologic risk factors. Further clarification of the epidemiology of constipation will be beneficial in suggesting potential risk factors and also in identifying populations who are at highest risk of developing this condition. If high-risk populations are identified, they can be targeted for treatment or possibly even interventions that might prevent the development of this often debilitating condition.

References

1. Borum ML. Constipation: evaluation and management. *Prim Care* 2001;**28**:577.
2. Connell AM *et al.* Variation of bowel habit in two population samples. *Br Med J* 1965;**5470**:1095.
3. Paré P *et al.* An epidemiological survey of constipation in Canada: definitions, rates, demographics, and predictors of health care seeking. *Am J Gastroenterol* 2001;**96**:3130.
4. Longstreth GF *et al.* Functional bowel disorders. *Gastroenterology* 2006;**130**:1480.
5. Higgins PDR *et. al.* Epidemiology of constipation in North America: a systematic review. *Am J Gastroenterol* 2004;**99**:750.
6. Talley NJ *et al.* Onset and disappearance of gastrointestinal symptoms and functional gastrointestinal disorders. *Am J Epidemiol* 1992;**136**:165.
7. Everhart JE *et al.* A longitudinal survey of self-reported bowel habits in the United States. *Dig Dis Sci* 1989;**34**:1153.
8. Robson KM *et al.* Development of constipation in nursing home residents. *Dis Colon Rectum* 2000;**43**:940.
9. Talley NJ *et al.* Epidemiology of colonic symptoms and the irritable bowel syndrome. *Gastroenterology* 1991;**101**:927.
10. Talley NJ *et al.* Functional constipation and outlet delay: a population-based study. *Gastroenterology* 1993;**105**:781.
11. Sonnenberg A *et al. Constipation.* Peters, UK: Wrightson Biomedical Publishing, 1994:19.
12. Harari D *et al.* Bowel habit in relation to age and gender. Findings from the National Health Interview Survey and clinical implications. *Arch Intern Med* 1996;**156**:315.
13. Johanson JF *et al.* Clinical epidemiology of chronic constipation. *J Clin Gastroenterol* 1989;**11**:525.
14. Johanson JF. Constipation. In: Everhart JE (ed.) *Digestive Diseases in the United States: Epidemiology and Impact.* NIH publication no. 94–1447. Washington, DC: US Government Printing Office, 1994.

15. Sandler RS *et al.* Demographic and dietary determinants of constipation in the US population. *Am J Public Health* 1990;**80**:185.

16. Johanson JF. Geographic distribution of constipation in the United States. *Am J Gastroenterol* 1998:**93**:188.

17. Johanson JF *et al.* Association of constipation with neurologic diseases: an epidemiologic study of the concordant occurrence of diseases in the Medicare population. *Dig Dis Sci* 1992;**37**:179.

18. Hinds JP *et al.* Prevalence of bowel dysfunction in multiple sclerosis. A population survey. *Gastroenterology* 1990;**98**:1538.

19. Han TR *et al.* Chronic gastrointestinal problems and bowel dysfunction in patients with spinal cord injury. *Spinal Cord* 1998;**36**:485.

20. Bohmer CJ *et al.* The prevalence of constipation in institutionalized people with intellectual disability. *J Intellect Disabil Res* 2001;**45**:212.

21. Dennison C *et al.* The health-related quality of life and economic burden of constipation. *Pharmacoeconomics* 2005;**23**:461.

22. Bracco K *et al.* Burden of chronic constipation must include estimates of work productivity and activity impairment in addition to traditional healthcare utilization. *Am J Gastroenterol* 2004;**99**:S233.

23. Irvine EJ *et al.* Health-related quality of life in functional GI disorders: focus on constipation and resource utilization. *Am J Gastroenterol* 2002;**97**:1986.

24. Damon H *et al.* Impact of anal incontinence and chronic constipation on quality of life. *Gastroenterol Clin Biol* 2004;**28**:16.

25. O'Keefe EA *et al.* Bowel disorders impair functional status and quality of life in the elderly – a population based study. *J Gerontol A Biol Sci Med Sci* 1995;**50**:184.

26. Cheng C *et al.* Coping strategies, illness perception, anxiety and depression of patients with idiopathic constipation: a population based study. *Aliment Pharmacol Ther* 2003;**18**:319.

27. Hammond E. Some preliminary findings on physical complaints from a prospective study of 1,064,004 men and women. *Am J Public Health* 1964;**54**:11.

26 Infectious Diarrhea

Crenguta Stepan and Christina M. Surawicz

Key points

- There occurs about one episode of infectious diarrhea per person-year in the USA.
- 80% of infectious diarrhea worldwide is caused by viruses.
- Each year more than 3 million people die worldwide as a result of infectious diarrhea.
- Prevention through education, medication and vaccination is a high priority.

From sporadic cases to familial outbreaks or epidemics, diarrheal disease is a common public health problem worldwide and is one of the leading causes of morbidity and mortality among infants and children in developing countries.

Definition

Acute diarrhea is defined as three or more stools per day (or at least 200 g of stool per day), lasting for 14 days or less; persistent diarrhea lasts for more than 14 days and chronic diarrhea lasts longer than 30 days. Chronic diarrhea does not commonly have an infectious etiology.

Clinical summary

Most acute infectious diarrhea is due to viruses such as noroviruses (formerly Norwalk agent), **rotaviruses, astroviruses** and **enteric adenoviruses**. Viral illnesses are typically associated with watery stools, nausea, vomiting, myalgia, fatigue, dehydration and low-grade fever. Bacteria can cause watery diarrhea, which can turn into bloody diarrhea. In general, invasive pathogens, such as *Shigella, Campylobacter, Yersinia, Aeromonas* and *Plesiomonas*, cause diarrhea with fever and signs of dehydration. Among the protozoa, *Giardia, Cryptosporidium, Entamoeba histolytica* and *Cyclospora* are the most common. Any enteric infection can have a prolonged course in immunosuppressed patients.

Immediate complications include most frequently dehydration but also rare cases of hemolytic uremic syndrome (HUS), usually associated with infection with Shiga toxin-producing *E. coli* (STEC). Other complications include postinfectious irritable bowel syndrome, persistent or chronic diarrhea, and uncommon complications such as Guillain–Barré syndrome and Reiter's syndrome.

Most diarrhea is self-limited, so diagnostic tests and treatment are not necessary. In some cases (e.g., extremes of age, severe diarrhea, bloody diarrhea, fever or immunocompromise) diagnostic tests such as stool lactoferrin, stool leukocytes, ova and parasites and stool culture may be indicated. In these cases, empiric therapy with appropriate antibiotics may be needed.

Incidence

USA
Adults

It is estimated that 211–270 million episodes of diarrhea occur annually in the USA, with about 0.72 episodes per adult-year [1]. Of these, 76 million cases of foodborne disease occur each year, 82% with an unknown etiology [2].

For pathogens, the incidence varies with the method used: stool culture, reports to the Centers for Disease Control, and reports to health department. In 2004, the incidence of diarrheal pathogens calculated using the laboratory-confirmed infections is shown in Table 26.1.

Etiology: pathogen	Frequency by stool culture (in USA)	Reference
Norovirus	8500 cases per 100 000 population	[3]
Rotavirus	1100 cases per 100 000 population	[3]
Giardia	750 cases per 100 000 population	[3]
Salmonella	14.7 cases per 100 000 population	[4]
Campylobacter	12.9 cases per 100 000 population	[4]
Shigella	5.1 cases per 100 000 population	[4]
E. coli O157: H7	0.9 cases per 100 000 population	[4]

Table 26.1 Common causes of infectious diarrhea

Children

The incidence of parent-defined diarrhea is 2.2 episodes per person-year. **Rotavirus** is the leading cause of hospitalization for diarrhea among children worldwide. The median detection rate for rotavirus among children hospitalized with diarrhea ranges from 29% to 45%, with a peak during the winter time [5]. Persistent diarrhea accounts for 8% of diarrheal illnesses during childhood and is associated with *Cryptosporidium, Giardia,* enteric adenoviruses and enterotoxigenic *E. coli.*

Developing countries

In developing countries, there is a median of 3.2 episodes of diarrhea per child-year in children under 5 years of age [6]. The etiology is mostly viral but the incidence of bacterial diarrhea is greater than in developed countries. An interesting difference has been noticed in the epidemiology of *Campylobacter*. In developing countries, *Campylobacter* infections are endemic among young children, asymptomatic infections are common and outbreaks are rare. In developed countries, asymptomatic *Campylobacter* infections are unusual and outbreaks are common [7]. However, worldwide, *Campylobacter* remains one of the most common bacterial causes of diarrhea.

Traveler's diarrhea

Among travelers to different areas of the world, the risk of traveler's diarrhea is about 7% in developed countries and 20–50% in the developing world, with a total of 15–20 million cases annually [8]. For travel to high-risk areas, such as Africa, Latin America and India, rates can vary from 20% to 90%. Low-risk areas such as southern Europe and North America have traveler's diarrhea rates of less than 8% [8]. **Enterotoxigenic *E. coli*** is the main cause. Tropical sprue can affect travelers in Asia, some Caribbean islands and parts of South America. It presents usually as

persistent diarrhea but can also be acute. It is likely that the disease is either initiated or sustained by a still-undefined infection because it responds to antibiotics.

Nosocomial diarrhea

Diarrhea is a common side effect of many antibiotic therapies (antibiotic-associated diarrhea, AAD, approximately 20%); of these, 10–15% will have *Clostridium difficile*-associated diarrhea (CDAD). The incidence in the USA is increasing, with an estimate for 2003 of about 61 per 100 000, and over 228 per 100 000 among patients aged 65 years or more [9]. The incidence of community-acquired *C. difficile* diarrhea appears to be substantially lower than rates observed in hospitals, with an estimated 12 cases per 100 000 person-years [10].

Immunocompromised patients

Human immunodeficiency virus (HIV) infection is frequently complicated by diarrhea. In patients with <200 CD4 cells/mm^3, the occurrence of chronic diarrhea ranges from 8% to 10% per year. Worldwide, the most common causes of diarrhea in HIV-infected patients are enteric bacteria including *Shigella flexneri, Salmonella enteritidis* and *Campylobacter jejuni*. As immunodeficiency advances, cytomegalovirus (CMV), cryptosporidiosis, microsporidia and *Mycobacterium avium* complex (MAC) are more common. *C. difficile* is a pathogen typically reported in developed countries, whereas tuberculosis is a common complication of AIDS in developing countries [11].

Risk factors

For any case of diarrhea, the epidemiological history may reveal important clues about the etiology. Specific pathogens can be associated with some specific risk factors, as shown in Table 26.2.

Table 26.2 Common risk factors for specific pathogens causing infectious diarrhea

Pathogen	Risk factors
E. coli O157: H7	Undercooked beef, unpasteurized milk, apple cider, visits to animal farms, petting zoos
Shigella	Contaminated water and vegetables, day-care centers, custodial institutions
Campylobacter	Undercooked poultry, contaminated milk, tuna salad
Salmonella	Raw eggs, undercooked poultry and turkey, unrefrigerated dressing, reptiles as a pet, family members with *Salmonella*
Non-cholera vibrio	Raw/undercooked seafood
Giardia	Contaminated water, recreational exposure in lakes, rivers or swimming pools, day-care centers
Cryptosporidium	International travel, contact with cattle, freshwater swimming
Rotavirus	Winter outbreaks, in children under 2 years
Norovirus	Winter outbreaks in adults, raw oyster consumption, cruise ships

Epidemiological surveys have revealed several factors that may influence the risk and incidence of infectious diarrhea. For some of these factors, data remain very limited.

• **Age:** Infants, toddlers and young adults (15–35 years old) are prone to develop traveler's diarrhea, which may be related to hygiene and dietary habits. Younger age is also a risk factor for rotavirus diarrhea and rotavirus-related hospitalization; its incidence decreases with age by presumably developing an antibody response. Children under 5 years also have the highest rate of HUS.

• **Gender:** There is no significant difference in diarrhea incidence rate according to gender; women and men have the same risk of developing infectious diarrhea or traveler's diarrhea. Female gender might have a higher incidence rate for HUS [12], although the incidence rates of *E. coli* O157:H7 showed no differences by gender.

• **Ethnicity:** Because data on ethnicity are incomplete, conclusions cannot be made about differences in the epidemiology of infectious diarrhea. However, Caucasians have a higher incidence of diarrhea-related HUS and ethnicity-specific hospitalization rates for rotavirus diarrhea [13].

• **Geography and socioeconomic status:** The country of origin and host country are important determinants for traveler's diarrhea. Coming from developed countries and traveling to developing countries is associated with highest attack rates. Although the pathogens causing diarrhea are the same worldwide, the incidence of specific pathogens varies.

• **Seasonality:** Rotavirus and norovirus infections occur more frequently during winter months. Bacterial diarrhea is most common during the summertime (because of traveling, swimming, food choices). The higher rate of

HUS during summer and fall reflects the exposure to *E. coli* O157:H7 infections.

• **Genetics:** Among blood types, certain ABO phenotypes have been reported to be associated with susceptibility to some enteric pathogens. Type O phenotype presents a greater susceptibility to *Vibrio cholerae* [14] and possibly also to norovirus [15] infection. Reiter's syndrome, as a complication of *S. flexneri* infection, occurs especially in persons with the genetic predisposition human leukocyte antigen (HLA) B27. There is also evidence of genetic factors associated with EAEC diarrhea and increased level of fecal interleukin 8 (IL-8) [16].

• **Environmental:** Behavioral risk factors associated with diarrhea include dietary habits (consumption of "risky" food or beverages, unpasteurized milk), or environmental exposure (animal exposure, poor hygiene); these are important determinants for traveler's diarrhea.

• **Medication:** Acid suppression medication increases the risk of traveler's diarrhea, and recently it has been shown that proton pump inhibitors, in particular, may be associated with an increased risk of community-acquired *C. difficile* [17]. Non-steroidal anti-inflammatory drugs should be investigated further in order to assess their possible role as a risk factor in community-acquired *C. difficile* infection [17]. Some antibiotics (clindamycin and the second- and third-generation cephalosporins, and more recently quinolones) predispose to nosocomial infection with *C. difficile*.

• **Medical conditions:** Conditions associated with decreased acid secretion (post-surgery or immunological) predispose to infectious diarrhea, including traveler's diarrhea, by decreasing the infective dose of pathogen. Immunodeficiency conditions, inherited or acquired, increase the risk of infections. A compromised immune system, abdominal surgery, comorbidity and length of hospitalization increase the risk of *C. difficile*-associated diarrhea.

For chronic diarrhea, the most important epidemiological risk factor is malnutrition. In children, other associated conditions are zinc deficiency, lack of breastfeeding, and a history of intrauterine growth retardation. Common variable immunodeficiency (CVID) presents with frequent bacterial infections, persistent diarrhea and malabsorption caused by *Giardia lamblia* infection.

Natural history, prognosis and mortality

The natural history and the prognosis of infectious diarrhea depend on etiology and host factors.

Adults

For norovirus infections, the symptoms typically abate in less than 3 days, but the shedding of the virus in stools may continue for longer than a week. Norovirus infection may lead to an increased duration of diarrhea and severe consequences in the elderly, patients with cardiovascular disease, and recipients of renal transplant or immunosuppressive therapy [18]. Asymptomatic infection is very common. The case-fatality rate varies from 0.01% in the USA to 0.075% in England or as high as 2% in Israel [19]. The highest mortality rate is associated with outbreaks in hospitals and residential-care facilities so infection in hospitalized persons might be more severe than that in other groups. Rotaviruses, enteric adenoviruses and astroviruses sometimes cause gastroenteritis in adults; however, they are less common, perhaps because protective immunity for these viruses often develops in childhood, whereas the immune response to noroviruses is generally short-lived or ineffective.

Children

Most childhood diarrhea is mild, with complete recovery. However, about 50 000 hospitalizations in the USA may be attributable to rotavirus [20]. Rotavirus gastroenteritis requiring hospitalization occurs most frequently in infants and young children, aged from 6 months to 2 years. In developed nations, rotavirus infection rarely results in death (a total of about 20–40 cases in the USA). In developing countries overall, diarrhea accounts for 21% of all deaths of children aged under 5 years, with 2.5 million

deaths per year [21]. Of these, about 500 000 children die every year from rotavirus gastroenteritis, with >80% of these deaths occurring in these countries [22]. For any etiology, interventions that can decrease morbidity and mortality rates are breastfeeding up to 6 months, improved sanitation and use of oral rehydration therapy. The number of deaths of children that could be prevented worldwide each year by breastfeeding alone has been estimated to be more than 1 million [23]. Oral rehydration reduces the diarrheal mortality, especially among children under 1 year of age, in whom acute dehydration is the greatest cause of death.

Traveler's diarrhea

International travel is often accompanied by gastroenteritis due to bacterial pathogens. Up to 80% of the cases of traveler's diarrhea are caused by bacteria. Most cases are benign and resolve in 1–2 days without treatment. Traveler's diarrhea is rarely life-threatening. The natural history is that 90% of cases resolve within 1 week, and 98% resolve within 1 month.

C. difficile-associated diarrhea

This presents a wide spectrum of clinical manifestations, from asymptomatic or mild, to severe necrotizing colitis. Most treated patients improve, but about 20% relapse. Patients with relapsing *C. difficile* colitis are prone to further relapses, which are more difficult to eradicate after each recurrence. Fulminant colitis occurs in 3% of patients, but accounts for most of the serious complications such as toxic megacolon, perforation and death [24]. In Canada, the fatality rate is estimated at 1.5%, with others reporting rates from 0.8% to 2% for nosocomial *C. difficile* diarrhea [25].

Chronic infectious diarrhea

Chronic diarrhea is rarely infectious. Infectious chronic diarrhea is associated with intestinal parasites, notably *C. difficile, Y. enterocolitica, Shigella* sp. and cytomegalovirus. The populations at risk for this are travelers returning from tropical countries and immunocompromised patients, especially patients with acquired immunodeficiency syndrome (AIDS) whose CD4 cell counts are below 50/µL [26]. In AIDS patients, chronic diarrhea is a common finding; the introduction of highly active antiretroviral therapy (HAART) has decreased the diarrhea caused by organisms such as microsporidia and cryptosporidia by improving the immune system. In children, persistent diarrhea accounts for 36–54% of all diarrhea-related deaths [27].

Disability and quality of life

Acute diarrhea

Acute diarrhea variably affects quality of life, from the inconvenience of having symptoms to the inability to leave home and function normally. Uncontrolled diarrhea can lead to dehydration and chemical imbalances that might be life threatening in infants and the elderly. Other postinfectious complications of diarrhea are reactive arthritis and Reiter's syndrome, associated with 1–4% of the gastroenteritis caused by *Shigella, Salmonella* and *Campylobacter*. Guillain–Barré syndrome occurs in 1–2 cases per 100 000 population per year but its incidence is <1 per 1000 infections with *Campylobacter* [28]. HUS is caused in almost all cases by STEC in developing countries. In the USA, Shiga toxin-producing *E. coli* (STEC) is implicated in 72% of cases of HUS, and *E. coli* O157: O7 was the pathogen in over 80% of patients with STEC infection [29].

Chronic diarrhea

Chronic diarrhea can have a substantial impact on quality of life and health overall. In children, morbidity is related to malnutrition, and physical and cognitive abnormalities. Diarrheal illnesses occurring during the first two years of life could have a profound impact on growth, cognitive development and educational performance [30]. In adults, the condition can be an inconvenience or it can be disabling, causing malnutrition, weight loss and increased morbidity.

Postinfectious irritable bowel syndrome (PI-IBS) is defined as a change in bowel habits or an onset of new abdominal pain or discomfort following a recent exposure to infectious organisms. PI-IBS has been reported to occur after traveler's diarrhea with ETEC and EAEC [31] and after gastroenteritis caused by *Campylobacter, Shigella* and *Salmonella*, in 8–10% of cases [32]. The development of PI-IBS is influenced by host and microbial factors, and the duration and severity of the acute infection. The course of PI-IBS is mild, but probably prolonged. One study has shown that more than 50% of IBS patients remain symptomatic 6 years post-gastroenteritis [33].

Healthcare utilization and costs

Diarrhea is an extremely costly disease. The yearly cost of acute diarrhea in the USA is $5–6 billion in direct medical expenses and lost productivity [34].
- **Indirect costs:** With an estimate of 50 000 hospitalizations attributable to rotavirus each year in the USA, the average nonmedical cost per case of rotavirus disease is about $448.77. The nonmedical costs of severe rotavirus infections may exceed $22 million annually, with 80% of the cost attributable to missed work [35].
- **Medication:** According to an Australian study, the average cost of prescribed medication per visit was A$6.83 and the estimated cost of over-the-counter medication was A$8.76 [36]. It has been estimated that in the USA more than 30% of the population with infectious diarrhea receives antidiarrheal medication [37]. There are no data available for medication costs in the USA.
- **Ambulatory care:** A survey of a sample of the US population found that each year 12% of persons with diarrhea (about 25 million) visited a medical provider for their illness, and another 20% (about 42 million) consulted a provider by telephone. The estimate for the median cost of diarrhea outpatient visits is $47–57 [38].
- **Hospitalization:** Diarrhea-associated hospitalization has been decreasing, with an estimate of 1.5% of all hospitalizations among adults in the USA. In children under 5 years of age, diarrhea accounts for 2% of all hospitalizations. The median cost of diarrhea-associated hospitalization was $2307 according to a study from 2001 [38]. *C. difficile*-associated diarrhea causes death in 1–2% of affected patients, and the estimate for the US healthcare costs attributable to *C. difficile*-associated diarrhea is over $600 million in excess healthcare costs and over 600 000 excess hospital days in nonfederal facilities [39].

Prevention

For developed countries, the use of vaccination against rotavirus and norovirus would decrease the incidence of diarrheal illnesses in children and adults and would ease the economic burden. Improvement in hygiene, use of available vaccines and self-medication with rifaximin or bismuth subsalicylate are the best prevention for traveler's diarrhea.

For developing countries, prevention should target sanitation and vaccination. These would have a great impact not just on acute illness, but on the high rate of mortality and morbidity as well.

Topical issues

Certain aspects of infectious diarrhea continue to pose intriguing questions for the epidemiologist.

• The epidemiology of tropical sprue remains obscure. Antibiotic treatment in combination with folate normalizes the mucosal structure and favors the hypothesis of an infectious etiology. Further studies may clarify its cause and the risk factors associated with the high incidence of relapses.

• Recently, community-acquired *C. difficile* diarrhea has been increasing in incidence. Given its cost and its impact on quality of life, early diagnostic strategies and better therapy for severe cases are needed.

• "Brainerd" diarrhea is another example of diarrhea that is thought to be infectious but for which no agent has been identified. Six outbreaks have been reported in the USA, but this may be an underestimate. Further investigations to identify the etiology and the risk factors would help in treating and preventing the condition.

Recommendations for future studies

There is still much to do in areas of clinical research, epidemiology and public health in order to combat infectious diarrhea more effectively.

• Controlling the incidence of infectious diarrhea in developing countries through educational programs to promote hygienic behavior and food processing.

• Developing an enteric vaccine coupled with studies of immunoprophylaxis.

• Defining rates and risk factors for PI-IBS as well as the most common associated pathogens, and determining whether medical treatment makes a difference to incidence or prevention.

• Investigating probiotics as a promising option in treating a variety of diarrheal disorders, including rotavirus diarrhea, *C. difficile* diarrhea and traveler's diarrhea. Future studies should determine their efficacy over the long term for prevention and treatment.

Conclusions

There are 2 to 4 billion cases of food-borne and diarrheal disease worldwide, resulting in 3.1 million deaths, mostly of children living in developing countries. Despite expensive stool tests, most are of unknown etiology. Identify-

ing the risk factors and the susceptible persons can lead to better strategies of prevention. In recent years, a global effort has tried to decrease the burden of this disease by improving hygiene, developing vaccines and formulating prophylaxis guidelines. However, diarrheal diseases are still a major challenge.

References

1. Guerrant RL *et al*. Practice guidelines for the management of infectious diarrhea. *Clin Infect Dis* 2001;**32**:331.
2. Flint JA *et al*. Estimating the burden of acute gastroenteritis, foodborne disease, and pathogens commonly transmitted by food: an international review. *Clin Infect Dis* 2005;**41**:698.
3. Mead PS *et al*. Food-related illness and death in the United States. *Emerg Infect Dis* 1999;**5**:607
4. Anon. Preliminary foodnet data on the incidence of infection with pathogens transmitted commonly through food – 10 sites, United States, 2004. *MMWR Morb Mortal Wkly Rep* 2005;**54**:352.
5. Parashar UD *et al*. *Rotavirus* and severe childhood diarrhea. *Emerg Infect Dis* 2006;**12**:304.
6. Kosec M *et al*. The global burden of diarrhoeal disease, as estimated from studies published between 1992 and 2000. *Bull World Health Organ* 2003;**81**:391.
7. Allos BM. *Campylobacter jejuni* infections: update on emerging issues and trends. *Clin Infect Dis* 2001;**32**:1201.
8. Steffen R. Epidemiology of traveler's diarrhea. *Clin Infect Dis* 2005;**41**:S536.
9. McDonald LC *et al*. *Clostridium difficile* infection in patients discharged from US short-stay hospitals, 1996–2003. *Emerg Infect Dis* 2006;**12**:409.
10. Levy DG *et al*. Antibiotics and *Clostridium difficile* diarrhea in the ambulatory care setting. *Clin Ther* 2000;**22**:91.
11. Wilcox CM. Etiology and evaluation of diarrhea in AIDS: a global perspective at the millennium. *World J Gastroenterol* 2000;**6**:177.
12. Chang HG *et al*. Hemolytic uremic syndrome incidence in New York. *Emerg Infect Dis* 2004;**10**:928.
13. Ford-Jones EL *et al*. Hospitalization for community-acquired, rotavirus-associated diarrhea: a prospective, longitudinal, population-based study during the seasonal outbreak. The Greater Toronto Area/Peel Region PRESI Study Group. Pediatric Rotavirus Epidemiology Study for Immunization. *Arch Pediatr Adolesc Med* 2000;**154**:578.
14. Harris JB *et al*. Blood group, immunity, and risk of infection with *Vibrio cholerae* in an area of endemicity. *Infect Immun* 2005;**73**:7422.
15. Hutson AM *et al*. Norwalk virus infection and disease is associated with ABO histo-blood group type. *J Infect Dis* 2002;**185**:1335.

16. Jiang Z-D *et al.* Genetic susceptibility to enteroaggregative *Escherichia coli* diarrhea: polymorphism in the interleukin-8 promotor region. *J Infect Dis* 2003;**188**:506.

17. Dial S *et al.* Use of gastric acid-suppressive agents and the risk of community-acquired *Clostridium difficile*-associated disease. *JAMA* 2005;**294**:2989.

18. Mattner F *et al.* Risk groups for clinical complications of norovirus infections: an outbreak investigation. *Clin Microbiol Infect* 2006;**12**:69.

19. Calderon-Margalit R *et al.* A large-scale gastroenteritis outbreak associated with *Norovirus* in nursing homes. *Epidemiol Infect* 2005;**133**:35.

20. Zimmerman CM *et al.* Cost of diarrhea-associated hospitalizations and outpatient visits in an insured population of young children in the United States**.** *Pediatr Infect Dis J* 2001;**20**:14.

21. Kosec M *et al.* The global burden of diarrhoeal disease, as estimated from studies published between 1992 and 2000. *B World Health Organ* 2003;**81**:391.

22. Parashar UD *et al.* Global illness and deaths caused by rotavirus disease in children. *Emerg Infect Dis* 2003;**9**:565.

23. Morrow AL *et al.* Human milk protection against infectious diarrhea: implications for prevention and clinical care. *Semin Pediatr Infect Dis* 2004;**15**:221.

24. Poutanen SM *et al. Clostridium difficile*-associated diarrhea in adults. *Can Med Assoc J* 2004;**171**:47.

25. Loo VG *et al. Clostridium difficile*: a formidable foe. *Can Med Assoc J* 2004;**171**:

26. Kist M. Chronic diarrhea: value of microbiology in diagnosis. 2000;**89**:1559.

27. Bhutta ZA *et al.* Persistent and chronic diarrhea and malabsorption: Working Group Report of the Second World Congress of Pediatric Gastroenterology, Hepatology, and Nutri-

tion. *J Pediatr Gastr Nutr* 2004;**39**(Suppl. 2):S711.

28. Allos BM. *Campylobacter jejuni* infections: update on emerging issues and trends. *Clin Infect Dis* 2001;**32**:1201.

29. Banatvala N *et al.* The United States National Prospective Hemolytic Uremic Syndrome Study: microbiologic, serologic, clinical, and epidemiologic findings. *J Infect Dis* 2001;**183**:1063.

30. Guerrant RL *et al.* Updating the DALYs for diarrhoeal disease. *Trends Parasitol* 2002;**18**:191.

31. Okhuysen PC *et al.* Post-diarrhea chronic intestinal symptoms and irritable bowel syndrome in North American travelers to Mexico. *Am J Gastroenterol* 2004;**99**:1774.

32. Collins SM *et al.* East meets West: infection, nerves, and mast cells in the irritable bowel syndrome. *Gut* 2004;**53**:1068.

33. Neal KR *et al.* Prognosis in post-infective irritable bowel syndrome: a six year follow up study. *Gut* 2002;**51**:410.

34. Foodborne disease. National Institute of Allergy and Infectious Disease, February 2005.

35. Lee BP *et al.* Nonmedical costs associated with rotavirus disease requiring hospitalization. *Pediatr Infect Dis J* 2005;**24**:984.

36. Hellard ME. Cost of community gastroenteritis. *J Gastroenterol Hepatol* 2003;**18**:322.

37. Guerrant RL. Practice guidelines for the management of infectious diarrhea. *Clin Infect Dis* 2001;**32**:331.

38. Zimmerman CM *et al.* Cost of diarrhea-associated hospitalizations and outpatient visits in an insured population of young children in the United States. *Pediatr Infect Dis J* 2001;**20**:14.

39. McDonald LC *et al. Clostridium difficile* infection in patients discharged from US short-stay hospitals, 1996–2003. *Emerg Infect Dis* 2006;**12**:409.

27 Inflammatory Bowel Disease

Edward V. Loftus Jr

Key points
- Crohn's disease and ulcerative colitis, the two major subtypes of inflammatory bowel disease, remain idiopathic.
- The incidence of these conditions continues to rise in both industrialized and developing countries, and as many as 1 in 200 persons has a form of inflammatory bowel disease.
- Crohn's disease and ulcerative colitis result in substantial morbidity, with up to 30% of colitis patients requiring colectomy and 60–80% of Crohn's disease patients requiring at least one intestinal resection.

Clinical summary

Ulcerative colitis is a chronic inflammatory bowel disease (IBD) characterized by mucosal inflammation of the rectum and/or colon. Crohn's disease, the other major subtype of idiopathic IBD, is characterized by transmural and sometimes granulomatous inflammation of the gastrointestinal tract, most commonly in the ileum and colon. Typical symptoms of ulcerative colitis include diarrhea, rectal bleeding, tenesmus, and increased stool urgency and frequency, while the most common symptoms of Crohn's disease are abdominal pain, fatigue and diarrhea. Complications of ulcerative colitis include toxic megacolon and colorectal dysplasia or cancer. Complications of Crohn's disease include intestinal stenosis, fistulas, abscesses and, rarely, intestinal cancer. The pathogenesis of these conditions remains unclear, but they are thought to arise due to a combination of defective mucosal immune regulation in the gut combined with exposure to as-yet-undetermined environmental factors or luminal antigens. The diagnosis of colitis is typically made by endoscopy and biopsy of the colorectum. The diagnosis of Crohn's disease may be difficult, as there are no pathognomonic features, and a host of modalities may be required, including colonoscopy with ileoscopy, small bowel radiography – barium-, CT (computed tomography)- or MR (magnetic resonance)-based – capsule endoscopy or serologic markers. Treatment of these diseases consists of one or more of the following medication classes: aminosalicylates, corticosteroids, antibiotics, immunosuppressive agents (thiopurines, methotrexate, or calcineurin inhibitors), or biologic (anticytokine or antiadhesion molecule) agents.

Disease definition

The idiopathic inflammatory bowel diseases (IBDs) consist of two major subtypes – ulcerative colitis and Crohn's disease (aka "regional enteritis" or "granulomatous colitis"). Disease classification can be troublesome, because these diagnoses are clinical ones and there is no single test that is pathognomonic for either condition. Ulcerative colitis is characterized by a continuous, confluent mucosal inflammation of the large intestine, almost always with rectal involvement, in the absence of infection, ischemia and radiation exposure [1]. Crohn's disease, a more heterogeneous disorder, requires one or more of the following for diagnosis:
- granulomatous transmural inflammation of the gastrointestinal tract (anywhere from mouth to anus);
- discontinuous involvement with "skip areas";
- a propensity for intestinal stenosis and/or fistula [1].

One of the challenges in interpreting epidemiologic research in IBD is that disease definitions have not been consistent. Further compounding the classification problem is the use of "indeterminate colitis" in some epidemiologic studies. Originally a term used by pathologists to describe surgical resection specimens with features of both ulcerative colitis and Crohn's disease, "indeterminate colitis" is now used by some clinicians and epidemiologists to describe chronic colitis that does not readily fall into either one of the two classic IBD subtypes. In some population-based investigations, cases of indeterminate colitis are tracked separately, while in other studies these are "forced" into one of two categories.

Incidence and prevalence

In high-incidence areas such as North America, the incidence of ulcerative colitis ranges from 8.8 cases per 100 000 person-years [2] to 14.6 per 100 000 [3], and the incidence of Crohn's disease ranges from 7.9 per 100 000 [2] to 14.8 per 100 000 [3]. In other words, if we assume that the combined population of the USA and Canada is 333 million persons, between 29 000 and 49 000 Americans and Canadians are diagnosed with ulcerative colitis annually, while between 26 000 and 49 000 are diagnosed each year with Crohn's disease.

The prevalence of ulcerative colitis in North America in 2001 ranged from 191 cases per 100 000 persons [4] to 241 per 100 000 (AJE Green, 2006), and the prevalence of Crohn's disease ranged from 129 cases per 100 000 [4] to 270 per 100 000 [3]. The overall prevalence of IBD was approximately 0.4% in Olmsted County, Minnesota [2], 0.4% in a study of nine health maintenance organizations (HMOs) in the USA [4], and approximately 0.5% in Canada [5]. If these estimates from 2001 are extrapolated to the current population of the USA and Canada, they imply that between 636 000 and 803 000 Americans and Canadians suffer from ulcerative colitis and that between 430 000 and 899 000 carry a diagnosis of Crohn's disease, for a combined total of between 1.1 and 1.7 million persons.

In general, the incidence of inflammatory bowel disease has continued to rise since these clinical entities were first recognized. There was a suggestion in some high-incidence areas of a rapid postwar rise in incidence until the late 1960s and early 1970s, and then a stabilizing of the incidence rate in the 1980s and 1990s [6,7], but the finding of a "plateau in incidence" was not universal. Furthermore, several recent studies in areas with excellent longitudinal data have demonstrated a continued increase in incidence rates [8,9]. As a consequence of rising incidence rates and normal or near-normal life expectancy with these conditions, the prevalence of both Crohn's disease and ulcerative colitis has continued gradually to rise.

Risk factors for disease

Age and gender

In a systematic review of the epidemiology of Crohn's disease from population-based cohorts from North America, the mean age at diagnosis ranged from 33 to 39 years [10]. The median age at diagnosis of Crohn's disease among Olmsted County residents in 2000 was 29 years (range 4–91 years) [2]. Whether there still exists a "bimodal distribution" in the age of onset of Crohn's disease is controversial, because a number of population-based studies no longer demonstrate this [2,11]. For ulcerative colitis, the average age at diagnosis tends to be slightly higher – in Olmsted County, median age of colitis diagnosis was 33 years (range 1–88 years). Some (but not all) recent studies have demonstrated a gender divergence in incidence of ulcerative colitis later in life [2,11], in that men are significantly more likely to be diagnosed with colitis in the sixth or seventh decades of life than women. The mechanism for the divergence remains undiscovered, but some have speculated that differential patterns of cigarette smoking status might play a role.

There may exist slight differences in IBD incidence by gender. Males are more likely than females to develop ulcerative colitis [7], while there may be a very slight female predominance in Crohn's disease.

Geography

Ulcerative colitis and Crohn's disease have been classically described most often in developed countries in northern climates, such as northern Europe and Scandinavia, the UK and North America. However, both ulcerative colitis and Crohn's disease are being described more often in other regions, such as southern and eastern Europe [12], Asia [13], Africa and Latin America [14]. The major subtypes of IBD are truly worldwide diseases. A north–south gradient of incidence has been described in Europe, but a multicenter study from the early 1990s suggested that this has to some extent dissipated [11]. Geographic differences in incidence from east to west have recently been identified in Canada – in general, the highest incidence rates and prevalence are noted in the maritime province of Nova Scotia, while the lowest are seen in the far western province of British Columbia [5]. However, these differences may be attributable to the higher proportion of ethnic minorities residing in British Columbia. One interesting phenomenon that has been observed in several areas with formerly low incidence rates is that ulcerative colitis is first observed in a region, followed a decade or two later by Crohn's disease [13].

Race/ethnicity

Differences in incidence and prevalence of IBD between Caucasians and other racial and ethnic groups seem to have lessened over time. A hospital-based study from Baltimore in the mid-1970s suggested that hospitalization rates for IBD among African Americans and Caucasians were becoming more similar [15]. The prevalence rate of Crohn's disease among African Americans was two-thirds that of White people in a study from a southern California HMO [16]. In a referral center-based study from Georgia, it was suggested that African American children were equally likely as Caucasian children to develop Crohn's disease [17].

Less data are available for Hispanic people and Asian Americans. The southern California HMO study suggested that both groups were significantly less likely to develop Crohn's disease [16]. There is an anecdotal sense that IBD, especially ulcerative colitis, is becoming more common among Mexican Americans [18], but the exact risk has not yet been quantified. In Manitoba, Canada, it is clear that aboriginal Canadians are significantly less likely to develop IBD [19].

In military veteran studies that are now almost 50 years old, those of Jewish ancestry had a markedly increased risk of IBD relative to non-Jewish Caucasians. A study from Wales later confirmed this difference [20]. Population-based investigations in Israel suggested that Ashkenazi Jews from Europe and the USA were more likely to develop IBD than Sephardic Jews from the Mediterranean region, but these differences have narrowed in succeeding generations [21,22].

Studies of migrant populations yield clues that environmental factors and/or lifestyle play a role in risk differences. South Asians who move to the UK are within one generation actually at greater risk of developing ulcerative colitis than people of European descent, and within the South Asian population Sikhs may be at greater risk for colitis than Hindus and Muslims [23,24]. Furthermore, South Asians who move to Singapore are at increased risk of colitis relative to ethnic Chinese and Malays [25].

Socioeconomic factors

The data are mildly conflicting, but in general there is a positive correlation between socioeconomic class and the risk of inflammatory bowel disease. For example, in a study from Manitoba, incidence rates from postal codes in the top tertile of income were 20% higher than rates from postal codes in the lowest tertile of income [19]. Another study from Manitoba incorporating census data on education and income could not demonstrate a relationship between these variables and IBD risk [26]. Nevertheless, the bulk of available data suggests that those of higher socioeconomic status are at increased risk for IBD.

Familial aggregation/genetics

Both familial aggregation studies and twin studies suggest that genetic factors play a role in susceptibility to these conditions. The relative risk of IBD for a sibling of a proband with IBD ranges from 15 to 35 for Crohn's disease and from 7 to 17 for ulcerative colitis [27]. Twin studies from Scandinavia and the UK demonstrate a concordance for Crohn's disease ranging from 20% to 50% for monozygotic twins versus 0% to 7% for dizygotic twins [28]. For ulcerative colitis, the concordance ranges from 14% to 19% for monozygotic twins and from 0% to 7% for dizygotic twins. Both types of studies suggest that genetic influences are stronger in Crohn's disease than in ulcerative colitis.

The search for susceptibility genes in IBD has employed both candidate gene investigations and genome-wide scans. Several susceptibility loci have been identified. In 2001, several groups reported that *NOD2/CARD15* was the gene at the IBD1 susceptibility locus, and this association has been confirmed in numerous populations [29–31]. Up to 30–40% of Crohn's disease patients carry at least one of three polymorphisms of this gene, which encodes a protein that recognizes muramyl dipeptide, a bacterial antigen. The relative risk of Crohn's disease in heterozygotes for one of the mutations is 2–3, while the risk in homozygotes or compound heterozygotes may be 40 times that of the general population. Other genes, such as *OCTN1* and *OCTN2*, are strongly suspected, but not proven, to be IBD susceptibility genes [32]. A recent genome-wide scan suggested that a polymorphism in the interleukin-23 receptor (*IL23R*) gene may be strongly protective against the development of Crohn's disease [33].

Cigarette smoking

The curious inverse relationship between cigarette smoking and ulcerative colitis has been recognized for 25 years. Current smokers are 20–90% less likely to develop ulcerative colitis than non-smokers. A recent meta-analysis using rigorous criteria pooled the results of 13 studies and estimated a pooled risk reduction of 42% [34]. Conversely, former smokers have an 80% greater risk of ulcerative colitis than never-smokers [34]. The mechanism behind this association remains unclear, but effects on rectal blood flow, colonic mucus production, mucosal IgA production, and synthesis of prostaglandins, leukotrienes and cytokines have been variously implicated. Smoking status may affect the clinical course of ulcerative colitis. Current smokers are half as likely to require hospitalization, while ex-smokers are twice as likely to undergo colectomy [35]. Transdermal nicotine is superior to placebo for clinical improvement of ulcerative colitis, but it does not appear to be superior to placebo for induction of clinical remission [36,37].

A number of studies have suggested that cigarette smoking is a risk factor for Crohn's disease. The aforementioned meta-analysis pooled the results of nine studies and estimated that current smokers are 76% more likely than non-smokers to develop Crohn's disease [34]. Moreover, active smokers who have Crohn's disease have a more severe clinical course than non-smokers, as measured by need for additional surgery after resection and need for immunosuppressive drugs [38,39]. Indeed, patients who quit smoking actually have an improved clinical course, with fewer exacerbations and less need for corticosteroids or immunosuppressives than those who continued to smoke [40].

Appendectomy

Next to cigarette smoking, a history of appendectomy is the best-established risk modifier in IBD. The inverse association between appendectomy and ulcerative colitis was first noted 20 years ago [41], and this relationship has been confirmed numerous times. A 2002 meta-analysis of 17 case-control studies yielded a pooled relative risk of 0.3; in other words, a nearly 70% risk reduction in ulcerative colitis following an appendectomy [42]. A large Swedish cohort study suggested that the indication for appendectomy influenced the magnitude of protective effect [43]. The incidence of ulcerative colitis among the 212 000 people who had undergone appendectomy was approximately 75% that of the controls who had not undergone the procedure, but there was no protective effect if appendectomy had been performed for abdominal pain (i.e., no clear-cut evidence of appendicitis). Several reports have also suggested that ulcerative colitis occurring after appendectomy has a milder clinical course, with lower likelihood of requiring immunosuppressive therapy or colectomy [44,45], but data are conflicting [46].

The relationship between appendectomy and risk of Crohn's disease is less clear [47]. Although most studies suggest that appendectomy increases the risk of Crohn's disease, one has to take into account the fact that the highest risk is seen in the first year after appendectomy, suggesting that the results may be confounded by patients presenting with acute abdominal pain, undergoing appendectomy, but in actuality having Crohn's ileitis. If patients developing Crohn's disease within one year of appendectomy are eliminated from analyses, the relative risks are still elevated, but not to the same magnitude [48].

Oral contraceptives

Analyses of oral contraceptives as a risk factor for IBD have yielded conflicting results, with some studies suggesting as much as a five-fold elevated risk of Crohn's disease in women who had used oral contraceptives for at least 6 years [49], but other studies demonstrating no association. An outdated meta-analysis estimated the pooled relative risk to be 1.4 for Crohn's disease and 1.3 for ulcerative colitis (the latter value was not statistically significant). Most subsequent studies have demonstrated similarly weak associations, but the most notable recent study, employing 444 incident cases of IBD and 10 000 controls from the UK, suggested a stronger association [50]. Users of oral contraceptives were two to three times more likely than non-users to develop IBD. In the same study, women on hormone replacement therapy were more than twice as likely to develop Crohn's disease as women not on such therapy, but no association with ulcerative colitis was detected [50]. Data on the effect of oral contraceptives on the clinical course of IBD are conflicting.

Antibiotics

Perhaps alteration of the intestinal microenvironment could serve as a trigger for inflammation in susceptible individuals. The role of antibiotics in the risk of IBD has been explored in several studies, and significant associations have been observed [41,51]. The strongest of these studies was a nested case-control study from a large database in the UK, where all prescriptions were recorded prospectively [52]. The use of antibiotics in the preceding 2–5 years increased the risk of Crohn's disease by 32%, after adjusting for age, gender and smoking.

Diet

Although it is logical and tempting to blame dietary factors on the increasing incidence of IBD, to date there is no definitive proof that a particular diet is protective or a risk factor. Studies examining this relationship are difficult to perform, because attempts to recall prediagnosis dietary intake are inaccurate. The most consistent relationship has been between Crohn's disease and sugar – numerous case-control studies have detected significant associations between Crohn's disease and intake of refined sugar [53], but there has always been concern that this association may be skewed by the fact that patients with Crohn's disease may have altered their diet in an attempt to control their symptoms. A recent Japanese case-control study suggested that higher consumption of sweets was significantly associated with the risk of ulcerative colitis, while higher consumption of sugars, sweets, fats and fish were associated with Crohn's disease risk [54].

Hygiene hypothesis

It has been observed that the incidence of allergic and immune-mediated diseases (e.g., asthma, multiple sclerosis) has risen in industrialized countries. There exists in the asthma and diabetes literature a "hygiene hypothesis," such that lack of exposure to pathogens predisposes one to disease, perhaps because of a failure to induce tolerance. Such a hypothesis might explain a higher incidence of IBD in developed countries as well as the association between higher socioeconomic status and risk of IBD. Several recent studies have examined the influence of a clean household environment during childhood on the risk of IBD and have yielded conflicting results [55–58].

Infection

The role of infection in promoting IBD risk is confusing, because a number of studies suggest that certain childhood infections may actually increase, not decrease, IBD risk. Recurrent respiratory infections in childhood, perinatal infections, recurrent pharyngitis in childhood, periodontitis and hand-foot-mouth disease have all been associated with Crohn's disease [41,51,59,60]. A large cohort study from the UK found that the risk of IBD, especially Crohn's disease, was at least twice as high among those developing acute gastroenteritis compared with healthy controls [61].

Mycobacterium avium paratuberculosis (MAP) causes a granulomatous wasting disease in cattle called Johne's disease. MAP was first cultured from the intestinal tissue of Crohn's disease patients over 20 years ago, but confirmatory reports have been inconsistent. Concerns about a lack of specificity of this finding have been raised, because atypical mycobacteria can be recovered from healthy controls. Polymerase chain reaction (PCR) technology has been utilized to recover mycobacterial DNA from the intestinal tissue of Crohn's disease patients, but the relatively high rate of recovery from controls again raises questions about the specificity of this finding. In a provocative study from Florida, MAP DNA could be extracted from buffy coat preparations of 46% of Crohn's patients compared with 20% in controls, and viable MAP could be cultured from the blood of 50% of Crohn's disease patients versus none of the controls [62]. What cannot be explained by the MAP theory of Crohn's disease is why patients seem to improve, not worsen, with infliximab, which is known to cause reactivation of latent *Mycobacterium tuberculosis*.

Natural history and mortality

Ideally, natural history studies should be performed in a population-based fashion, patients should be followed from time of diagnosis, and follow-up should be long enough and complete enough to measure the outcome of interest. Because ulcerative colitis and Crohn's disease are diseases of a lifetime, and important events such as surgery occur relatively infrequently, well-designed natural history studies are scarce.

For Crohn's disease, after the first 2 years post-diagnosis, the course is waxing and waning [63]. At any given point in time after the first 2 years, approximately 30% of patients have moderate to high disease activity, 15% have low disease activity, and 55% are in symptomatic remission. For individual patients, of course, the disease activity may change from year to year. Roughly 25% have continuously active disease, 20% remain in prolonged remission, and the other 55% have a waxing and waning course [63]. Estimates of the cumulative probability of at least one surgical resection range from 64% at 30 years post-diagnosis [64] to 82% at 20 years [65].

For ulcerative colitis, at any given point in time, 40–50% of patients who have not undergone colectomy are in remission, and the remainder have active disease [66]. Only about 10% of patients will experience prolonged symptomatic remission, but only 1% have continuously active disease. Ninety percent have a waxing and waning course. For ulcerative colitis, estimates of the cumulative risk of requiring colectomy range from 28% at 30 years post-diagnosis [67] to 30% at 30 years [68].

Colorectal cancer risk is increased in ulcerative colitis, but recent studies indicate that the risk has decreased markedly [68,69], but it is not yet clear if this is due to more widespread use of aminosalicylates, more frequent colonoscopic surveillance, judicious use of colectomy, or other factors [70]. In Crohn's disease, the relative risk of small bowel cancer is elevated, as is the risk of colorectal cancer in those with colonic involvement [69,71].

Recent mortality rates in Crohn's disease, with few exceptions, are higher than those seen in the general population, ranging from 20% higher than expected [72] to almost twice as high as expected [73]. There is as yet no satisfactory explanation for these differences in relative mortality. Approximately one-third of Crohn's disease patients die from disease-related complications. In ulcerative colitis, mortality rates have decreased significantly over time, such that several recent studies have found either similar or decreased mortality compared with the general population [72,74,75]. Roughly 20% of patients die from colitis-related complications, and there is a suggestion that colitis patients are less likely to die from cardiovascular causes, perhaps due to the inverse association with cigarette smoking [72,75].

Disability and quality of life

Patients with IBD have higher rates of disability than the general population, and quality of life for many patients is diminished. A case-control study from the Netherlands showed a full-time employment rate of 61% for male Crohn's disease patients and 65% for those with ulcerative colitis, compared with 75% for controls [76]. Overall disability rates for males were 33% for Crohn's, 28% for colitis and 12% for the controls, resulting in disability rates that were more than twice that expected. In Norway, 25% of women with Crohn's disease were collecting disability pensions [77]. Among participants in the ACCENT I trial of maintenance infliximab for Crohn's disease, 39% were unemployed and 25% were receiving disability compensation [78]. Numerous studies have indicated that health-related quality of life is diminished in both Crohn's disease and ulcerative colitis, and that this is largely driven by disease activity.

Healthcare utilization and costs

Several reports indicate that IBD patients are more likely than members of the general population to have an outpatient visit, to see a specialist, and to require an emergency room visit or overnight hospitalization [79,80]. They are more likely than non-IBD patients to use prescription medication. Much of the resource utilization seems to occur in the first 5 years after diagnosis [79,80]. The average annual direct costs of Crohn's disease have ranged from $6561 in 1990 to $12 417 in 1994 [81]. Furthermore, in Sweden it was estimated that indirect costs of these conditions (lost work productivity, early retirement) account for two-thirds of the total costs [82].

Recommendations for future studies

Many of the observations made in these retrospective studies ideally should be confirmed in different populations. We need to understand better the reasons for disparities in outcomes between different regions or countries – are these due to differences in disease severity (and if so, why?), treatment strategy or quality of care? There are hints in the recent literature that biologic agents may be able to alter the occurrence of "hard outcomes" such as hospitalization and surgery, and further studies are required to confirm definitively these observations.

Conclusions

Although etiopathogenic hypotheses abound, Crohn's disease and ulcerative colitis remain idiopathic. The incidence and prevalence of these conditions continue to increase. Cigarette smoking and appendectomy are well-established risk modifiers. The hygiene hypothesis is intriguing but remains unproven. Over time these conditions result in hospitalization, surgery, disability and sometimes mortality. There is hope that newer treatment agents might be able to alter the natural history of IBD.

References

1. Lennard-Jones JE. Classification of inflammatory bowel disease. *Scand J Gastroenterol Suppl* 1989;**170**:2.
2. Loftus CG *et al.* Update on the incidence and prevalence of Crohn's disease and ulcerative colitis in Olmsted County, Minnesota, 1940–2000. *Inflamm Bowel Dis* 2007;**13** (in press).
3. Green C *et al.* A population-based ecologic study of inflammatory bowel disease: searching for etiologic clues. *Am J Epidemiol* 2006;**164**:615; discussion 624.
4. Herrinton LJ *et al.* Estimation of the period prevalence of inflammatory bowel disease among nine health plans using computerized diagnoses and outpatient pharmacy dispens-

ings. *Inflamm Bowel Dis* 2007;**13** (in press).

5. Bernstein CN *et al.* The epidemiology of inflammatory bowel disease in Canada: a population-based study. *Am J Gastroenterol* 2006;**101**:1559.

6. Loftus EV Jr *et al.* Crohn's disease in Olmsted County, Minnesota, 1940–1993: incidence, prevalence, and survival. *Gastroenterology* 1998;**114**:1161. [Published erratum appears in *Gastroenterology* 1999;**116**:1507.]

7. Loftus EV Jr *et al.* Ulcerative colitis in Olmsted County, Minnesota, 1940–1993: incidence, prevalence, and survival. *Gut* 2000;**46**:336.

8. Lapidus A. Crohn's disease in Stockholm County during 1990–2001: an epidemiological update. *World J Gastroenterol* 2006;**12**:75.

9. Vind I *et al.* Increasing incidences of inflammatory bowel disease and decreasing surgery rates in Copenhagen City and County, 2003–2005: a population-based study from the Danish Crohn colitis database. *Am J Gastroenterol* 2006;**101**:1274.

10. Loftus EV Jr *et al.* The epidemiology and natural history of Crohn's disease in population-based patient cohorts from North America: a systematic review. *Aliment Pharmacol Ther* 2002;**16**:51.

11. Shivananda S *et al.* Incidence of inflammatory bowel disease across Europe: is there a difference between north and south? Results of the European Collaborative Study on Inflammatory Bowel Disease (EC-IBD). *Gut* 1996;**39**:690.

12. Lakatos L *et al.* Is the incidence and prevalence of inflammatory bowel diseases increasing in Eastern Europe? *Postgrad Med J* 2006;**82**:332.

13. Ouyang Q *et al.* The emergence of inflammatory bowel disease in the Asian Pacific region. *Curr Opin Gastroenterol* 2005;**21**:408.

14. Loftus EV Jr. Clinical epidemiology of inflammatory bowel disease: Incidence, prevalence, and environmental influences. *Gastroenterology* 2004;**126**:1504.

15. Calkins BM *et al.* Trends in incidence rates of ulcerative colitis and Crohn's disease. *Dig Dis Sci* 1984;**29**:913.

16. Kurata JH *et al.* Crohn's disease among ethnic groups in a large health maintenance organization. *Gastroenterology* 1992;**102**:1940.

17. Ogunbi SO *et al.* Inflammatory bowel disease in African-American children living in Georgia. *J Pediatr* 1998;**133**:103.

18. Basu D *et al.* Impact of race and ethnicity on inflammatory bowel disease. *Am J Gastroenterol* 2005;**100**:2254.

19. Blanchard JF *et al.* Small-area variations and sociodemographic correlates for the incidence of Crohn's disease and ulcerative colitis. *Am J Epidemiol* 2001;**154**:328.

20. Mayberry JF *et al.* Crohn's disease in Jewish people – an epidemiological study in south-east Wales. *Digestion* 1986;**35**:237.

21. Fireman Z *et al.* Epidemiology of Crohn's disease in the Jewish population of central Israel, 1970–1980. *Am J Gastroenterol* 1989;**84**:255.

22. Odes HS *et al.* Epidemiology of Crohn's disease in southern Israel. *Am J Gastroenterol* 1994;**89**:1859.

23. Probert CS *et al.* Epidemiological study of ulcerative proctocolitis in Indian migrants and the indigenous population of Leicestershire. *Gut* 1992;**33**:687.

24. Carr I *et al.* The effects of migration on ulcerative colitis: A three-year prospective study among Europeans and first- and second-generation South Asians in Leicester (1991–1994). *Am J Gastroenterol* 1999;**94**:2918.

25. Lee YM *et al.* Racial differences in the prevalence of ulcerative colitis and Crohn's disease in Singapore. *J Gastroenterol Hepatol* 2000;**15**:622.

26. Bernstein CN *et al.* The relationship between inflammatory bowel disease and socioeconomic variables. *Am J Gastroenterol* 2001;**96**:2117.

27. Tamboli CP *et al.* What are the major arguments in favour of the genetic susceptibility for inflammatory bowel disease? *Eur J Gastroenterol Hepatol* 2003;**15**:587.

28. Halme L *et al.* Family and twin studies in inflammatory bowel disease. *World J Gastroenterol* 2006;**12**:3668.

29. Hugot JP *et al.* Association of NOD2 leucine-rich repeat variants with susceptibility to Crohn's disease. *Nature* 2001;**411**:599.

30. Ogura Y *et al.* A frameshift mutation in NOD2 associated with susceptibility to Crohn's disease. *Nature* 2001;**411**:603.

31. Hampe J *et al.* Association between insertion mutation in NOD2 gene and Crohn's disease in German and British populations. *Lancet* 2001;**357**:1925.

32. Noble CL *et al.* The contribution of OCTN1/2 variants within the IBD5 locus to disease susceptibility and severity in Crohn's disease. *Gastroenterology* 2005;**129**:1854.

33. Duerr RH *et al.* A genome-wide association study identifies IL23R as an inflammatory bowel disease gene. *Science* 2006;**314**:1461.

34. Mahid SS *et al.* Smoking and inflammatory bowel disease: A meta-analysis. *Mayo Clinic Proc* 2006;**81**:1462.

35. Boyko EJ *et al.* Effects of cigarette smoking on the clinical course of ulcerative colitis. *Scand J Gastroenterol* 1988;**23**:1147.

36. Pullan RD *et al.* Transdermal nicotine for active ulcerative colitis. *N Engl J Med* 1994;**330**:811.

37. Sandborn WJ *et al.* Transdermal nicotine for mildly to moderately active ulcerative colitis – a randomized, double-blind, placebo-controlled trial. *Ann Intern Med* 1997;**126**:364.

38. Timmer A *et al.* Oral contraceptive use and smoking are risk factors for relapse in Crohn's disease. The Canadian Mesalamine for Remission of Crohn's Disease Study Group. *Gastroenterology* 1998;**114**:1143.

39. Cosnes J *et al.* Effects of current and former cigarette smoking on the clinical course of Crohn's disease. *Aliment Pharmacol Ther* 1999;**13**:1403.

40. Cosnes J *et al.* Smoking cessation and the course of Crohn's disease: An intervention study. *Gastroenterology* 2001;**120**:1093.

41. Gilat T *et al.* Childhood factors in ulcerative colitis and Crohn's disease. An international cooperative study. *Scand J*

Gastroenterol 1987;**22**:1009.

42. Koutroubakis IE *et al*. Role of appendicitis and appendectomy in the pathogenesis of ulcerative colitis: a critical review. *Inflamm Bowel Dis* 2002;**8**:277.

43. Andersson RE *et al*. Appendectomy and protection against ulcerative colitis. *N Engl J Med* 2001;**344**:808.

44. Radford-Smith GL *et al*. Protective role of appendicectomy on onset and severity of ulcerative colitis and Crohn's disease. *Gut* 2002;**51**:808.

45. Cosnes J *et al*. Effects of appendicectomy on the course of ulcerative colitis. *Gut* 2002;**51**:803.

46. Selby WS *et al*. Appendectomy protects against the development of ulcerative colitis but does not affect its course. *Am J Gastroenterol* 2002;**97**:2834.

47. Radford-Smith GL. The role of the appendix and appendectomy in patients with IBD. *IBD Monitor* 2003;**4**:120.

48. Andersson RE *et al*. Appendectomy is followed by increased risk of Crohn's disease. *Gastroenterology* 2003;**124**:40.

49. Boyko EJ *et al*. Increased risk of inflammatory bowel disease associated with oral contraceptive use. *Am J Epidemiol* 1994;**140**:268.

50. Garcia Rodriguez LA *et al*. Risk factors for inflammatory bowel disease in the general population. *Aliment Pharmacol Ther* 2005;**22**:309.

51. Wurzelmann JI *et al*. Childhood infections and the risk of inflammatory bowel disease. *Dig Dis Sci* 1994;**39**:555.

52. Card T *et al*. Antibiotic use and the development of Crohn's disease. *Gut* 2004;**53**:246.

53. Riordan AM *et al*. A review of associations between Crohn's disease and consumption of sugars. *Eur J Clin Nutr* 1998;**52**:229.

54. Sakamoto N *et al*. Dietary risk factors for inflammatory bowel disease – A multicenter case-control study in Japan. *Inflamm Bowel Dis* 2005;**11**:154.

55. Baron S *et al*. Environmental risk factors in paediatric inflammatory bowel diseases: a population based case control study. *Gut* 2005;**54**:357.

56. Amre DK *et al*. Investigating the hygiene hypothesis as a risk factor in pediatric onset Crohn's disease: A case-control study. *Am J Gastroenterol* 2006;**101**:1005.

57. Bernstein CN *et al*. A population-based case control study of potential risk factors for IBD. *Am J Gastroenterol* 2006;**101**:993.

58. Lashner BA *et al*. True or false? The hygiene hypothesis for Crohn's disease. *Am J Gastroenterol* 2006;**101**:1003.

59. Ekbom A *et al*. Perinatal risk factors for inflammatory bowel disease: a case-control study. *Am J Epidemiol* 1990;**132**:1111.

60. Van Kruiningen HJ *et al*. Environmental factors in familial Crohn's disease in Belgium. *Inflamm Bowel Dis* 2005;**11**:360.

61. Garcia Rodriguez LA *et al*. Acute gastroenteritis is followed by an increased risk of inflammatory bowel disease. *Gastroenterology* 2006;**130**:1588.

62. Naser SA *et al*. Culture of *Mycobacterium avium* subspecies *paratuberculosis* from the blood of patients with Crohn's disease. *Lancet* 2004;**364**:1039.

63. Munkholm P *et al*. Disease activity courses in a regional cohort of Crohn's disease patients. *Scand J Gastroenterol* 1995;**30**:699.

64. Dhillon S *et al*. The natural history of surgery for Crohn's disease in a population-based cohort from Olmsted County, Minnesota (abstract). *Am J Gastroenterol* 2005;**100**:S305.

65. Munkholm P *et al*. Intestinal cancer risk and mortality in patients with Crohn's disease. *Gastroenterology* 1993;**105**:1716.

66. Langholz E *et al*. Course of ulcerative colitis: analysis of changes in disease activity over years. *Gastroenterology* 1994;**107**:3.

67. Dhillon S *et al*. The natural history of surgery for ulcerative colitis in a population-based cohort from Olmsted County, Minnesota (abstract). *Am J Gastroenterol* 2005;**100**:S303.

68. Winther KV *et al*. Long-term risk of cancer in ulcerative colitis: a population-based cohort study from Copenhagen County. *Clin Gastroenterol Hepatol* 2004;**2**:1088.

69. Jess T *et al*. Risk of intestinal cancer in inflammatory bowel disease: a population-based study from Olmsted County, Minnesota. *Gastroenterology* 2006;**130**:1039.

70. Loftus EV. Epidemiology and risk factors for colorectal dysplasia and cancer in ulcerative colitis. *Gastroenterol Clin N* 2006;**35**:517.

71. Jess T *et al*. Intestinal and extra-intestinal cancer in Crohn's disease: follow-up of a population-based cohort in Copenhagen County, Denmark. *Aliment Pharmacol Ther* 2004;**19**:287.

72. Jess T *et al*. Survival and cause specific mortality in patients with inflammatory bowel disease: a long term outcome study in Olmsted County, Minnesota, 1940–2004. *Gut* 2006;**55**:1248.

73. Wolters FL *et al*. Crohn's disease: increased mortality 10 years after diagnosis in a Europe-wide population based cohort. *Gut* 2006;**55**:510.

74. Winther KV *et al*. Survival and cause-specific mortality in ulcerative colitis: follow-up of a population-based cohort in Copenhagen County. *Gastroenterology* 2003;**125**:1576.

75. Masala G *et al*. Divergent patterns of total and cancer mortality in ulcerative colitis and Crohn's disease patients: the Florence IBD study 1978–2001. *Gut* 2004;**53**:1309.

76. Boonen A *et al*. The impact of inflammatory bowel disease on labor force participation: Results of a population sampled case-control study. *Inflamm Bowel Dis* 2002;**8**:382.

77. Bernklev T *et al*. Relationship between sick leave, unemployment, disability, and health-related quality of life in patients with inflammatory bowel disease. *Inflamm Bowel Dis* 2006;**12**:402.

78. Feagan BG *et al*. Unemployment and disability in patients with moderately to severely active Crohn's disease. *J Clin Gastroenterol* 2005;**39**:390.

79. Longobardi T *et al*. Utilization of health care resources by individuals with inflammatory bowel disease in the United

States: a profile of time since diagnosis. *Am J Gastroenterol* 2004;**99**:650.

80. Longobardi T *et al*. Health care resource utilization in inflammatory bowel disease. *Clin Gastroenterol Hepatol* 2006;**4**:731.

81. Bodger K. Cost of illness of Crohn's disease. *Pharmacoeconomics* 2002;**20**:639.

82. Blomqvist P *et al*. Inflammatory bowel diseases: health care and costs in Sweden in 1994. *Scand J Gastroenterol* 1997;**32**:1134.

28 Fecal Incontinence

Adil E. Bharucha

Key points

- Fecal incontinence is a common symptom among nursing-home residents and also in the community, where the prevalence varies from 2.2% to 15%.
- Though most attention has focused on women, the prevalence of fecal incontinence in men is comparable with that in women.
- Fecal incontinence results from weakness of the pelvic floor muscles (i.e., the anal sphincters and/or the levator ani) and/or

diarrhea. Anal sphincter weakness, often attributable to obstetric anal sphincter injury and/or a pudendal neuropathy, and functional diarrhea are the commonest predisposing causes of fecal incontinence in women.

- Though the symptom significantly impacts on quality of life and is associated with psychosocial distress, only a minority of patients will discuss the symptom with family members or a physician, partly due to embarrassment.

Introduction

Fecal incontinence (FI) is the involuntary loss of feces – solid or liquid. Anal incontinence includes involuntary loss of feces and flatus. Although incontinence for flatus can be embarrassing, patients find it difficult to quantify flatus incontinence, and there is no cut-off to discriminate inadvertent expulsion of gas from incontinence. Most epidemiologic studies and the Rome criteria [1] are based on fecal rather than anal incontinence. Some epidemiologic studies on FI have excluded leakage during short-term diarrheal illnesses (e.g., acute gastroenteritis) [2,3].

Our understanding of the epidemiology and pathophysiology of FI is predominantly derived from selected populations (e.g., tertiary care centers) rather than community patients. These studies suggest that FI occurs in conditions associated with pelvic floor weakness and/or altered bowel habits, particularly diarrhea [4], and can impact on nearly every aspect of daily life [5]. At the extreme, individuals with FI may withdraw from social contact and remain tethered to the toilet in an attempt to minimize incontinence [6]. FI may also contribute to institutionalization: up to 50% of nursing-home residents in one survey had FI [7]. Despite these potentially devastating consequences, it is unclear why only a small proportion of incontinent patients discuss the symptom with a physician [2,8,9]. Therefore, physicians tend to underestimate the personal impact of FI [6]. Moreover, results of clinic-based studies on FI cannot be extrapolated to the entire

population, and community-based studies are essential to understand the risk factors, clinical spectrum and personal impact of FI. Where possible, this chapter will focus on evidence derived from large population-based studies on the epidemiology of FI.

Methodologic considerations

Survey techniques

Most studies on the epidemiology of FI have used a mailed questionnaire. Two large studies were conducted by telephone [8,10]. In the Chicago Health and Aging Project (CHAP) survey, subjects were interviewed at home [11]. Patients with FI are reluctant, perhaps embarrassed, to discuss the symptom [9], not only with physicians but also with family members and friends, which perhaps explains why the prevalence of FI was lower in surveys conducted by interviewing only one member of the household by phone (e.g., the Wisconsin survey) [10] compared with a mailed questionnaire [2,12].

Assessing severity of fecal incontinence and its impact on quality of life

There are several instruments for rating the severity of FI. However, these scales suffer from one or more limitations and there is no agreed threshold to identify clinically significant FI. First, most scales for rating symptom severity in FI incorporate the frequency and type, but not the amount of leakage [13–16]. Without the latter, FI severity would be identical for two subjects, one of whom had minor staining and the other a large liquid bowel movement once a week. Second, only one questionnaire (i.e., the St Marks severity rating system) incorporates urgency, assigning a score of 0 to 4 for patients who can or cannot defer defecation for 15 minutes, respectively [15]. It is important to incorporate rectal urgency in assessing the severity of FI because patients with urge FI and rectal hypersensitivity have more frequent stools, use more pads, and report more lifestyle restrictions compared with patients with normal rectal sensation [17]. However, this threshold (i.e., 15 minutes) for discriminating normal from excessive rectal urgency is relatively liberal, because clinical observations suggest a majority of incontinent patients are unable or reluctant to defer defecation for 15 minutes. Third, concerns have been raised about the weighting of variables in existing scales, which assume that different components (e.g., amount and frequency) are equally important in determining the severity of FI [16]. However, patients and colorectal surgeons disagree on the relative impact of different symptoms. For example, patients assigned a higher severity score to incontinence for flatus compared with physicians; conversely, physicians assigned a higher severity score for solid stool incontinence compared with patients. Finally, most symptom severity scales do not shed light on the impact of FI on quality of life (QOL). Thus, separate scales have been devised for assessing the impact of FI on QOL [18].

To overcome these limitations, we developed and validated a scale for rating symptom severity in FI that includes four components – frequency of FI, type of FI, amount of FI and circumstances surrounding FI (i.e., urge or passive FI) – derived from a self-report questionnaire – the Fecal Incontinence and Constipation Assessment (FICA) [19] (Table 28.1) The symptom-severity score was devised *a priori* to be user friendly by assigning arbitrary weights (i.e., 0, 1, 2 and 3) for symptoms within each category (e.g., frequency of FI). Subjects who reported they often (i.e., >25% of time) or usually (i.e., >75%) experienced an "urgent need to empty their bowels" making them rush to the toilet were considered to have rectal urgency. Subjects who often (i.e., >25% of time) or usually (i.e., >75%) "leaked liquid or solid stool without any warning" were considered to have passive incontinence. Patients who did not report symptoms of urge or passive incontinence were classified as "neither," while those who had symptoms of urge and passive incontinence were classified as "combined" incontinence. In contrast to urinary incontinence [20], this

FI symptom severity scale was strongly correlated with a QOL-weighted symptom severity score, suggesting that the symptom severity score, which is simple to use in the office, is a reasonable indication not only of the physical manifestations of FI (i.e., symptom severity), but also of its impact on quality of life [21]. This strong correlation dispels the concern that measures of stool leakage may underestimate the severity of FI in people who avoid FI by staying close to a toilet (e.g., by staying at home) [22].

Perry *et al.* characterized the severity of FI as rare or no FI, minor FI and major FI [23]. Those who leaked several times a year or less were characterized as rare incontinence regardless of the extent of soiling. Infrequent leakage was attributed to a coincident acute illness rather than a chronic condition. Minor incontinence was defined as staining of underwear several times a month or more often. Major FI was defined as soiling of underwear, outer clothing, furnishing or bedding several times a month or more often. However, the reliability and validity of this simple and rational approach has not been evaluated.

Perineal protective devices

It is possible to quantify the use of devices worn to protect underclothes from FI by evaluating the type of device (i.e., panty liner, pad or diaper), the duration for which the device was worn (i.e., all the time, when awake away from home, when awake at home or when asleep), and the number of devices worn when awake (i.e., none, about one device/day, two to four devices/day, five or more devices/day) [2]. Because FI is associated with urinary incontinence, it is important to specify that devices worn only to protect against leakage of urine be excluded when responding to these items. Because the use of perineal protective devices may reflect coping strategies rather than severity of FI *per se*, this factor should not be used to gauge the severity of FI. For example, it is conceivable that fastidious people are more likely to use perineal protective devices even with mild FI.

Prevalence of FI in the community

Nelson comprehensively reviewed epidemiologic studies in FI up to 2004 [24]. Only 8 of 34 surveys in that review were community based and sampled the entire population, i.e., were unrestricted by age, residence or underlying disease. However, four of these eight studies surveyed <750 subjects, and only two studies, conducted in a market mailing sample and Wisconsin households [8,10], were

Table 28.1 Symptom-severity scale in fecal incontinence (after Bharucha *et al.* [19])

Symptoms	Score			
	1	2	3	4
Frequency	<1/month	>1/month to several times/week	Daily	
Composition	Mucus/liquid stool	Solid stool	Liquid and solid stool	
Amount	Small (i.e., staining only)	Moderate (i.e., requiring change of underwear)	Large (i.e., requiring change of all clothes)	
Urgency or passive incontinence	Neither	Passive incontinence	Urge incontinence	Combined urge and passive incontinence

The symptom severity score (maximum score = 13) is calculated by summing scores for individual components in this scale.

from the USA. Since that review, there have been three large studies on the epidemiology of FI [2,11,25].

The prevalence of FI in the population has varied among studies. Estimates range from 2.2% in Wisconsin households and 7% in a sample of US householders, to ~11–15% in Australia, in Sweden, and in Olmsted County, Minnesota (Table 28.2). Different prevalence rates among studies probably reflect varying definitions of FI, differences in survey methods, and in the age distribution of the population surveyed. Although most attention has focused on FI in women, at least one study suggests that the prevalence in men is comparable with that in women [23].

The prevalence of FI among nursing-home residents (i.e., up to 50%) is much higher compared with the general population [24]. FI is one of the commonest reasons for admission to a nursing home, perhaps explaining the strong association between nursing-home residence and FI. Community-based studies demonstrate that the prevalence of FI increases with age. However, age-related trends in the prevalence of FI vary across studies. For example, in Leicestershire, UK, the prevalence increased steadily from ~4% for any incontinence in women aged 40–49 years to 7.8% in subjects aged 70–79 years, and sharply thereafter to 11.6% in women aged 80 years and older [23]. However, in Olmsted County, the age-specific prevalence in the past year increased with age from 7% in the third decade to 22% in the sixth decade and was steady thereafter [2].

Severity of FI and its impact on quality of life

Severity

A majority of people with FI in the community have mild

symptoms. In Olmsted County, most women with FI reported infrequent symptoms (55% less than monthly), and most reported only staining of underwear (60% of those with FI) [2]. Thus, 50% of women had mild, 45% had moderate, and 5% had severe symptoms. In contrast to the prevalence of the condition, the severity of FI was not related to age.

Impact on quality of life

FI was associated with anxiety, depression and physical disability in a community-based study of subjects aged >65 years from the UK [26]. In the Wisconsin Family Health Study, 33% of subjects restricted their activities due to incontinence [10]. Studies from Leicestershire, UK, Olmsted County, Minnesota, indicate that FI impacts on quality of life (QOL) in the community. In Leicestershire, 32% of all subjects with FI and over 50% of those reporting major FI (i.e., soiling of underwear, outer clothing, furnishing or bedding several times a month or more often) reported that the symptom had "a lot of impact" on their QOL [23]. In Olmsted County, 23% of women with FI reported that the symptom had a moderate to severe impact on one or more domains of QOL [2]. Moreover, the impact of FI on QOL was clearly related to symptom severity. Thus, 6% of women with mild symptoms, 35% of women with moderate symptoms, and 82% of women with severe symptoms reported a moderate or severe impact on one or more domain of QOL. The proportion reporting moderate to severe impact for a given domain ranged from 3–4% (e.g., for family relationships, employment, sex life) to 12% (for the ability to eat outside home or going out to eat). However, differences in the impact of FI on specific domains of QOL were not significant.

Table 28.2 Epidemiology of fecal incontinence: community-based studies

Survey (year of survey)	Respondents; instrument	Response rate (no. of respondents)	Prevalence
Talley et al. [36] (1990)	Olmsted County residents ≥65 years; mailed questionnaire	66% (328)	FI once per week over past year: 3.1% (F); 4.5% (M)
Drossman et al. [8] (1990)	US householder marketing list; mailed questionnaire	66% (5430)	Soiling: 6.9%(F); 7.4%(M) Gross incontinence: 0.9% (F); 0.5% (M)
Nelson et al. [10] (1993)	Wisconsin residents of all ages; phone interview with one member in each household	73% (6959)	Any FI over past year: 2.2% (overall); 7.5% (aged ≥65)
Reilly et al. [3] (1994)	Olmsted County residents ≥50 years; mailed questionnaire	64% (1540)	Any FI: 17.8% (F); 12.8% (M)
Walter et al. [37] (2002)	County of Ostergotland (Sweden); aged 31–76 years; mailed questionnaire	81% (1610)	Liquid FI >1/month: 10.9% (F); 9.7% (M) Solid FI >1/month: 1.4% (F); 0.4% (M)
Perry et al. [23] (2002)	Leicestershire Health Authority (UK) patient register; mailed questionnaire	70% (10 226)	Any FI: 5.7% (F); 6.2% (M)
Bharucha et al. [2] (2005)	Olmsted County residents ≥20 years; mailed questionnaire	53% (2800)	Any FI: 14% (F)
Melville et al. [38] (2005)	HMO population, 30–90 years, Washington State; mailed questionnaire	64% (3536)	Loss of liquid or solid stool once/month: 7.7% (F)
Quander et al. [11] (2006)	Chicago Health and Aging Project, ≥65 years, door-to-door survey (1one member of household)	79% (6158)	

Prevalence rates for males (M) and females (F) are provided separately where available.
FI = fecal incontinence.

Risk factors for FI

FI occurs in conditions associated with pelvic floor weakness and/or altered bowel habits, particularly diarrhea [4] (Box 28.1). Few epidemiologic studies have comprehensively evaluated the multiple putative risk factors for FI (Table 28.3). In the Wisconsin Family Health Study, age, female gender, poor general health and physical limitations were risk factors for FI [10], whereas in an Australian community loose stools, urgency, perianal injury and surgery were risk factors for FI [12]. However, neither study evaluated obstetric risk factors for FI, nor the interactions among bowel symptoms, obstetric risk factors and other risk factors (e.g., prior anal surgery) for FI. We assessed individual risk factors and the interaction among risk factors (e.g., between risk factors for anal sphincter injury, rectal urgency and bowel symptoms) for FI in Olmsted County [27]. The symptom of rectal urgency was the single most important risk factor for FI in women. The risk of FI was higher among women with rectal urgency whether or not they also had bowel disturbances (i.e., constipation, diarrhea or abdominal pain) (odds ratio (OR), 8.3; 95% confidence interval (CI), 4.8–14.3) or had a vaginal delivery with forceps or stitches (OR 9.0; 95% CI, 5.6–14.4). Though rectal urgency was associated with loose stools as previously reported [28], this symptom was an independent, and much stronger risk factor for FI compared with loose stools (i.e., functional diarrhea), extending previous observations that in patients with functional bowel disorders, rectal urgency is not always associated with loose stools [28]. Indeed, the symptom of rectal urgency is associated with reduced rectal capacity, and reduced rectal

capacity is associated with rectal hypersensitivity among women with FI [29].

Because vaginal delivery can damage the anal sphincters and the pudendal nerve, up to 10% of women develop FI after a vaginal delivery [4]. The incidence of postpartum FI is considerably higher (i.e., 15–59%) in women who sustain a third-degree (i.e., anal sphincter disruption) or a fourth-degree tear (i.e., a third-degree tear with anal epithelial disruption) [30]. The only prospective study demonstrated that anal sphincter defects and pudendal nerve injury after vaginal delivery were often clinically occult and that forceps delivery was the single independent factor associated with anal sphincter damage during vaginal delivery [31]. A systematic Cochrane review concluded that maternal morbidity was lower for assisted deliveries conducted with a vacuum extractor than with forceps [32]. Another Cochrane review concluded that restrictive **episiotomy** policies were beneficial (i.e., less posterior perineal trauma, less suturing and fewer complications) compared with routine **episiotomy** policies [33]. However, there is an increased risk of anterior perineal trauma with restrictive **episiotomy.**

Based on these data, current guidelines suggest endoanal imaging to identify anal sphincter injury in women with FI. However, among unselected women with FI in the community, the symptom began before the age of 40 years in 31%, between 41 and 60 years in 37%, and between 61 and 80 years in 32% [2], suggesting that obstetric pelvic floor injury is not the only risk factor for FI among women in the community. In that study, compared with nulliparous women without anorectal injury, rectal urgency or abnormal bowel habits, the risk for FI was not significantly different among women with cesarean section or vaginal delivery without forceps or stitches (OR, 0.6; 95% CI, 0.3–1.1) and vaginal delivery with forceps or stitches (OR, 1.0; 95% CI, 0.6–1.6) [27]. In a study of female HMO enrollees from Washington state, self-reported operative (i.e., forceps or vacuum-assisted) vaginal deliveries were associated with an increased (OR, 1.52; 95% CI, 1.09–2.12) risk of FI. Because self-reported data on details (e.g., operative intervention) about vaginal deliveries are subject to recall bias, these data need to be confirmed by reviewing obstetric records. In contrast to urinary incontinence, the risk of FI was not significantly lower among women who had a cesarean section only compared with a vaginal delivery [24,34]. Further studies are necessary to clarify the risk of pelvic floor injury relative to the type of cesarean section (i.e., emergency or elective) because women who have an emergency cesarean section for stalled labor may not, in

---

Box 28.1 Common causes of fecal incontinence
- **Anal sphincter weakness:**
  –**traumatic:** obstetric, surgical (e.g., hemorrhoidectomy, internal sphincterotomy);
  –**nontraumatic:** scleroderma, internal sphincter degeneration of unknown etiology.
- **Neuropathy:** peripheral (e.g., pudendal) or generalized (e.g., diabetes mellitus).
- **Disturbances of pelvic floor:** rectal prolapse, descending perineum syndrome.
- **Inflammatory conditions:** radiation proctitis, Crohn's disease, ulcerative colitis.
- **Central nervous system disorders:** dementia, stroke, brain tumors, multiple sclerosis, spinal cord lesions.
- **Diarrhea:** irritable bowel syndrome, post-cholecystectomy diarrhea.
- **Other:** fecal retention with overflow, behavioral disorders.

Table 28.3 Risk factors for fecal incontinence (FI) in community-based studies

Survey	Risk factors significantly associated with FI	Risk factors not significantly associated with FI
Talley *et al.* [36]	None	Age and gender
Drossman *et al.* [8]	Employment (OR, 0.8; 95% CI, 0.6–1.0)	Risks associated with other sociodemographic features (e.g., income) not specified
Nelson *et al.* [10]	Age, male sex, poor general health, physical limitations	Race, marital status, employment status, educational level, launderer respondent
Reilly *et al.* [3]	Urgency, pelvic radiation and rectal/anal trauma	Unclear – published in abstract form only
Kalantar *et al.* [12]	Poor general health, perianal injury, perianal surgery	Radiation treatment to abdomen and pelvis (OR, 2.7; 95% CI, 0.8–8.9), diabetes mellitus (OR, 2.1; 95% CI, 0.7–6.3)
Bharucha *et al.* [26]	Age, rectal urgency, prior anal surgery, history of anal fissure, cholecystectomy	Vaginal delivery with forceps/stitches alone (i.e., without bowel symptoms), hysterectomy (OR, 1.3; 95% CI, 1.0–1.7), contraceptive use (OR, 1.4; 95% CI, 1.0–1.9)
Melville *et al.* [38]	Age, major depression, urinary incontinence, medical comorbidity, operative vaginal delivery	Body mass index, h/o cesarean delivery only, nulliparity
Quander *et al.* [11]	Age, low income and education, diabetes, stroke, certain medications	Gender, certain medications

Odds ratios are specified when the mean risk factor is >1.0 but the lower bound of the 95% CI is ≤1.0.

contrast to women who have an elective section, be protected against pelvic floor injury.

The risk factors for FI are strongly influenced by the age distribution of the population. In a population aged 65 years and older, self-reported diabetes mellitus (OR, 1.7; 95% CI, 1.4–2.1), self-reported stroke (OR, 2.8; 95% CI, 2.2–3.5) and certain medications were also risk factors for FI after adjusting for age, sex and race [11]. It is unclear if FI preceded or followed diabetes mellitus or stroke. Because other medical conditions and other putative risk factors for FI were not assessed, it is unclear if the increased risk was attributable to diabetes mellitus or stroke, or if these conditions were merely markers for other risk factors. In the same study, anti-Parkinsonian, hypnotic and antipsychotic medications were also associated with a 3–4-fold increased risk for FI even after adjusting for age, sex, race, stroke and diabetes. On the other hand, calcium channel blockers decreased the risk of FI whereas estrogens, diuretics, antacids, beta-blockers and benzodiazepines did not affect the risk of FI.

FI is well documented to occur even after "minor" operations (e.g., lateral internal anal sphincterotomy) [4]. In Olmsted County, prior anal surgery, a history of anal inflammation (e.g., abscess, fistula), and a cholecystectomy increased the risk for FI [24].

Health-seeking for FI

In one study, only 10% of women with FI had discussed the symptom with a physician in the preceding year [2]. Although this estimate may not include subjects who had discussed the symptom with a physician at an earlier time, it confirms other studies in which only ~20–25% of subjects with FI or irritable bowel syndrome (IBS) had discussed the symptom with a physician [8,35]. However, 48% of women with severe FI had consulted a physician for the symptom. In addition to symptom severity, general health status also independently predicted physician consulting behavior for FI. Taken together, these factors explained 15% of the variance in consulting behavior, which is similar to previous population-based studies in IBS that have addressed this issue [35,36].

Summary and a look to the future

Population-based studies in FI are important because they: (i) avoid the bias accompanying studies on the epidemiology of FI in selected populations; (ii) underscore that the symptom is common not only in nursing homes but also in the community; (iii) quantify the impact of FI on quality of life; and (iv) demonstrate that the symptom generally begins two to three decades after the initial insult to the pelvic floor, namely, vaginal delivery. While most studies have focused on women, there are limited data to suggest that the prevalence of FI is comparable in men and in women. Epidemiologic studies have also provided insights into the etiology of FI. Further studies are necessary to define the relationship between obstetric history, pelvic floor injury and FI, to evaluate the incidence and natural history of FI, and to explore the factors that influence health-seeking behavior in FI.

Acknowledgments

This work was supported in part by Grant R01 HD41129 from the National Institutes of Health, US Public Health Service.

References

1. Bharucha AE *et al.* Functional anorectal disorders. *Gastroenterology* 2006;**130**:1510.
2. Bharucha AE *et al.* Prevalence and burden of fecal incontinence: A population based study in women. *Gastroenterology* 2005;**129**:42.
3. Reilly W *et al.* Fecal incontinence: prevalence and risk factors in the community. *Gastroenterology* 1995;**108**:A32.
4. Bharucha A. Fecal incontinence. *Gastroenterology* 2003;**124**:1672.
5. Norton NJ. The perspective of the patient. *Gastroenterology* 2004;**126**:S175.
6. Miner PB Jr. Economic and personal impact of fecal and urinary incontinence. *Gastroenterology* 2004;**126**:S8.
7. Nelson R *et al.* Fecal incontinence in Wisconsin nursing homes: prevalence and associations. *Dis Colon Rectum* 1998;**41**:1226.
8. Drossman DA *et al.* U.S. householder survey of functional gastrointestinal disorders. Prevalence, sociodemography, and health impact. *Dig Dis Sci* 1993;**38**:1569.
9. Leigh RJ, Turnberg LA. Faecal incontinence: the unvoiced symptom. *Lancet* 1982;**i**:1349.
10. Nelson R *et al.* Community-based prevalence of anal incontinence. *JAMA* 1995;**274**:559.
11. Quander CR *et al.* Prevalence of and factors associated with fecal incontinence in a large community study of older individuals. *Am J Gastroenterol* 2005;**100**:905.
12. Kalantar JS *et al.* Prevalence of faecal incontinence and associated risk factors; an underdiagnosed problem in the Australian community? *Med J Aust* 2002;**176**:54.
13. Jorge JM, Wexner SD. Etiology and management of fecal in-

continence. *Dis Colon Rectum* 1993;**36**:77.
14. Pescatori M *et al.* New grading and scoring for anal incontinence. Evaluation of 335 patients. *Dis Colon Rectum* 1992;**35**:482.
15. Vaizey CJ *et al.* Prospective comparison of faecal incontinence grading systems. *Gut* 1999;**44**:77.
16. Rockwood TH *et al.* Patient and surgeon ranking of the severity of symptoms associated with fecal incontinence: the fecal incontinence severity index. *Dis Colon Rectum* 1999;**42**:1525.
17. Chan CL *et al.* Rectal hypersensitivity worsens stool frequency, urgency, and lifestyle in patients with urge fecal incontinence. *Dis Colon Rectum* 2005;**48**:134.
18. Rockwood TH *et al.* Fecal incontinence quality of life scale: quality of life instrument for patients with fecal incontinence. *Dis Colon Rectum* 2000;**43**:9; discussion 16.
19. Bharucha AE *et al.* A New Questionnaire for Constipation and Fecal Incontinence. *Aliment Pharmacol Ther* 2004;**20**:355.
20. Naughton MJ *et al.* Symptom severity and QOL scales for urinary incontinence. *Gastroenterology* 2004;**126**:S114.
21. Bharucha AE *et al.* Symptoms and quality of life in community women with fecal incontinence. *Clin Gastroenterol Hepatol* 2006;**4**:1004.
22. Rockwood TH. Incontinence severity and QOL scales for fecal incontinence. *Gastroenterology* 2004;**126**:S106.
23. Perry S *et al.* Prevalence of faecal incontinence in adults aged 40 years or more living in the community. *Gut* 2002;**50**:480.
24. Nelson RL. Epidemiology of fecal incontinence. *Gastroenterology* 2004;**126**:S3.
25. Melville JL *et al.* Fecal incontinence in US women: a population-based study. *Am J Obstet Gynecol* 2005;**193**:2071.
26. Edwards NI, Jones D. The prevalence of faecal incontinence in older people living at home. *Age Ageing* 2001;**30**:503.
27. Bharucha AE *et al.* Risk factors for fecal incontinence: a population-based study in women. *Am J Gastroenterol* 2006;**101**:1305..
28. Heaton KW *et al.* How bad are the symptoms and bowel dysfunction of patients with the irritable bowel syndrome? A prospective, controlled study with emphasis on stool form. *Gut* 1991;**32**:73.
29. Bharucha AE *et al.* Relationship between symptoms and disordered continence mechanisms in women with idiopathic fecal incontinence. *Gut* 2005;**54**:546.
30. Mostwin J *et al.* Pathophysiology of urinary incontinence, fecal incontinence and pelvic organ prolapse. In: Abrams P *et al.* (eds), *Incontinence*, vol. 1. Paris: Health Publication Ltd, 2005:425.
31. Sultan AH *et al.* Anal-sphincter disruption during vaginal delivery. *N Engl J Med* 1993;**329**:1905.
32. Johanson RB *et al.* Vacuum extraction versus forceps for assisted vaginal delivery. *Cochrane Database of Systematic Reviews* 2006.
33. Carroli G, Belizan J. Episiotomy for vaginal birth. *Cochrane Database of Systematic Reviews* 2006.
34. Rortveit G *et al.* Urinary incontinence after vaginal delivery

or cesarean section. *N Engl J Med* 2003;**348**:900.

35. Talley NJ *et al.* Epidemiology of colonic symptoms and the irritable bowel syndrome. *Gastroenterology* 1991;**101**:927.

36. Koloski NA *et al.* Predictors of conventional and alternative health care seeking for irritable bowel syndrome and functional dyspepsia. *Aliment Pharmacol Ther* 2003;**17**:841.

37. Talley NJ *et al.* Prevalence of gastrointestinal symptoms in the elderly: a population-based study. *Gastroenterology* 1992;**102**:895.

38. Walter S *et al.* A population-based study on bowel habits in a Swedish community: prevalence of faecal incontinence and constipation. *Scand J Gastroenterol* 2002;**37**:911.

29 Gallstones

Torben Jørgensen

Key points
- Gallstone disease covers a clinical spectrum from an asymptomatic condition to biliary pain to acute complications.
- Gallstone disease affects a substantial proportion of the general population in Europe and the USA.
- Gallstones are caused by an interaction between genetic susceptibility and a number of risk factors as lifestyle and biomarkers linking the disease to the metabolic syndrome.
- Among asymptomatic individuals, complications occur in less than 1% annually.

Clinical summary

Gallstone disease is a chronic condition that starts – and usually ends – as an asymptomatic condition. The disease spectrum varies from an asymptomatic state to pain to severe complications.

Intense, steady pain that arises in the right upper quadrant of the abdomen and last for several hours, eventually radiating to the back, is generally attributed to gallstones; but the pain is not specific for gallstones. When treatment is indicated, cholecystectomy is the treatment of choice. Acute cholecystitis, which is the most common complication with stones in the gallbladder, should be expected if the pain lasts longer than a few hours and is combined with tenderness under the right curvature and fever. Cholecystectomy within 72 hours is recommended. Stones that migrate from the gallbladder to the common bile duct can cause jaundice, acute cholangitis or acute pancreatitis. Diagnostic tools are ultrasonography, liver function tests and ERCP (endoscopic retrograde cholangiopancreatography). Treatment is either with cholecystectomy and surgical removal of choledochal stones or ERCP with bile duct stone clearance followed by cholecystectomy. In very rare cases gallbladder stones can cause a chronic inflammation, which erodes into the common bile duct or causes fistulation to the bile duct or intestine.

Disease definition

Gallstones refer to the presence of cholesterol or pigment stones in the gallbladder or bile duct. **Cholesterol stones** are made primarily of cholesterol crystals and calcium, and their formation is facilitated by hypersaturation of biliary cholesterol, nucleation of cholesterol monohydrate crystals, and gallbladder hypomotility. **Pigment stones** are primarily composed of calcium and bilirubin and appear in two major forms: black and brown. **Black pigment stones** are caused by hypersecretion of bilirubin, whereas **brown pigment stones** are associated with infection of the biliary tract. Cholesterol stones account for about 80–90% of all gallstones in Europe and the USA. Whereas cholesterol stones and black pigment stones are formed in the gallbladder, brown pigment stones can be formed in the common bile duct [1].

Prevalence and incidence

Earlier knowledge of prevalence came from autopsy studies showing prevalence rates higher than today. With the development of ultrasonography, a number of population-based screening studies for gallstones have been performed since the 1980s (Table 29.1). In general the greatest prevalence is found in America, followed by Europe, whereas Asia and Africa have the lowest occurrence [2], but there are great variations within the continents. In particular, the greater prevalence among Native Americans and South Americans compared with non-Hispanic White people in the USA, and the big difference between Western and Eastern Europe (except for Norway) is noteworthy. Interpretation of these prevalence rates should be done with care, as age intervals and participation rates differ between studies.

Table 29.1 Prevalence of gallstone disease in different populations in Europe, America and Asia. Only cross-sectional studies of entire or random samples of populations with at least 1000 individuals screened by ultrasonography for gallstone disease are included. Studies dealing with selected populations (e.g., blood donors, employed, children) are not included

Geography	Study	Year	Age	Number	Prevalence in % (range) Male	Female	Overall
Europe							
UK (Barry)[a]	Bainton, 1976	–	45–69	1127	6.3 (5.0–8.0)	12.1 (10.1–14.1)	9.2
Italy (Sirmione)	Barbera, 1987	1982	18–65	1911	6.7 (1.1–11.0)	14.6 (2.9–27.0)	11.0
Norway (Bergen)	Glambek, 1987	–	20–70	1371	20.3 (4.9–37.0)	23.3 (6.0–41.3)	21.9
Denmark (Copenhagen)	Jørgensen, 1987	1982–84	30–60	3608	5.7 (1.8–12.9)	11.9 (4.8–22.4)	8.8
German Democratic Republic (Schwedt)	Berndt, 1989	1986–87	All	1400	14.0 (0–24.4)	22.6 (0–53.8)	18.3
UK (Bristol)	Heaton, 1991	1987–89	25–69 (men: 40–69)	1896	6.9 (4.7–11.5)	8.0 (3.9–22.4)	7.5
Czechoslovakia (Trencin)	Bielik, 1992	–	15–92	1952	–	17.2 (0.2–58.6)	–
Czechoslovakia (Bruntal)	Zoubek, 1992	1989–90	20–59	1186	12.6	28.5 (17.6–41.4)	22.1
Italy (Chianciano)	Loria, 1994	1985–86	15–65	1804	3.7 (0–16.6)	8.4 (0–30.9)	5.9
Italy (10 regions)	Attili, 1995	1984–87	30–69	29739	9.5 (2.3–19.4)	18.9 (7.4–31.6)	14.2
Poland	Tomecki, 1995	–	16–70	10133	8.2	18	10.7
Germany (Römerstein)	Kratzer, 1999	–	10–65	2498	4.9	10.5	7.8
Spain (Valencia)	Devesa, 2001	1991–93	20–75	1268	5.7	13.9	10.0
Germany (Pomerania)	Völzke, 2005	1999–01	20–79	4202	(3–33)	(5–57)	21.2
Germany (south)	Walcher, 2005	–	10–65	2147	4.8	10.9	8.0
North America							
USA	Maurer, 1989	1982–84	20–74	2293	7.1 (0–15.5)	16.6 (9.0–44.1)	11.9
USA (Texas)	Hanis, 1993	1985–86	15–74	1004	8.0 (0–25.8)	22.2 (3.5–45.8)	15.1
Mexico (Mexico City)	Villalpando, 1997	–	35–64	1735	5.8	19.7	14.1
USA (National)	Everhart, 1999	1988–94	20–74	14000			
Mexican Americans					8.9	26.7	17.8
Non-Hispanic, White					8.6	16.6	12.6
Non-Hispanic, Black					5.3	13.9	9.6
USA (Native Americans)	Everhart, 2002	1989–	45+	3296	29.5	64.1	46.8
South America							
Chile (Santiago)	Covarrubias, 1995	–	20+	1811	14.5	37.4	28.5
Argentina (Rosario City)	Brasca, 2000	–	20+	1173	15.5 (1.9–26.1)	23.8 (6.3–48.6)	20.5
Peru (Lima)	Moro, 2000	–	15+	1534	10.7	16.1	13.4
Asia							
Taiwan (south)	Yuan, 1987	1981–82	10+	3004	2.3	2.7	2.5
Japan (Okinawa)	Nomura, 1988	1982	All	2584	2.4	4.0	3.2
India (Srinagar)	Khuroo, 1989	–	15+	1104	3.1 (0–8.1)	9.6 (2.0–29.1)	6.1
China	Zhao, 1990	–	7–70	15856	2.3	4.7	3.5
Thailand (Chiang Mai)	Prathnadi, 1992	1987	20–70	6146	2.5	3.7	3.1
Russia (northern Siberia)	Tsukanov, 1997	–	Adults		–	–	
Migrants				3420			8.7
Aboriginals				1445			3.0
Bangladesh	Dhar, 2001	–	15+	1058	3.3	7.7	5.4
Russia (Novosibirsk)	Reshetnikov, 2002	1989–95	25–64	1712	2.2	10.3	6.3
Taiwan (Shengang)	Chen, 2005	2003–04	18+	3333	4.6	5.4	5.0

[a]Prevalence assessed by cholecystography.

Table 29.2 Incidence of gallstones in different populations in Europe. Only studies of entire or random samples of populations screened by ultrasonography for gallstone disease on at least two occasions with years apart are included. Studies dealing with selected populations (e.g., diabetics) are not included

Geography	Study	Year	Age	Number	Annual incidence (%)		
					Males	Females	Overall
Italy (Sirmione)	Barbara, 1988	1982/1987	18–65	1325	0.7	0.5	0.6
Denmark (Copenhagen)	Jensen, 1991	1987–88	30–60	2987	0.4 (0.1–0.7)	0.6 (0.3–0.7)	0.5
Italy (south of Rome)	Angelico, 1997	1985/1995	20–69	<426	–	0.6	–
Italy (Bari)	Misciagna, 1999	1985–86/1992–93	30–69	2235	–	–	0.8

The incidence of gallstones (i.e., the development of stones in persons with a formerly normal gallbladder verified by ultrasonography) is only sparsely analyzed, most probably because two screening studies of the same population with years apart is needed. Results show a yearly incidence rate of 0.5–0.8% with trends toward higher rates in females and among the elderly (Table 29.2).

Risk factors for gallstones

Age

Gallstones have historically been rare among young children and adolescents [2], but the increasing prevalence of obesity in childhood may change this. Gallstone prevalence increases with increasing age, reaching more than 50% in some elderly populations. After puberty gallstone prevalence becomes twice as common in women as in men.

Genetics

Family and twin studies in humans, and genetic studies in mice, indicate that gallstone disease is a complex disease caused both by genetic and environmental factors [3]. In this respect, gallstone disease is similar to many other chronic diseases. From a twin study it has been calculated that genetic factors account for 25% of gallstone prevalence [4]. Due to the complex pathogenesis of cholesterol stones, several genes are suspected to be involved.

Demographic risk factors

Gallstone prevalence is greater among lower compared with higher socioeconomic classes in Western countries [5]. The sex difference in gallstone prevalence seems to be explained by female hormone use and pregnancy. While the association between use of oral contraceptives and gallstone disease is very weak, if existing at all, both cohort studies and randomized controlled trials show that estrogen replacement therapy increases the risk of gallstone formation [6,7]. Most studies find a positive association between number of pregnancies and gallstone prevalence [8], which is in accordance with changes in the lithogenic index in bile and the contractility of the gallbladder during pregnancies. Nulliparous women seem to have the same prevalence of gallstones as age-matched men.

Lifestyle risk factors

There is general agreement that alcohol intake [5,9,10] and physical activity [5,11,12] are associated with a lower risk of gallstones, whereas smoking shows varying results [5]. Regarding diet, a raised intake of saturated fat is associated with increased gallstone occurrence, whereas greater intake of fiber, fruit, vegetables, and poly- and monounsaturated fat is associated with reduced occurrence of gallstones [10,11,13]. Furthermore, a high carbohydrate intake, glycemic load and glycemic index seem to be associated with increased occurrence of gallstones [11,14]. Studies on caffeine intake show both positive and negative associations. High body mass index and large waist circumference are also associated with gallstones [5,8,11,15]. With respect to plasma lipids, the picture is unclear, as different studies show both positive and negative associations between gallstones and total cholesterol and high-density lipoprotein (HDL) cholesterol [5,8,16], whereas there is general agreement about a positive association between high triglyceride concentrations and gallstones. The association with high fasting insulin [17] connects gallstones to the metabolic syndrome and insulin resistance [15,18]. Gallstones are more common in individuals with diabetes, cardiovascular diseases [15] and colonic cancer, which seems reasonable from the above-mentioned risk profile.

Race and ethnic groups

Our current knowledge of risk factors and genetic susceptibility (Box 29.1) gives some clues to the vast variation in gallstone prevalence among populations. Populations with a certain admixture of "thrifty" genes like the Native Americans will – given a westernized lifestyle – experience a high prevalence, which is not seen in populations without these "thrifty" genes (such as people from China and Taiwan), where the effect of a westernized lifestyle can still be observed, but where so far there has been only a moderate increase in gallstone prevalence (e.g., in Taiwan; Table 29.1). Non-Hispanic White people in the USA are not thought to have a major admixture of Native American genes and their gallstone prevalence is similar to that of Europeans.

Risk factors for pigment stones

Although epidemiologic risk factor studies cannot distinguish between cholesterol stones and pigment stones, the risk factor profile will be that of cholesterol stones, as these are the most dominant. Less is known about risk factors for pigment stones, but hemolytic conditions, chronic liver diseases and infections play a role.

Box 29.1 Risk factors for cholesterol stones

- Increasing age
- Female sex:
  –(oral contraceptive)
  –estrogen replacement therapy
  –pregnancies
- Genes (several genes are involved)
- Social factors:
  –low social classes in Western countries
  –high social classes in Asian countries
- Lifestyle factors:
  –abstinence from alcohol
  –low level of physical activity
  –diet rich in saturated fat and refined sugars and low in fibers
  (inconclusive results for smoking and coffee intake)
- Biomarkers:
  –obesity (high BMI and high waist/hip ratio)
  –high fasting insulin
  –high triglycerides
  (inconclusive results for total cholesterol and HDL cholesterol)

Natural history and mortality

In general, gallstone disease is an uneventful condition. Persons with asymptomatic gallstones develop biliary colic with an annual rate of 1–2% [19] and complications with a rate of 0.2–0.8% per year [19,20]. Patients with symptomatic gallstones have an annual complication rate of 1–2% [20,21]. Small gallstones can disappear spontaneously. Gallstone disease is an indicator of increased mortality, shown both in nationwide cohorts of cholecystectomized patients [22] and in a population of Native Americans screened for gallstones. The excess mortality was mainly due to cardiovascular diseases, gastrointestinal diseases and certain cancers, which is in accordance with the risk factor profile among persons with gallstones.

Disability and quality of life

Biliary pain affects quality of life. Randomized trials comparing patients treated with watchful waiting, ESWL (extracorporeal shock-wave lithotripsy), or cholecystectomy by minilaparotomy and by laparoscopy all showed an increase in quality of life after treatment or start of observation [20,23]. After cholecystectomy about one-fifth of patients complain of persistent symptoms. Only a minor proportion of these are as severe as before surgery, and some of them will be new symptoms, possibly the result of gastritis caused by increased bile reflux after cholecystectomy [20]. Bile duct lesions, which occur in 0.25–1% [20,24], rarely lead to permanent disability (e.g., liver cirrhosis).

Healthcare utilization and costs

There is international consensus that persons with asymptomatic gallstones should not be offered treatment. Because both abdominal symptoms and gallstones are very common in the population, it is a challenge to select patients who need treatment. Despite attempts to reach international consensus, there is still considerable disagreement about the indications for cholecystectomy. This is evident from the substantial regional variation in the cholecystectomy rate and the fact that the introduction of the laparoscopic technique around 1990 increased the cholecystectomy rate considerably [20].

More than 700 000 cholecystectomies are performed annually in the USA and the number most probably is similar in Europe, which makes it a very common procedure in surgical departments. Like many other surgical procedures, the number of days of admission after a cholecystectomy has decreased during the last 30 years, and since the introduction of minimally invasive procedures a certain proportion are treated as day-care procedures. Costs per treatment have decreased due to the decreasing length of hospital stay, but the greater number of operations has increased the total cost [20]. In the USA the total cost of treating gallstone patients is close to $6bn [25]. The length of convalescence depends on the prevailing attitudes in society, but since the introduction of minimally invasive procedures it has decreased and now varies between 2 and 4 weeks [20,26].

Prevention

There are no studies aimed at primary prevention of gallstone disease. However, taking the risk factors into consideration, preventive strategies against obesity, type 2 diabetes and cardiovascular diseases also should prevent gallstone formation. In a clinical setting medical treatment with bile acid in patients undergoing rapid weight loss has been proposed to avoid gallstone formation. Secondary prevention in terms of prophylactic cholecystectomy in persons with asymptomatic gallstones has been suggested, but decision analyses have questioned the benefit, and it is not recommended by international guidelines.

Issues and gaps in epidemiologic knowledge

Most screening studies have been cross-sectional, so incidence studies are needed to get a better understanding of the risk factors for gallstone formation. The association between gallstone formation and lipid and glucose metabolism in particular needs further attention. Cohort studies only aiming at clinical gallstones are valuable, but are hampered by problems with selection bias. More knowledge is needed on the natural history of gallstone disease to identify those who are at risk for complications, and finally a better understanding of the reasons for the big variation in cholecystectomy rates both nationally and regionally is warranted.

Recommendations for future studies

Some recommendations for the future direction of gallstone research include:
- Large-scale cohort studies including ultrasonography screening for gallstones on two or more occasions separated by an interval of several years and with long-term follow-up.
- Pooling of different national cohorts should be facilitated to analyze whether differences in risk factors can explain national variations.
- Priority should be given to observational patient cohorts and clinical randomized trials focusing on the outcomes of cholecystectomy versus watchful waiting, to obtain more precise indications for cholecystectomy.

Conclusions

Gallstone disease is a common condition in Europe and the USA and is caused by an interaction of genes and lifestyle. Gallstone disease seems to be linked to the metabolic syndrome and shares many risk factors with type 2 diabetes and cardiovascular disease. Most stones are asymptomatic and the condition is rather uneventful with an annual incidence of biliary colic of 1–2% and a complication rate of less than 1%. Gallstones are one of the most common gastrointestinal disorders, with more than a million treatments annually in Europe and the USA, but with a substantial regional variation.

References

1. Portincasa P *et al*. Cholesterol gallstone disease. *Lancet* 2006;**368**:989.
2. Kratzer W *et al*. Prevalence of gallstones in sonographic surveys worldwide. *J Clin Ultrasound* 1999;**27**:1.
3. Lammert F, Sauerbruch T. Mechanisms of disease: the genetic epidemiology of gallbladder stones. *Nat Clin Pract Gastroenterol Hepatol* 2005;**2**:423.
4. Katsika D *et al*. Genetic and environmental influences on symptomatic gallstone disease: A Swedish study of 43,141 twin pairs. *Hepatology* 2005;**41**:1138.
5. Völzke H *et al*. Independent risk factors for gallstone formation in a region with high cholelithiasis prevalence. *Digestion* 2005;**71**:97.
6. Uhler ML *et al*. Estrogen replacement therapy and gallbladder disease in postmenopausal women. *Menopause* 2000;**7**:162.

7. Cirillo DJ *et al.* Effect of estrogen therapy on gallbladder disease. *JAMA* 2005;**293**:330.

8. Devesa F *et al.* Cholelithiasic disease and associated factors in a Spanish population. *Dig Dis Sci* 2001;**46**:1424.

9. Okamoto M *et al.* The relationship between gallbladder disease and smoking and drinking habits in middle-aged Japanese. *J Gastroenterol* 2002;**37**:455.

10. Cuevas A *et al.* Diet as a risk factor for cholesterol gallstone disease. *J Am Coll Nutr* 2004;**23**:187.

11. Misciagna G *et al.* Diet, physical activity, and gallstones – a population-based, case-control study in southern Italy. *Am J Clin Nutr* 1999;**69**:120.

12. Storti K *et al.* Physical activity and decreased risk of clinical gallstone disease among post-menopausal women. *Prev Med* 2005;**41**:772.

13. Tsai C-J *et al.* Long-term intake of dietary fiber and decreased risk of cholecystectomy in women. *Am J Gastroenterol* 2004;**99**:1364.

14. Tsai C-J *et al.* Dietary carbohydrates and glycaemic load and the incidence of symptomatic gall stone disease in men. *Gut* 2005;**54**:823.

15. Méndez-Sánches N *et al.* Strong association between gallstones and cardiovascular disease. *Am J Gastroenterol* 2005;**100**:827.

16. Duque MX *et al.* Inverse association between plasma cholesterol and gallstone disease. *Arch Med Res* 1999;**30**:190.

17. Ruhl CE, Everhart JE. Association of diabetes, serum insulin, and C-peptide with gallbladder disease. *Hepatology* 2000;**31**:299.

18. Nakeeb A *et al.* Insulin resistance causes human gallbladder dysmotility. *J Gastrointest Surg* 2006;**10**:940.

19. Halldestam I *et al.* Development of symptoms and complications in individuals with asymptomatic gallstones. *Br J Surg* 2004;**91**:734.

20. Jørgensen T. *Treatment of Gallstone Patients. A Health Technology Assessment.* Copenhagen County: National Institute of Public Health and Danish Institute for Health Technology Assessment, 2000 (www.rcph.dk).

21. Vetrhus M *et al.* Symptomatic, non-complicated gallbladder stone disease. Operation or observation? A randomized clinical study. *Scand J Gastroenterol* 2002;**37**:834.

22. Andersen TF *et al.* Survival until 6 years after cholecystectomy: female population of Denmark, 1977–83. *World J Surg* 1995;**19**:609.

23. Vetrhus M *et al.* Pain and quality of life in patients with symptomatic, non-complicated gallbladder stones: results of a randomized controlled trial. *Scand J Gastroenterol* 2004;**39**:270.

24. Gentileschi P *et al.* Bile duct injuries during laparoscopic cholecystectomy. *Surg Endosc* 2004;**18**:232-6.

25. Anon. *The Burden of Gastrointestinal Diseases.* Bethesda, MD: American Gastroenterological Association, 2001.

26. Keus F *et al.* Laparoscopic versus small-incision cholecystectomy for patients with symptomatic cholecystolithiasis. The Cochrane Library, 2006 (ISSN 1464-780X).

30 Pancreatitis

Santhi Swaroop Vege, Dhiraj Yadav and Suresh T. Chari

Key points
- The incidence of acute pancreatitis appears to be increasing worldwide.
- The natural history of alcoholic chronic pancreatitis differs from idiopathic forms.
- Future studies on pancreatitis should focus on host–environment interactions, factors determining quality of life and healthcare costs, and better disease estimates in general and in high-risk populations.

Acute pancreatitis

Clinical summary

Patients with acute pancreatitis (AP) typically present with severe, continuous upper abdominal pain radiating to the back. Severe cases may develop organ failure, and local complications such as fluid collections and pancreatic necrosis may occur. Treatment is predominantly conservative in the form of pain relief by narcotics and aggressive fluid resuscitation. Patients with severe AP may require monitoring and treatment in the intensive care unit, prophylactic antibiotics, enteral nutrition and debridement of infected necrotic pancreatic tissue.

Disease definition

Clinically, AP is diagnosed when patients with upper abdominal pain have a threefold elevation of serum amylase and lipase and/or evidence of pancreatic inflammation on imaging studies (e.g., computerized tomography scan). AP can recur.

Incidence and prevalence

Based on several studies conducted before 2000, the incidence of AP was low in England and the Netherlands (approximately 5–10 per 100 000 inhabitants), higher in Scotland and Denmark (approximately 25–35 per 100 000 inhabitants) and highest in the USA and Finland (approximately 70–80 per 100 000 inhabitants) [1]. However, in studies conducted after 2000, the annual incidence of AP per 100 000 population has ranged from 4.9 to 35 [2–9]. According to the National Inpatient Sample, a database of hospital inpatient stays in the USA, there were 210 188 admissions for AP in the year 2000 and AP was the second most common principal gastrointestinal diagnosis among hospitalized patients [10]. Because AP is not usually a chronic condition, all the population-based studies of AP [1–12] describe incidence and not prevalence.

Temporal trends in incidence

Many studies [4,6,7,9,11] have reported a significant increase in the incidence of AP over time. This was suggested to be due to increased testing for pancreatitis among patients with abdominal pain. One study did not find this to be the case [11]. It is more likely to represent a real increase in gallstone-induced pancreatitis in some studies [9] and an increase in alcohol-related AP in others [7]. AP based on administrative codes without review of medical records may overestimate its incidence. In one such study of 99 patients, the diagnosis code of AP was not confirmed on review of medical records in ~20% [6].

Demographics and risk factors

Increased risk of AP has been linked to particular sections of the population or certain factors .
- **Gender:** While most studies report a higher incidence in males [3–5,7–9,11], a Danish study reported a higher incidence in women [6]. Temporal trends in Danish and British studies show a more pronounced increase in incidence rates in females compared with males [4,6]; the

British study also observed an increase in the proportion of women who drank >14 units of alcohol per week [4].

• **Age:** Many studies have observed increasing incidence of AP with increasing age; the incidence reported per 100 000 population was <5–10, 10–30 and >20–30 in age groups <25 years, 25–60 years and >60 years, respectively [3,4,7,11]. In southern England, the more pronounced increase in AP in younger men and women is, at least in part, due to an increase in alcohol-related AP [7].

• **Gallstones and alcohol:** Gallstones are the commonest cause of AP [3,5,8,9], and with alcohol abuse, account for >60% of cases. Gallstone-induced AP is more common in women whereas alcohol-induced AP is more often seen in men. Lindkvist *et al.* observed an increase of 7.6% per year in gallstone-induced AP in Sweden and correlated this finding with increased obesity and gallstone-related diseases [9]. The same authors also found a decrease in alcohol-related AP of 5.1% per year and correlated this finding with a decrease in the incidence of delirium tremens and mortality from cirrhosis, both markers of alcohol-induced diseases [9].

• **Drugs:** A Danish study showing increasing incidence of AP over time [6] also observed an increase in the number of prescriptions for potentially pancreatitis-causing drugs such as azathioprine, estrogens and estrogen-progesterone combinations during the study period. However, it is not clear that the patients with AP in this population were exposed to these drugs [6].

Natural history and mortality

Approximately 80% of patients with AP will have mild disease and recover without sequelae. The remaining 20% with severe AP will have a prolonged hospital stay due to organ failure, local complications and sepsis. While overall mortality in AP is reported to be 1.8% [10], in severe AP it is 15–25%, with most deaths (65%) occurring in the first 14 days [6]. In recent studies reporting trends, decreasing case-fatality rate over time was observed [4,6,11]. Mortality increased with age [11]. There was no difference in the mortality due to different etiologies [5]. Recurrent attacks are associated with lower mortality compared with a first attack of AP [5,11].

Issues and gaps in the epidemiology

The very few prospective studies cover only a short period of time and hence trends in incidence and outcomes cannot be accurately determined. Hospital-based studies may not accurately reflect incidence in the population; they may overestimate incidence because sicker patients are transferred to tertiary hospitals from outside the population base of the hospital. Hospital-based studies are less likely to underestimate the incidence of AP as most patients with AP are hospitalized [2], although not necessarily in the area hospitals.

Recommendations for future studies

In defined populations, excluding cases transferred from hospitals outside the area, recurrent attacks and flares of chronic pancreatitis, all cases of confirmed AP should be prospectively studied for temporal trends, etiology, clinical outcomes and healthcare utilization costs. Such studies could perhaps be done in centers with well-defined catchment areas and limited number of healthcare facilities.

Conclusions

Based on available epidemiologic studies (which are mostly retrospective and hospital-based), it appears that the incidence of AP is increasing (especially that due to gallstones and alcohol in some areas), and that the case-fatality rate is decreasing. Prospective, preferably population-based, studies are needed to confirm these findings.

Chronic pancreatitis (CP)
Disease definition

Chronic pancreatitis (CP) is a progressive fibroinflammatory disease of the pancreas that, in its end stages, is characterized by permanent loss of pancreatic parenchyma and consequent functional insufficiency (diabetes and steatorrhea) [12]. Three forms of CP are currently recognized.

• **Usual CP, or calcifying CP (CCP):** This is characterized by severe abdominal pain, recurrent bouts of clinical acute pancreatitis (AP) and eventual development of intraductal calculi in a high proportion of cases. On histology, there is perilobular fibrosis and acinar destruction with acute and chronic inflammatory cells [13]. The most frequent cause of CCP is alcohol and tobacco use.

• **Obstructive CP:** This form of CP develops upstream from an area of ductal obstruction, often due to a tumor or postinflammatory AP pancreatic duct stricture. It is usually painless but occasionally causes clinical AP. Persistent obstruction leads to pancreatic atrophy upstream from the area of ductal narrowing. The development of steatorrhea and diabetes depends on the amount of pancreas that becomes atrophied. Intraductal calculi are generally absent.

• **Autoimmune CP (lymphoplasmacytic sclerosing pancreatitis):** This systemic autoimmune fibroinflammatory disorder afflicts the pancreas as well as other organs [14]. Affected organs show a lymphoplasmacytic infiltrate rich in IgG4-positive cells that responds to steroid therapy. Intense fibrosis may lead to permanent structural damage and functional insufficiency. It is a relatively painless disorder and clinical AP is not a common presentation [14]. Intraductal calculi are uncommon, but may develop in the late "burnt-out" stage.

Epidemiology of usual CP (or CCP)

Almost all literature on the epidemiology of CP relates to CCP, mostly from Western countries [3,4,15–18] and Japan [19], with little information on the epidemiology of other forms. The annual incidence varies widely (1.9–14.1 per 100 000) in Western countries depending on the study design, year of study and risk factor prevalence [3,4,15–18]. Prevalence estimates are available from Copenhagen [16] (27.4 per 100 000 in 1979) and Japan [19] (28.9 per 100 000 in 1994). Longitudinal studies indicate a trend toward an increase in incidence over time [4,15].

Risk factors and etiology

In Western countries, heavy **alcohol use** and **smoking** account for the majority (55–80%) of CP cases. In 20% of cases, no cause can be identified (idiopathic CCP) [12]. Among alcoholics the risk of developing pancreatitis increases with the duration and amount of alcohol intake [20]. The exact risk is unknown but is believed to be ~2–3% in alcoholics who consume large amounts of alcohol [21]. Data on **racial predisposition** for CP are limited but important observations indicate that Black people may have a greater risk for alcoholic pancreatitis compared with White people [22]. The exact role of diet in CP is still unclear. Smoking is an independent risk factor for development [20] and progression of CP [23]. **Genetic susceptibility** to CCP is conferred by mutations in the cationic trypsinogen, *CFTR* and *SPINK1* genes (reviewed in ref. [11]) [12]. Hereditary pancreatitis is an autosomal dominant disorder with high (80%) penetrance caused by mutations in the cationic trypsinogen

gene. Mutations in the *CFTR* and *SPINK1* genes are associated with apparently idiopathic CCP. Other less common associations of CP are **hypertriglyceridemia** and **hypercalcemia** [12].

Presentation

Alcoholic CCP, which is more common in middle-aged men with a long history of heavy alcohol and tobacco use, usually presents in the fifth decade of life with attacks of pain or AP. The presentation of the idiopathic form of CCP, which affects both sexes equally, is bimodal: the juvenile form (early-onset) is painful, while over 50% of subjects with senile-onset idiopathic CP have painless disease [24]. Most patients with hereditary pancreatitis are symptomatic by age 20 years, with pain and clinical AP [12]. Tropical pancreatitis is an early-onset form of idiopathic CP that is endemic in south Asia, particularly southern India, and in Africa and South America. It is characterized by a high prevalence of pancreatic calcification, diabetes and pancreatic cancer [25].

Natural history

Described mainly from centers specializing in pancreatic disease [24,26,27], the natural history of alcoholic CP may be different from idiopathic CP. Patients with early-onset idiopathic CP have a much slower progression toward requiring pain relief, and to experiencing exocrine and endocrine insufficiency compared with alcoholic and late-onset idiopathic CP [23]. Approximately 50–60% of patients undergo surgery at some point, primarily to achieve pain relief or to treat complications from CP [23,26]. The mortality in CP subjects is significantly higher than expected (SMR 3.6, 95% CI 3.3–3.9) [27] and is mostly from nonpancreatic causes. The cumulative risk of developing pancreatic cancer is much greater in hereditary pancreatitis (40%) than in other forms of CP [28].

Disability and quality of life

Abdominal pain, which can be continuous and intractable, is the most important determinant of quality of life in CP [29]. However, disability data are lacking in this field.

Prevention

Apart from modification of risk factors (smoking, alcohol), no preventive strategies are currently available.

Issues and gaps in the epidemiology

Despite the progress made in recent years in understanding the pathogenesis of CP, especially its inherited forms, several questions remain unanswered. For example, why do only a small proportion of heavy-drinking alcoholics develop CP? What is the role of cofactors (host, environmental or both) in individual susceptibility to develop CP? What is the mechanism of pain in CP? Limited information is available on healthcare costs and utilization by subjects with CP. In addition, diagnosis codes for CP do not differentiate between etiologies, indicating the need for etiology-based diagnosis codes. The current classification of CP is based on morphology rather than etiology. Because biopsy from the pancreas is rarely obtained, classification systems providing an improved understanding of both the etiology and progression of the disease are needed.

Recommendations for future studies

Future studies should focus on establishing incidence and prevalence estimates and trends in general and high-risk populations, factors determining individual susceptibility to CP, mechanisms of pain in CP, and determinants of quality of life and healthcare utilization by subjects with CP.

Conclusions

Significant advances have been made in our understanding of the etiology, mechanisms and natural history of CP. Most epidemiological studies on CP have originated from specialized centers and are not population-based. Well-designed, preferably prospective, population-based studies are needed to understand better the disease estimates and trends.

References

1. Banks PA. Epidemiology, natural history, and predictors of disease outcome in acute and chronic pancreatitis. *Gastrointest Endosc* 2002;**56**:S226.
2. Eland IA *et al.* Incidence of acute pancreatitis. *Scand J Gastroenterol* 2002;**37**:124.
3. Lankisch PG *et al.* Epidemiology of pancreatic diseases in Luneburg County. A study in a defined German population. *Pancreatology* 2002;**2**:469.
4. Tinto A *et al.* Acute and chronic pancreatitis – diseases on the rise: a study of hospital admissions in England 1989/90–1999/2000. *Aliment Pharmacol Ther* 2002;**16**:2097.
5. Birgisson H *et al.* Acute pancreatitis: a prospective study of its incidence, aetiology, severity, and mortality in Iceland. *Eur J Surg* 2002;**168**:278.
6. Floyd A *et al.* Secular trends in incidence and 30-day case fatality of acute pancreatitis in North Jutland County, Denmark: a register-based study from 1981–2000. *Scand J Gastroenterol* 2002;**37**:1461.
7. Goldacre MJ *et al.* Hospital admission for acute pancreatitis in an English population, 1963–98: database study of incidence and mortality. *Br Med J* 2004;**328**:1466.
8. Gislason H *et al.* Acute pancreatitis in Bergen, Norway. A study on incidence, etiology and severity. *Scand J Surg* 2004;**93**:29.
9. Lindkvist B *et al.* Trends in incidence of acute pancreatitis in a Swedish population: is there really an increase? *Clin Gastroenterol Hepatol* 2004;**2**:831.
10. Russo MW *et al.* Digestive and liver diseases statistics, 2004. *Gastroenterology* 2004;**126**:1448.
11. Eland IA *et al.* Incidence and mortality of acute pancreatitis between 1985 and 1995. *Scand J Gastroenterol* 2000;**35**:1110.
12. Etemad B *et al.* Chronic pancreatitis: diagnosis, classification, and new genetic developments. *Gastroenterology* 2001;**120**:682.
13. Kloppel G *et al.* Pathology of acute and chronic pancreatitis. *Pancreas* 1993;**8**:659.
14. Lara LP *et al.* Autoimmune pancreatitis. *Curr Gastroenterol Rep* 2005;**7**:101.
15. O'Sullivan JN *et al.* Acute and chronic pancreatitis in Rochester, Minnesota, 1940 to 1969. *Gastroenterology* 1972;**62**:373.
16. Copenhagen pancreatitis study. An interim report from a prospective epidemiological multicentre study. *Scand J Gastroenterol* 1981;**16**:305.
17. Schmidt DN. Apparent risk factors for chronic and acute pancreatitis in Stockholm county. Spirits but not wine and beer. *Int J Pancreatol* 1991;**8**:45.
18. Jaakkola M *et al.* Pancreatitis in Finland between 1970 and 1989. *Gut* 1993;**34**:1255.
19. Lin Y *et al.* Nationwide epidemiological survey of chronic pancreatitis in Japan. *J Gastroenterol* 2000;**35**:136.
20. Talamini G *et al.* Cigarette smoking: an independent risk factor in alcoholic pancreatitis. *Pancreas* 1996;**12**:131.
21. Lankisch PG *et al.* What is the risk of alcoholic pancreatitis in heavy drinkers? *Pancreas* 2002;**25**:411.
22. Lowenfels AB *et al.* Racial factors and the risk of chronic pancreatitis. *Am J Gastroenterol* 1999;**94**:790.
23. Maisonneuve P *et al.* Cigarette smoking accelerates progression of alcoholic chronic pancreatitis. *Gut* 2005;**54**:510.
24. Layer P *et al.* The different courses of early- and late-onset idiopathic and alcoholic chronic pancreatitis. *Gastroenterology* 1994;**107**:1481.
25. Mohan V *et al.* Tropical chronic pancreatitis: an update. *J Clin*

Gastroenterol 2003;**36**:337.

26. Ammann RW *et al.* The natural history of pain in alcoholic chronic pancreatitis. *Gastroenterology* 1999;**116**:1132.

27. Lowenfels AB *et al.* Prognosis of chronic pancreatitis: an international multicenter study. International Pancreatitis Study Group. *Am J Gastroenterol* 1994;**89**:1467.

28. Lowenfels AB *et al.* Epidemiology and risk factors for pancreatic cancer. *Best Pract Res Clin Gastroenterol* 2006;**20**:197.

29. Pezzilli R *et al.* The quality of life in patients with chronic pancreatitis evaluated using the SF-12 questionnaire: a comparative study with the SF-36 questionnaire. *Dig Liver Dis* 2006;**38**:109.

31 Pancreatic Cancer

Suresh T. Chari

Key points
- Pancreatic cancer is the fourth commonest cause of cancer death in the USA.
- Mortality from pancreatic cancer exceeds 95% because it is unresectable in >85% by the time diagnosis is made, it recurs in 80% of patients who undergo resection, and it is not very responsive to chemoradiation therapy.
- Detecting asymptomatic pancreatic cancer remains a challenge as no high-risk groups for sporadic cancer are known and there is no serologic test for early cancer.
- New-onset diabetes is a promising clue for presence of pancreatic cancer, but it needs further study as a marker of early cancer.

The problem of pancreatic cancer

Pancreatic cancer is a devastating and poorly understood cancer. It arises from a noninvasive precursor lesion called pancreatic intraepithelial neoplasia (PanIN). Approximately 75% of all pancreatic cancers occur within the proximal pancreas (head and neck), 15–20% occur in the body of the pancreas, and 5–10% occur in the tail.

Despite widespread use of imaging studies, it is unusual for pancreatic cancer to be diagnosed in an asymptomatic patient. The most common presentation of pancreatic cancer is with obstructive jaundice accompanied by itching and pale stools. Epigastric abdominal pain, back pain, early satiety and weight loss are the other common symptoms in patients with pancreatic cancer. Development of new-onset diabetes in the elderly can herald pancreatic cancer; however, the cancer is not usually diagnosed until after more specific cancer-related symptoms (noted above) develop.

The only hope of cure for pancreatic cancer is successful surgical resection. This involves removal of the duodenum and head of the pancreas (pancreaticoduodenectomy) for proximally located tumors, and resection of the body and tail of the pancreas along with the spleen (distal pancreatectomy) for distally located cancers. However, most (>85%) pancreatic cancers are unresectable (i.e., incurable) by the time diagnosis is made. This is because at diagnosis most patients already have distant metastases or involvement of adjacent arteries (commonly celiac and superior mesenteric arteries) and/or veins (occlusion or extensive involvement of portal and superior mesenteric veins), which precludes resection. The tumor is not very responsive to chemoradiation therapy.

The median survival of unresected pancreatic cancer is 4–6 months. Once symptomatic, pancreatic cancer patients rapidly develop severe cachexia (almost complete loss of appetite, marked muscle wasting, rapid weight loss and fatigue), which is the principal reason for early death in pancreatic cancer. Chemotherapy in unresected cancer improves 1-year survival from <5% to 20% but not long-term survival. Following resection, the median survival increases to 18–22 months; only 20% survive 5 years. Adjuvant chemoradiation has marginal benefit and is frequently not curative. Thus, for most patients, resection is palliative and not curative.

Epidemiology: incidence and burden of cancer-related death

The lifetime risk of developing pancreatic cancer for men and women born today is 1.27%; in other words ~1 in 80 men and women will develop pancreatic cancer in their lifetime [1]. In the USA in 2005 an estimated 32 180 cases of pancreatic cancer were diagnosed [2], and an estimated 31 800 deaths from pancreatic cancer occurred in the same time period [2], making it the fourth most common cause of cancer death in humans, surpassing prostate cancer in the number of cancer-related deaths in 2005 [2] (Fig. 31.1). As can be seen from these statistics, the incidence and mortality of pancreatic cancer are nearly identical; less than 5% of individuals survive 5 years [2]. Even more sobering is the fact that the survival in pancreatic cancer has not improved dramatically over the past 40 years [3].

Risk factors

Age

The median age at diagnosis of pancreatic cancer is 69 years in White people and 65 years in Black people [1]. The incidence of pancreatic cancer is relatively low in individuals up to age 50, after which it increases significantly. At age 70, the incidence of pancreatic cancer is approximately 60 deaths per 100 000 persons per year [1].

Estimated New Cases*

			Males	Females			
Prostate	234 460	33%		Breast	212 920	31%
Lung and bronchus	92 700	13%		Lung and bronchus	81 770	12%
Colon and rectum	72 800	10%		Colon and rectum	75 810	11%
Urinary bladder	44 690	6%		Uterine corpus	41 200	6%
Melanoma of the skin	34 260	5%		Non-Hodgkin lymphoma	28 190	4%
Non-Hodgkin lymphoma	30 680	4%		Melanoma of the skin	27 930	4%
Kidney and renal pelvis	24 650	3%		Thyroid	22 590	3%
Oral cavity and pharynx	20 180	3%		Ovary	20 180	3%
Leukemia	20 000	3%		Urinary bladder	16 730	2%
Pancreas	17 150	2%		Pancreas	16 580	2%
All sites	**720 280**	**100%**		**All sites**	**679 510**	**100%**

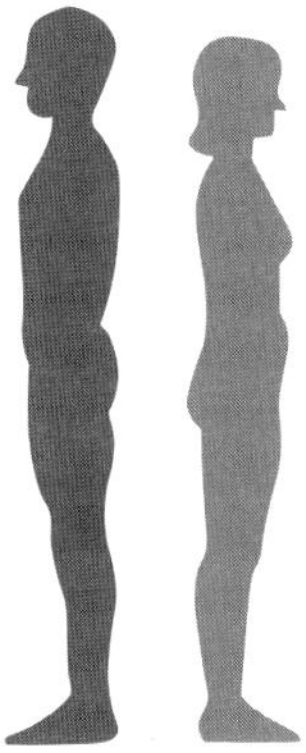

Estimated Deaths

			Males	Females			
Lung and bronchus	90 330	31%		Lung and bronchus	72 130	26%
Colon and rectum	27 870	10%		Breast	40 970	15%
Prostate	27 350	9%		Colon and rectum	27 300	10%
Pancreas	16 090	6%		Pancreas	16 210	6%
Leukemia	12 470	4%		Ovary	15 310	6%
Liver and intrahepatic bile duct	10 840	4%		Leukemia	9 810	4%
Esophagus	10 730	4%		Non-Hodgkin lymphoma	8 840	3%
Non-Hodgkin lymphoma	10 000	3%		Uterine corpus	7 350	3%
Urinary bladder	8 990	3%		Multiple myeloma	5 630	2%
Kidney and renal pelvis	8 130	3%		Brain and other nervous system	5 560	2%
All sites	**291 270**	**100%**		**All sites**	**273 560**	**100%**

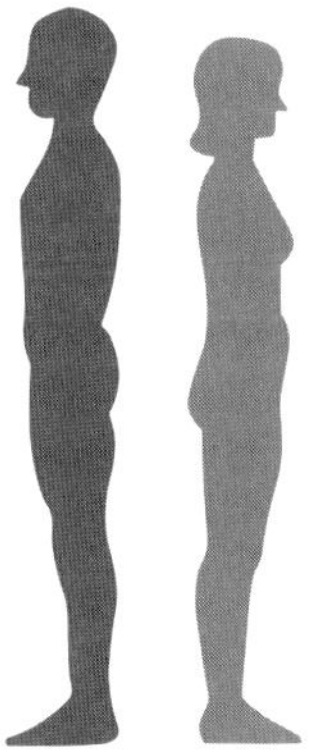

Fig. 31.1 The ten leading cancer types in the USA for estimated new cancer cases and deaths, by gender, for 2006. Excludes basal and squamous cell skin cancers and *in situ* carcinoma except urinary bladder. Estimates are rounded to the nearest 10. Note: percentages may not total 100% due to rounding. (Reproduced from Jemal A *et al. CA Cancer J Clin* 2006;**56**:106–130, with permission from Lippincott Williams and Wilkins.)

Gender

There is slight preponderance of males in patients with pancreatic cancer (male-to-female ratio 1.2–1.5:1)

Race

The incidence of pancreatic cancer for Black males in the USA is 11.9–13.7 cases per 100 000 persons per year, and the incidence for Black females is 10.5–11.9 cases per 100 000 persons per year. For White males in the USA, the incidence is 8.2 cases per 100 000 persons per year, and for females the incidence is 6 cases per 100 000 persons per year. The reason for the higher incidence in Black people is unclear.

Environmental factors

Smoking is the most common and consistently identified environmental risk factor for pancreatic carcinoma [4]. Epidemiologic studies, both cohort and case-control studies, have found an increased relative risk of pancreatic cancer in smokers, with the risk increasing in a dose-dependent manner. Moreover, after cessation of smoking, the excess risk level only returns to baseline in about 15 years [4].

Habits, dietary factors and obesity

Alcohol consumption does not appear to be an independent risk factor for pancreatic cancer unless it is associated with chronic pancreatitis [5]. Despite early reports to the contrary, coffee consumption does not appear to be an independent risk factor for pancreatic carcinoma [5]. The incidence of pancreatic cancer appears to be greater in people with increased energy consumption and lower in those with a diet rich in fresh fruits and vegetables. The risk of pancreatic cancer increases with increasing body mass index [6].

Diabetes mellitus

Numerous studies have examined the relative risk of pancreatic cancer in persons with diabetes mellitus. A meta-analysis of 30 studies concluded that patients with diabetes mellitus of at least 5 years' duration have a twofold increased risk of developing pancreatic carcinoma [7].

Chronic pancreatitis

Long-standing chronic pancreatitis is a substantial risk factor for the development of pancreatic cancer. A multi-center study of more than 2000 patients with chronic pancreatitis showed a 26-fold increase in the risk of developing pancreatic cancer [8]. This risk increased linearly with time, with 4% of patients who had chronic pancreatitis of 20 years' duration developing pancreatic cancer. The risk of pancreatic cancer is even higher in patients with hereditary pancreatitis [9]. The mean age of development of pancreatic cancer in these patients is approximately 57 years. The relative risk of pancreatic cancer in hereditary pancreatitis is increased more than 50-fold, and the cumulative risk rate of pancreatic cancer by age 70 years is 40%. This cumulative risk increases to 75% in those families with a paternal inheritance pattern [9].

Genetic factors

Approximately 5–10% of patients with pancreatic carcinoma have some genetic predisposition to developing the disease [10]. The inherited disorders that increase the risk of pancreatic cancer include hereditary pancreatitis, multiple endocrine neoplasia, hereditary nonpolyposis colorectal cancer, familial adenomatous polyposis and Gardner syndrome, familial atypical multiple mole melanoma syndrome, von Hippel–Lindau syndrome and germline mutations in the *BRCA2* gene.

Screening for pancreatic cancer

Because pancreatic cancer patients seldom exhibit disease-specific symptoms until late in the course of the disease, it is critically important to identify and develop surveillance strategies for early detection of asymptomatic pancreatic cancer. The detection of small pancreatic cancers is likely to increase resectability rates and presumably long-term survival. In a study of 99 pancreatic cancer patients with small tumors (<20 mm), all tumors were resectable and in the 37% in whom the tumor was confined to the pancreas, long-term survival was 35% [11].

There are two major obstacles to screening for pancreatic cancer. Pancreatic cancer is relatively uncommon and it would not be cost-effective to screen for it in the general population. For example, if a test with 99% specificity for pancreatic cancer were used to screen the general population, the false positives would far outnumber the true pancreatic cancer cases identified by the test. The solution to this problem is to identify groups at higher than average risk of having or developing pancreatic cancer. So far two high-risk groups have been targets of screening for pancreatic cancer; one approach relies on detecting high-grade preinvasive lesions in **familial pancreatic cancer** kindreds and other focuses on detecting early invasive cancer in subjects with **new-onset diabetes**.

The second major problem in screening for pancreatic cancer is lack of a serologic marker of early (resectable) pancreatic cancer. Currently, genetic syndromes with a high incidence of pancreatic cancer are being targeted for screening [12–14] using invasive endoscopic procedures such as endoscopic ultrasound and endoscopic retrograde cholangiopancreatography [12]. Though successful in the setting of high-risk families, these expensive and invasive procedures cannot be used to screen for sporadic pancreatic cancer.

High-risk groups for pancreatic cancer

Familial pancreatic cancer

These kindreds have been defined as families having at least one pair of first-degree relatives with pancreatic cancer. The risk of pancreatic cancer in **familial pancreatic cancer** kindreds was best assessed in a study from Johns Hopkins University [15] in which the observed-to-expected rate of pancreatic cancer was evaluated in 5179 individuals from 838 **familial pancreatic cancer** kindreds. In this group, the risk of pancreatic cancer increased as the number of first-degree relatives with pancreatic cancer increased. Kindreds having three or more affected first-degree relatives had a 32.0-fold increased risk of developing pancreatic cancer (95% CI, 10.4–74.7); those with two affected first-degree relatives with pancreatic cancer had a 6.4-fold increased risk (95% CI, 1.8–16.4), and those with a single affected first-degree relative had a 4.5-fold increased risk (95% CI, 0.54–16.3) [32]. Risk was not increased among 369 spouses and other genetically unrelated relatives or in those with sporadic pancreatic cancer [15].

A strategy of surveillance using endoscopic ultrasound and endoscopic retrograde cholangiopancreatography has been successfully used to detect precancerous lesions in one family with autosomal dominant familial pancreatic cancer with high penetrance [12]. Mapping of a susceptibility locus for pancreatic cancer in this family to chromosome 4q32-34 [16] adds further impetus to this approach to pancreatic cancer screening. This has led to further studies using endoscopic approaches to screening for high-grade precursor lesions and early cancer in familial pancreatic cancer kindreds. However, the limitation of this approach is that these groups with very high risk of pancreatic cancer collectively constitute <5% of all pancreatic cancer patients. Therefore, a different approach will be necessary to identify sporadic pancreatic cancer.

New-onset diabetes

The only significant clue to the presence of sporadic pancreatic cancer before it becomes symptomatic is the development of hyperglycemia and diabetes. When formally tested, up to 80% of pancreatic cancer patients have glucose intolerance [17,18]. While the association between diabetes and pancreatic cancer has long been recognized, the assessment of diabetes as a clinically relevant screening target for pancreatic cancer is complicated by the fact that although long-standing diabetes is an etiologic factor for pancreatic cancer, new-onset diabetes is a manifestation of the cancer. Though most studies show an elevated risk of pancreatic cancer among persons with long-standing diabetes, the strength of this association is modest at best [7]. In a meta-analysis of 20 epidemiologic studies, the pooled relative risk of pancreatic cancer for those whose diabetes was diagnosed at least 1 year prior to either diagnosis of pancreatic cancer or to pancreatic cancer death was 2.1 (95% CI, 1.6–2.8) [7]. Whereas the number of persons with pancreatic cancer in the population is small, the number of older persons with long-standing diabetes is large. Thus long-standing diabetes as a marker for pancreatic cancer is likely to have limited clinical utility.

Most diabetes in pancreatic cancer is new-onset. In a study of 66 consecutive pancreatic cancer patients with diabetes, in 88% the diabetes was new-onset, that is, it was diagnosed <24 months before diagnosis of pancreatic cancer [19]. In a case-control study of hospitalized pancreatic cancer patients, the frequency of new-onset diabetes (<24 months) was markedly higher in cases than controls (56.0 vs 13.3%, $P < 0.001$) [20]. These studies show that glucose intolerance is present in most patients with pancreatic cancer and is often of recent onset. Conversely, other studies have shown that subjects with new-onset diabetes have a higher than expected likelihood of having pancreatic cancer [21–23]. A recent population-based study showed that compared with the general population, subjects with new-onset diabetes are eight times more likely to be diagnosed with pancreatic cancer within 3 years of meeting criteria for diabetes [23]. Others have targeted selected subjects with recently diagnosed diabetes for screening and found an even higher prevalence of pancreatic cancer (5.2–13.6%) [21,22]. Thus, new-onset diabetes in subjects >50 years appears to define a high-risk group for pancreatic cancer.

Screening all new-onset diabetics for pancreatic cancer is unlikely to be cost-effective as the prevalence of pancreatic cancer in this population is <1%. To overcome this, two studies have targeted patients with new-onset diabetes with cancer-related symptoms for screening. While the prevalence of pancreatic cancer in this subset was clearly raised (5.2–13.6%) [21,22], pancreatic cancer identified in both studies was mostly unresectable. This is not surprising considering that cancer-related symptoms are associated with unresectable pancreatic cancer. The success of the strategy to use hyperglycemia as a screening tool to identify subjects with a high likelihood of having underlying undiagnosed pancreatic cancer will depend largely on our ability to differentiate pancreatic cancer-induced diabetes from type 2 diabetes using a serologic biomarker in patients without cancer-specific symptoms. Currently there is no such marker.

Summary

Pancreatic cancer is a devastating and poorly understood cancer. Environmental risk factors are inadequately understood. The prognosis is poor because the majority of patients have unresectable disease at diagnosis, and severe cachexia leads rapidly to death following diagnosis. Further research is needed into how best to identify high-risk groups that can be targeted for screening for high-grade precursor lesions or early cancer.

References

1. Surveillance, Epidemiology, and End Results (SEER) Program. SEER*Stat database. Incidence – SEER 9 Regs Public-Use, Nov 2003 Sub (1973–2001) (www. seer.cancer.gov). Released April 2004, based on the November 2002 submission. National Cancer Institute, DCCPS, Surveillance Research Program, Cancer Statistics Branch.
2. Jemal A *et al*. Cancer Statistics, 2005. *CA Cancer J Clin* 2005;**55**:10.
3. Cancer Registry of Norway. *Cancer in Norway* (http://www.kreftregisteret.no).
4. Lowenfels AB *et al*. Epidemiologic and etiologic factors of pancreatic cancer. *Hematol Oncol Clin North Am* 2002;**16**:1.
5. Lowenfels AB *et al*. Cigarette smoking as a risk factor for pancreatic cancer in patients with hereditary pancreatitis. *JAMA*

2001;**286**:169.
6. Larsson SC *et al*. Overall obesity, abdominal adiposity, diabetes and cigarette smoking in relation to the risk of pancreatic cancer in two Swedish population-based cohorts. *Br J Cancer* 2005;**93**:1310.
7. Everhart J *et al*. Diabetes mellitus as a risk factor for pancreatic cancer. A meta-analysis. *JAMA* 1995;**273**:1605.
8. Lowenfels AB *et al*. Pancreatitis and the risk of pancreatic cancer. International Pancreatitis Study Group. *N Engl J Med* 1993;**328**:1433.
9. Lowenfels AB *et al*. Risk factors for cancer in hereditary pancreatitis. International Hereditary Pancreatitis Study Group. *Med Clin North Am* 2000;**84**:565.
10. Lynch HT *et al*. Familial pancreatic cancer: a review. *Semin Oncol* 1996;**23**:251.
11. Tsuchiya R *et al*. Collective review of small carcinomas of the pancreas. *Ann Surg* 1986;**203**:77.
12. Brentnall TA *et al*. Early diagnosis and treatment of pancreatic dysplasia in patients with a family history of pancreatic cancer. *Ann Intern Med* 1999;**131**:247.
13. Goggins M *et al*. Can we screen high-risk individuals to detect early pancreatic carcinoma? *J Surg Oncol* 2000;**74**:243.
14. Canto M *et al*. Screening for pancreatic neoplasia in hgh-risk individuals: the Johns Hopkins experience. *Gastroenterology* 2002;**122**(Suppl. 1):A-17.
15. Klein AP *et al*. Prospective risk of pancreatic cancer in familial pancreatic cancer kindreds. *Cancer Res* 2004;**64**:2634.
16. Eberle MA *et al*. A new susceptibility locus for autosomal dominant pancreatic cancer maps to chromosome 4q32–34. *Am J Hum Genet* 2002;**70**:1044.
17. Permert J *et al*. Pancreatic cancer is associated with impaired glucose metabolism. *Eur J Surg* 1993;**159**:101.
18. Schwarts SS *et al*. A prospective study of glucose tolerance, insulin, C-peptide, and glucagon responses in patients with pancreatic carcinoma. *Am J Dig Dis* 1978;**23**:1107.
19. Chari ST *et al*. Islet amyloid polypeptide is not a satisfactory marker for detecting pancreatic cancer. *Gastroenterology* 2001;**121**:640.
20. Gullo L *et al*. Diabetes and the risk of pancreatic cancer. Italian Pancreatic Cancer Study Group. *N Engl J Med* 1994;**331**:81.
21. Ogawa Y *et al*. A prospective pancreatographic study of the prevalence of pancreatic carcinoma in patients with diabetes mellitus. *Cancer* 2002;**94**:2344.
22. Damiano J *et al*. Should pancreas imaging be recommended in patients over 50 years when diabetes is discovered because of acute symptoms? *Diabetes Metab* 2004;**30**:203.
23. Chari S *et al*. Probability of pancreatic cancer following diabetes: A population-based study. *Gastroenterology* 2005;**129**:504.

32 Alcoholic Liver Disease

Mary C. Dufour

Key points
- Alcoholic liver disease comprises a spectrum of liver pathology including alcoholic fatty liver, alcoholic hepatitis, alcoholic cirrhosis and hepatocellular carcinoma.
- In the general population, people with alcoholic liver disease are often asymptomatic.
- Alcoholic liver disease is a major cause of morbidity and mortality in most developed countries in the world.
- Alcoholic liver disease is preventable.
- Healthcare providers should routinely ask all their patients about alcohol use.

Clinical summary

The diagnosis of alcoholic liver disease (ALD) is established by a history of habitual intake of alcohol of sufficient duration and quantity, together with the physical signs and laboratory evidence of liver disease. Many studies have shown that the amount of alcohol consumed and the duration of consumption are closely associated with the type and degree of ALD. Alcohol dependence is not a prerequisite for the development of ALD, but because alcohol-dependent individuals tend to be the heaviest drinkers, they are most at risk for developing ALD.

Diagnosis of ALD may be difficult because patients frequently minimize their alcohol consumption or deny abuse. In addition, there may be no evidence of ALD from physical examination, and laboratory test abnormalities may not be specific for ALD. There are usually no symptoms in the early stages of disease. Alcoholic fatty liver is usually asymptomatic in ambulatory patients. Hepatomegaly is common in hospitalized patients. Alcoholic hepatitis also may be asymptomatic or present with isolated hepatomegaly [1].

The clinical presentation of alcoholic hepatitis varies greatly with the severity of disease. Common symptoms are fatigue, exhaustion, weakness, anorexia, weight loss, nausea, vomiting and diarrhea. Patients with alcoholic hepatitis are often malnourished and pyrexial. The classic clinical syndrome associated with alcoholic hepatitis includes fever, malaise, jaundice and tender hepatomegaly [2]. Cirrhosis may coexist with alcoholic hepatitis, and therefore in some people the first sign of disease may be due to complications of cirrhosis such as edema, ascites, bruising or bleeding, and jaundice. Portal hypertension can cause the formation of esophageal and gastric varices, which can cause life-threatening bleeds. Like patients with alcoholic fatty liver and alcoholic hepatitis, those with alcohol-induced cirrhosis may present with very few signs and symptoms of liver disease or they may present with jaundice, parotid enlargement, spider angiomas, gynecomastia, palmar erythema, Dupuytren's contracture and testicular atrophy [3]. Over time, most patients with cirrhosis develop evidence of portal hypertension as well as hepatocellular dysfunction (e.g., cachexia and jaundice).

There is no one blood test or imaging study that can be used to diagnose ALD reliably. The pattern of aminotransferase abnormalities may provide a clue that alcohol is the likely cause of liver injury [1]. Typically the serum aspartate aminotransferase (AST) level is two to three times greater than the serum alanine aminotransferase (ALT) level in alcoholic liver injury. Gamma-glutamyl transferase (GGT) and mean corpuscular volume (MCV), used in conjunction with the AST/ALT ratio, may provide a further indication of ALD. Sonography, computed tomography (CT) and magnetic resonance imaging (MRI) are useful for suggesting fatty liver (steatosis). Unfortunately these imaging techniques are not able to determine the cause of the steatosis or ascertain the presence of co-occurring alcoholic hepatitis. These tests can, however, detect the presence of portal hypertension even before the patient becomes symptomatic. On ultrasound, the features of cirrhosis and portal hypertension include liver nodules, sluggish or reversed portal vein blood flow, splenomegaly and intra-abdominal varices [3]. Liver biopsy is the most sensitive and specific way to determine the degree of alcoholic liver injury including liver cell injury and hepatic fibrosis. At present it is the only way reliably to detect alcoholic hepatitis and cirrhosis in asymptomatic individuals. Once evidence of portal hypertension becomes apparent, biopsy is less critical for this purpose [1].

Treatment strategies for ALD include lifestyle changes to reduce alcohol consumption, cigarette smoking and obesity; nutritional therapy; pharmacological therapy; and liver transplantation. Alcoholic cirrhosis is the most common underlying cause of hepatocellular carcinoma (HCC) in the USA. Abstinence from alcohol is a critical component of treatment for ALD. The outcome of ALD depends on not only whether the patient continues to drink, but also whether additional causes of liver injury are present such as hepatitis C, hemochromatosis or obesity [4].

Disease definition

The liver is one of the largest and most complex organs in the body. It performs multiple functions including the production of proteins and enzymes, detoxification, metabolic functions and the regulation of cholesterol and blood clotting. Because the liver is primarily responsible for alcohol metabolism, it is especially vulnerable to alcohol-related injury [5]. Liver cells (hepatocytes) are the site of alcohol oxidation and alcohol-induced injury. The nonparenchymal liver cells provide a supporting role in maintaining liver homeostasis and actively participate in alcohol-induced pathological processes [5].

Alcoholic liver disease (ALD) encompasses three conditions: alcoholic fatty liver, alcoholic hepatitis and alcoholic cirrhosis. Alcoholic fatty liver is the earliest stage of ALD and is marked by lipid accumulation in large and small droplets within the hepatocytes. Alcoholic hepatitis is a well-characterized histologic disease, defined by a constellation of features, including confluent parenchymal necrosis, varying degrees of steatosis, deposition of intrasinusoidal and pericentral collagen, and infiltration by polymorphonuclear cells, typically clustered around eosinophilic cytoplasmic structures known as Mallory bodies [6]. Lobular infiltration with polymorphonuclear leukocytes distinguishes alcoholic hepatitis from other forms of hepatitis in which the inflammatory infiltrate is predominantly periportal and mononuclear [1]. In cir-

rhosis, broad bands of connective tissue stretch between portal and central areas of adjacent liver lobules, dividing the liver tissue into nodules that contain injured and regenerating hepatocytes. Normal liver cells are replaced by scar tissue and consequently the liver is unable to perform many of its usual functions [6].

Although multiple mechanisms have been proposed, it is clear that the hepatotoxicity of alcohol is mediated by both direct and indirect mechanisms, balanced against the liver's ability to regenerate. In addition to the mechanisms of injury, any number of which may be occurring simultaneously, there are also a number of predisposing factors [6].

Incidence and prevalence

Alcohol use is pervasive in the USA. In 2004, over 86% of adults aged 18 and older reported ever consuming alcohol, and nearly two-thirds reported drinking in the past year [7]. However, only a fraction of drinkers are serious problem drinkers or drink sufficient quantities to suffer serious health consequences. The top 20% of current drinkers consume 80% of all alcohol, with the top 2.5% consuming 27% [8]. In 2001–2002, 8.46%, or 17.6 million Americans aged 18 and older, met *Diagnostic and Statistical Manual, Fourth Edition* (DSM-IV) criteria for alcohol abuse or dependence [9]. Although cirrhosis mortality has been researched for centuries, few studies of the incidence and prevalence of alcoholic liver disease have been done in the general population. Accurate estimates for the incidence and prevalence of ALD in the general population are difficult to make because many individuals with ALD are asymptomatic and national surveys (e.g., National Health Interview Survey, National Health and Nutrition Examination Survey) do not ask questions in sufficient detail to allow classification by specific causes of liver disease. The liver has an extensive reserve and often only after extensive damage has been done do patients become symptomatic. Unless they have decompensated cirrhosis, patients with ALD may not seek medical attention. Autopsy series have estimated the prevalence of cirrhosis to be between 5% and 10% of the US population [10]. Obviously alcohol consumption is required for the development of ALD; however, not all heavy drinkers develop serious alcoholic liver disease. Approximately 90–100% of heavy drinkers show evidence of fatty liver but only 10–35% develop alcoholic hepatitis, and 8–20% develop cirrhosis [4,6]. The probability of developing cirrhosis is approximately 10–20% per year, and approximately 70% of patients with alcoholic hepatitis will ultimately develop cirrhosis [11].

Based on data from the National Hospital Discharge Survey, in 2003 there were approximately 424 000 hospital discharge episodes for persons aged 15 and older that had a principal (first-listed) alcohol-related diagnosis, and approximately 1.6 million discharge episodes that had an any (all-listed) alcohol-related diagnosis. ALD accounted for 25% of the first-listed diagnoses and approximately 29% of the all-listed diagnoses [12]. In the USA in 2003, there were 27 503 deaths from cirrhosis and chronic liver disease, making it the 12th leading cause of death [13]. Approximately 44% of these deaths were coded as alcohol-induced [14].

Risk factors for disease

The association between alcohol intake and alcohol-induced liver disease is unquestionable, but the dose–response relation and its variations by sex and race/ethnicity remain unclear. In studies based on retrospective ascertainment of alcohol consumption at the time of diagnosis of ALD, it has been reported that the risk of developing liver damage increased with increasing alcohol consumption and that minimum alcohol intake associated with a significant increase in risk was 40–80 g daily (about four to eight drinks) among men and 20 g among women for at least 10 years [3,15]. Alcohol abuse and ALD are found primarily in men; however, women who do drink have a significantly greater risk of developing ALD than do men at any given level of alcohol consumption [16]. Compared with men, women develop alcohol-induced liver disease over a shorter period of time and after consuming less al-

cohol [11]. In addition, women are more likely than men to develop alcoholic hepatitis and to die from cirrhosis [11].

In the USA variations exist in ADL mortality according to race/ethnicity. The rank order of cirrhosis as a leading cause of death in the USA in 2003 by Hispanic origin, race and sex is shown in Table 32.1 [17]. Although alcohol consumption varies widely among tribes, ALD mortality rates are highest among American Indian and Alaska Native men and women [17]. In 2003, among Hispanic White men, the age-adjusted death rate from ALD was 12.2 per 100 000, more than double the rates for non-Hispanic White men (6.0 per 100 000) and non-Hispanic Black men (6.2) [14]. Mortality rates for Hispanic White women were similar (2.3) to those for non-Hispanic White women (2.1) and non-Hispanic Black women (2.1). In the past, ALD mortality rates for Black men were considerably higher than those for non-Hispanic White men, but in recent years these differences have disappeared [14]. The differences in cirrhosis mortality between Hispanic men and non-Hispanic Black and White men suggest differences in alcohol consumption, but studies of alcohol consumption patterns in these groups tend not to support this interpretation [18]. The higher prevalence of hepatitis C virus (HCV) infection in Hispanic men is one possible explanation for the increased alcoholic cirrhosis mortality rates in this population [18].

Adult per capita alcohol consumption is greatest in Europe followed by the Americas [19]. In recent years alcohol consumption has begun to increase in the countries of Southeast Asia and the Western Pacific. Worldwide, per capita pure alcohol consumption ranges from zero in countries such as Iran and Kuwait to 16.21 liters in the Czech Republic and 17.54 liters in Luxembourg. The USA

Table 32.1 Cirrhosis as a leading cause of death in 2003 by race/ethnicity and sex

Hispanic origin, race and sex	Rank order of cirrhosis as a leading cause of death
Non-Hispanic American Indian/Alaska Native males	5th
Non-Hispanic American Indian/Alaska Native females	6th
Hispanic males, all races	7th
Hispanic White males	7th
Non-Hispanic White males	11th
Hispanic females, all races	11th
Non-Hispanic Asian males	13th
Non-Hispanic White females	13th
Non-Hispanic Black males	14th
Non-Hispanic Black females	15th
Non-Hispanic Asian females	18th

Source: CDC Wonder http://webapp.cdc.gov/sas web/ncipc/leadcaus.html

ranks 41st in the world in per capita alcohol consumption at 8.51 liters [19]. Alcohol is considered to be the leading cause of liver cirrhosis in established market economies throughout the world [19]. Mortality rates per 100 000 for cirrhosis range from 4.0 in Kuwait to 26.29 in Slovenia, 37.09 in Romania and 45.79 in Hungary. France (11.45) and Germany (13.36) have rates nearly double that in the USA (7.47) [19].

The threshold of alcohol necessary for the development of advanced ALD varies substantially among individuals, and factors other than absolute alcohol consumption clearly play an important role in determining who will develop ALD. These factors may be genetic or environmental. The National Academy of Sciences/National Research Council twin registry of almost 16 000 male twin pairs reported concordance rates for cirrhosis of 16.9% in monozygotic twins and 5.3% in dizygotic twins, implying a genetic predisposition to this complication of alcohol abuse [20]. Several genetic factors may increase an individual's susceptibility to ALD. Various candidate genes for drinking behavior and alcohol dependence are beginning to be identified [4]. Early studies looking for candidate genes focused primarily on genes encoding ethanol-metabolizing enzymes but genetic variations in these enzymes seem to play a relatively minor role in Caucasian populations. Increasing evidence supports a role for cytokines and immune responses in the pathogenesis of ALD, thus suggesting an alternate set of candidate genes [21].

The fact that the concordance rate for alcoholic cirrhosis in monozygotic twins falls well below 100% highlights the fact that environmental factors such as diet and lifestyle also play a role in susceptibility to ALD. A diet high in polyunsaturated fatty acids appears to be a risk factor for ALD [6]. Some research suggests that there is a high degree of correlation between pork consumption and the development of ALD. Moreover, there appears to be a strong negative correlation between coffee consumption and the development of ALD [11]. Malnutrition is a key risk factor. Prolonged alcohol consumption induces dietary deficiencies, which have profound effects on the metabolic pathways that influence the stages of hepatic fat accumulation, oxidant liver injury and fibrosis. The fact that malnutrition is promoted by worsening liver function during the development of ALD supports a vicious cycle whereby alcohol causes specific nutritional deficiencies that promote mechanisms of liver injury that enhance the development of ALD [22]. Tobacco use may also be a risk factor; however, the research findings are mixed. In addition, because heavy drinkers are very likely to be heavy smokers, ascertaining an effect of tobacco independent of alcohol has been difficult [11].

Obesity is strongly associated with liver disease (see Chapter 34 on Nonalcoholic Fatty Liver Disease). In addition, obesity is an independent risk factor for alcohol-induced liver damage and seems to increase all stages of ALD [23].

One of the most important risk factors for ALD is the presence of concomitant infection with hepatitis C virus (HCV). The relationship between alcohol use and infection with HCV is complex. It is estimated that the prevalence of HCV in patients with ALD ranges from 14% to 43% [11]. Both alcohol and HCV are independent risk factors for the development of cirrhosis. In fact, in the USA in 2005, the most common indications for liver transplantation were HCV (30%) and ALD (18%) [24]. Research now suggests that the combination of the two risk factors may act synergistically to hasten the progression of liver disease. Alcoholics with HCV are more likely to develop fibrosis and cirrhosis, and to develop cirrhosis more rapidly than alcoholic patients without HCV [11]. The interaction between alcohol consumption and hepatitis B virus (HBV) infection is less well understood. Some studies have reported an increased risk of developing cirrhosis in HBV-infected individuals who drink alcohol. Others have not. Because many of these studies were performed prior to the discovery of HCV, the influence of HBV infection on ALD requires further clarification [11].

Natural history and mortality

Alcoholic fatty liver generally resolves within two weeks of discontinuing alcohol consumption; however, cirrhosis may develop in individuals with chronic alcoholic fatty liver who also have fibrosis [1]. The short-term prognosis of hospitalized patients with alcoholic hepatitis is extremely variable. Patients with severe alcoholic hepatitis may develop rapid liver failure and die or may recover with abstinence. In patients with severe disease, the 30-day mortality rate approaches 50% but in all patients with alcoholic hepatitis, the overall 30-day mortality rate is about 15%. The long-term prognosis of patients with less severe alcoholic hepatitis is primarily determined by drinking status, but abstinence from alcohol may not completely prevent the development of cirrhosis. Between a quarter and a third of patients with alcoholic hepatitis go on to develop cirrhosis [4]. The long-term prognosis for patients with cirrhosis improves with abstinence. The 5-year survival for patients who abstain can be as high as

90% compared with less than 70% for those who continue to drink. In patients with decompensated cirrhosis, the survival rate for abstainers is 60% but drops to less than 30% for those who continue to drink [3]. The overall 5-year survival in cirrhosis patients who continue to drink is approximately 35% [11]. The survival of patients after liver transplant secondary to alcoholic cirrhosis parallels that of patients with cirrhosis due to other causes [25]. Alcohol is both a primary cause of HCC and a cofactor for the development of HCC. The rates of HCC increase dramatically in patients having both alcohol consumption and HCV [11].

Disability and quality of life

The health-related quality of life in alcohol-dependent individuals is severely impaired; moreover, people associated with the problem drinker are also affected [26]. ALD is characterized by general tiredness and fatigue [27]. All domains of health-related quality of life, except pain, are altered in patients with cirrhosis [28]. Severity of disease and muscle cramps are the factors most often associated with poor health status perception [28]. Most areas of daily life are affected by perceived health problems. The major areas of concern for men are paid employment and sex life, while those for women are home life and social life. At the end stages of cirrhosis, ascites and encephalopathy, as well as muscle cramps, further decrease the quality of life [27]. Following recovery from surgery, the effect of liver transplantation is generally a dramatic improvement in quality of life [27].

Healthcare utilization and costs

Kim and colleagues recently summarized the burden of liver disease in the USA [29]. The data on the economic impact of chronic liver disease are derived from a report produced by the American Gastroenterological Association [30,31]. This report was published in 2001 and presents 1998 data. Although now somewhat dated, this information is the most current available. For chronic liver disease exclusive of HCV, the largest direct cost arose from 357 000 hospital inpatient stays. These visits were responsible for $134.0 million in physician fees and $1.1 billion in facility costs. The 758 000 visits to physician offices accounted for $64.8 million in direct costs. Hospital outpatient departments saw 186 000 cases at a cost

of $57.1 million. The cost of medications used to treat chronic liver disease and cirrhosis contributes another $16.9 million. Overall total direct costs were more than $1.4 billion. Adjusting for inflation yields over $1.5 billion in direct costs in year 2000 dollars [30]. Patients with chronic liver disease were hospitalized for over 2.3 million days with an average length of stay of 5.9 days. This translates to $185.9 million in the value of lost wages. Including the time associated with visits to physicians' offices, hospital emergency departments and outpatient departments, total indirect costs equal $221.5 million annually. Adjusting for inflation, this totals $234.0 million in 2000 dollars [30,31]. In 2003, 44% of deaths from chronic liver disease and cirrhosis were coded as alcohol-related [14]. Therefore the direct and indirect costs of ALD could be estimated to be 44% of the above-mentioned figures. Because ALD is known to be under-recorded, these estimates are conservative.

In 2005, 6444 liver transplants were performed in the USA and 18% of these were performed for ALD [24]. Liver transplant procedure costs can vary considerably but generally average between $100 000 and $400 000, depending on the time waiting in the intensive care unit (ICU) and the extent of liver disease before transplantation [32]. Costs can also vary due to rate of recovery, complications after surgery, severity of rejection and the number of medications or procedures needed after surgery [33]. The costs of medications after the patient goes home can be $700 to $1000 per month or more [33].

Prevention

ALD is entirely preventable. All healthcare providers need to be aware that most Americans are drinkers and therefore should routinely ask their patients about alcohol consumption. Men who drink five or more standard drinks in a day (or 15 or more per week) and women who drink four or in a day (or eight or more per week) appear to be at increased risk for alcohol-related problems including medical consequences [34]. The Healthy People 2010 goals include reducing the proportion of adults in the USA whose alcohol consumption exceeds recommended daily (no more than four standard drinks a day for men and no more than three a day for women) and weekly (no more than 14 standard drinks a week for men and seven for women) limits. Drinking at or below these daily and weekly limits would greatly reduce the occurrence of alcoholic liver disease.

Issues and gaps in epidemiologic knowledge

Better data on the incidence and prevalence rates of all types of ALD in the general population are needed as are updated estimates of the economic burden and resource utilization of ALD. Studies of the impact on health-related quality of life of ALD that take into consideration the impact of alcohol abuse and dependence as well as ALD are also needed. Most classic epidemiologic studies of ALD were done prior to the identification of HCV. The epidemiology of ALD in the general population needs to be reassessed in concert with HCV.

Recommendations for future studies

ALD is one of the most common causes of chronic liver disease in the world. Therefore research is urgently needed in a number of areas related to ALD. Research is needed to clarify further the environmental and genetic factors that modulate the severity of ALD. This information is urgently needed to identify the individuals most susceptible to ALD and to inform the development of targeted prevention strategies. Studies that ascertain levels of "safe" drinking in various vulnerable subpopulations would be especially informative. Research is needed to develop more sensitive and specific noninvasive means to diagnose and stage ALD, and to develop better therapies for ALD. We know that alcoholic fatty liver is reversible with abstinence from alcohol. The picture is far less clear for alcoholic hepatitis and especially for alcohol-induced cirrhosis. Therefore, research is needed to determine whether abstinence from alcohol promotes the regression of established alcoholic hepatitis and cirrhosis and what other factors would enhance the regression.

Conclusions

Alcoholic liver disease is a major cause of morbidity and mortality worldwide. ALD is largely preventable. Therefore it is paramount that healthcare providers routinely ask all patients about their alcohol consumption. Because ALD is frequently asymptomatic in the general population, better measures of the magnitude of the problem are needed as are more sensitive and specific noninvasive means of detecting ALD.

References

1. Diehl AM. Liver disease in alcohol abusers: clinical perspective. *Alcohol* 2002;**27**:7.
2. Arteel G *et al.* Advances in alcoholic liver disease. *Best Pract Res Cl Ga* 2003;**17**:625.
3. Mendez-Sanchez N *et al.* Alcoholic liver disease. An update. *Ann Hepatol* 2005;**4**:32.
4. Wilner *et al.* Alcohol and the liver. *Curr Opin Gastroenterol* 2005;**21**:323.
5. Marsano LS *et al.* Diagnosis and treatment of alcoholic liver disease and its complications. *Alcohol Res Health* 2003;**27**:247.
6. O'Shea RS *et al.* Treatment of alcoholic hepatitis. *Clin Liver Dis* 2005;**9**:103.
7. Substance Abuse and Mental Health Services Administration. *Results from the 2004 National Survey on Drug Use and Health: National Findings.* Office of Applied Studies, NSDUH Series H-28, DHHS Publication No. SMA 05–4062. Rockville, MD: Substance Abuse and Mental Health Services Administration, 2005 (http://oas.samhsa.gov/NSDUH/2k4Results/2k4results.pdf).
8. Greenfiled T *et al.* Who drinks most of the alcohol in the US? The policy implications. *J Studies Alcohol* 1999;**60**:78.
9. Grant BF *et al.* The 12-month prevalence and trends in DSM-IV alcohol abuse and dependence: United States, 1991–1992 and 2001–2002. *Drug Alcohol Depend* 2004;**74**:223.
10. Graudal N *et al.* Characteristics of cirrhosis undiagnosed during life: a comparative analysis of 73 undiagnosed cases and 149 diagnosed cases of cirrhosis, detected in 4929 consecutive autopsies. *J Intern Med* 1991;**230**:165.
11. Mandayam S *et al.* Epidemiology of alcoholic liver disease. *Semin Liver Dis* 2004;**24**:217.
12. Chen C *et al. Surveillance Report #72: Trends in Alcohol-Related Morbidity Among Short-Stay Community Hospital Discharges, United States, 1979–2003.* Rockville, MD: National Institute on Alcohol Abuse and Alcoholism, 2005.
13. Hoyert DL *et al.* Deaths: final data for 2003. *National Vital Statistics Reports* 2006;**54**:1.
14. Yoon Y *et al. Surveillance Report #75: Liver Cirrhosis Mortality in the United States, 1970–2003.* Rockville, MD: National Institute on Alcohol Abuse and Alcoholism, 2006.
15. Becker U *et al.* Prediction of risk of liver disease by alcohol intake, sex and age: A prospective population study. *Hepatology* 1996;**23**:1025.
16. Menon KVN *et al.* Pathogenesis, diagnosis, and treatment of alcoholic liver disease. *Mayo Clin Proc* 2001;**76**:1021.
17. Centers for Disease Control and Prevention (CDC). Leading causes of death reports http://webapp.cdc.gov/sasweb/ncicp/leadcaus.html
18. Mann RE *et al.* The epidemiology of alcoholic liver disease. *Alcohol Res Health* 2003;**27**:209.

19. World Health Organization. *Global Status Report on Alcohol 2004*. Geneva: World Health Organization, 2004.

20. Reed T *et al*. Genetic predisposition to organ-specific endpoints of alcoholism. *Alcohol Clin Exp Res* 1996;**20**:1528.

21. Grove J *et al*. Interleukin 10 promoter region polymorphisms and susceptibility to advanced alcoholic liver disease. *Gut* 2000;**46**:540.

22. Halstead CH. Nutrition and alcoholic liver disease. *Semin Liver Dis* 2004;**24**:289.

23. Diehl AM. Obesity and alcoholic liver disease. *Alcohol* 2004;**34**:81.

24. U.S. Department of Health and Human Services. *2005 Annual Report of the U.S. Organ Procurement and Transplantation Network and the Scientific Registry of Transplant Recipients: Transplant Data 1995–2004*. Rockville, MD: Health Resources and Services Administration, Healthcare Systems Bureau, Division of Transplantation (http://www.hrsa.gov/).

25. Wakim-Fleming J *et al*. Long-term management of alcoholic liver disease. *Clin Liver Dis* 2005;**9**:135.

26. Morgan M *et al*. Improvement in quality of life after treatment for alcohol dependence with acamprosate and psychosocial support. *Alcohol Clin Exp Res* 2004;**28**:64.

27. Glise H *et al*. Health-related quality of life and gastrointestinal disease. *J Gastroenterol Hepatol* 2002;**17**(Suppl.):S72.

28. Marchesini G *et al*. Factors associated with poor health-related quality of life of patients with cirrhosis. *Gastroenterology* 2001;**120**:170.

29. Kim WR *et al*. Burden of liver disease in the United States: Summary of a workshop. *Hepatology* 2002;**6**:227.

30. American Gastroenterological Association. *The Burden of Gastrointestinal Diseases*. Bethesda, MD: American Gastroenterological Association, 2001.

31. Sandler RS *et al*. The burden of selected digestive diseases in the United States. *Gastroenterology* 2002;**122**:1500.

32. American Liver Foundation. ALF Transplant Fund Program (http://www.liverfoundation.org/).

33. Emory Healthcare. Liver transplantation program (http://www.emoryhealthcare.org/departments/transplant_liver/patient).

34. Dawson DA *et al*. Quantifying the risks associated with exceeding recommended drinking limits. *Alcohol Clin Exp Res* 2005;**29**:902.

33 Cirrhosis and Hepatocellular Carcinoma

William Sanchez and Jayant A. Talwalkar

Key points

- Despite an increase in hospitalization rate and resource utilization, the mortality rate from cirrhosis has been stable in the USA. Recent increases in the death rate in the UK appear related to changing alcohol consumption patterns in this country.
- Much of the published literature regarding the epidemiology of cirrhosis comes from referral-based populations. Well-designed, contemporary, population-based studies of the incidence and prevalence rates for cirrhosis are needed.

- Globally, hepatocellular carcinoma is a leading cause of death, accounting for over half a million deaths in the year 2000. The development of hepatocellular carcinoma is closely associated with cirrhosis and chronic infection with viral hepatitis.
- In the USA the incidence of hepatocellular carcinoma has steadily increased over the past two decades, due mainly to chronic hepatitis C virus infection. The mortality rate and healthcare expenditures associated with hepatocellular carcinoma have also increased.

Clinical summary

Cirrhosis and hepatocellular carcinoma (HCC) are the final common endpoints of chronic liver disease from a variety of causes. Disruption of the normal hepatic architecture gives rise to portal venous hypertension manifested by ascites, gastroesophageal varices, hypersplenism and hepatic encephalopathy. Chronic injury and increased hepatocyte turnover are, in turn, risk factors for carcinogenesis within the diseased liver.

Many patients are asymptomatic or experience only nonspecific symptoms until advanced hepatic fibrosis is present. While specific complications of cirrhosis may be individually managed, the performance of liver transplantation is considered ideal therapy for patients with end-stage liver failure. The development of HCC often portends a grim prognosis related to advanced stage at diagnosis. Individuals with early-stage tumors, however, should be evaluated for curative surgical procedures (e.g., hepatic resection or liver transplantation) while palliative therapies (e.g., percutaneous ablation or hepatic artery chemoembolization) may be appropriate for patients with advanced disease.

Cirrhosis

Incidence and prevalence

Current, population-based studies focusing on the descriptive epidemiology of cirrhosis are lacking. Population-based data from Iceland describe the annual incidence of cirrhosis as between 2.2 and 2.5 cases per 100 000 population between 1971 and 1990. These are the lowest incidence rates in Europe, reflecting a low amount of alcohol consumption per capita and the low prevalence of chronic viral hepatitis in this country [1]. Higher rates in other European nations, such as those reported in England and Spain, are likely based on differences in alcohol consumption, a growing rate of ambulatory-based diagnoses and the increase in obesity and diabetes mellitus (see below). Based on limited information, the influence of gender on the incidence or prevalence of cirrhosis remains unknown. 1998 data found over 5.5 million prevalent cases of chronic liver diseases and cirrhosis in the USA, a rate of 2030 cases per 100 000 persons [2].

Direct comparisons of prevalence among various ethnic groups have been recently performed. In a population-based study, the ethnic differences in frequency of hepatic steatosis (45% in Hispanic people, 33% in White people, 24% in Black people) mirrored those observed previously for non-alcoholic cirrhosis [3]. From a population-based, case-control study, the prevalence rate for cirrhosis among Hispanic persons in Texas was estimated at 126 cases per 100 000 population. The prevalence of cryptogenic cirrhosis in Hispanic patients was 3.1-fold higher than among European American patients in a geographic area where only 26% of adult individuals seeking medical care were

Hispanic. In contrast, the prevalence rate for cryptogenic cirrhosis among African-American patients was 3.9-times lower than in European Americans [5].

Inciting exposures
Alcohol

In Europe and North America, alcohol is the most common exposure associated with the development of cirrhosis. The duration of use and dose–response relationship between alcohol and cirrhosis are established. In a case-control study of patients with cirrhosis evaluated between 1989 and 1996, the attributable risk for cirrhosis from alcohol was estimated at 68%, in contrast to 40% for hepatitis C and 4% for hepatitis B virus [6]. The effect of type of alcohol consumed (spirits vs beer or wine) on progression to cirrhosis remains unknown. While per capita consumption has remained stable, the possibility of periodic excessive (or binge) drinking is hypothesized as an explanation for increasing case rates in Great Britain [7].

Obesity

Data regarding the impact of obesity on the development of cirrhosis are emerging. While there does not appear to be an increased risk for liver-related hospitalization or death among overweight individuals (BMI ≥25) within the US general population, a nearly twofold increase in hospitalization and death was observed among obese individuals (BMI ≥30) compared with lean persons (adjusted hazard ratio 1.69, 95% CI 1.0–3.0) [8]. This result was adjusted for age, sex, race, alcohol consumption, education level and geographic region. Among patients who do not consume alcohol, this risk increased to fourfold in obese compared with lean individuals (adjusted hazard ratio 4.10, 95% CI 1.4–11.4) [9]. Additional data suggest that central obesity (defined by skinfold thickness ratio >1) rather than peripheral obesity is linked to an increased rate of liver-related hospitalization and death [10].

Cigarette smoking

There is no population-based study available to estimate accurately the impact of cigarette smoking on the prevalence of cirrhosis. A previous hospital-based geographic study observed a dose–response relationship between cigarette smoking and risk for cirrhosis. More recent studies from tertiary referral centers identify a significant relationship between smoking and fibrosis in hepatitis C virus (HCV) [11].

Coffee/tea consumption

There is mounting evidence that a protective association between coffee/tea consumption and risk for developing cirrhosis exists. From a geographic, hospital-based, case-control study [12], an inverse association was identified across various strata of age, sex, tobacco use, alcohol consumption and duration of cirrhosis. Two recent population-based investigations have shown longitudinal and dose–response evidence for this observation. In a defined population from Norway, a lower risk for both alcohol-related and all-cause mortality in coffee drinkers was reported [13]. Within the US general population [8], a 40% reduction in liver-related hospitalization or death was associated with the daily consumption of more than two cups of coffee or tea versus less than one cup per day. Notably, the cumulative risk for hospitalization in persons at high risk for cirrhosis was reduced by 60% when two or more cups were consumed.

Natural history
Complications of portal hypertension

The cumulative risk for developing complications of portal hypertension has not been described among contemporary, population-based cohorts to date. Available data come from recent studies from tertiary referral centers. Among 312 patients with compensated cirrhosis (75% from chronic hepatitis C) evaluated between 1986 and 1996, the cumulative incidence for developing at least one complication of cirrhosis was 32% over a median follow-up period of 93 months (range, 14–194 months). The 10-year cumulative incidence rates for individual complications, including ascites (28%), gastrointestinal bleeding (5%), hepatic encephalopathy (5%) and hepatocellular carcinoma (28%), were also reported [14]. Similar data are observed from contemporary European cohorts with co-infection with chronic hepatitis B and D [15] as well as alcoholic cirrhosis [16].

Among 212 patients hospitalized with their first episode of hepatic decompensation from chronic hepatitis C between 1998 and 2001, the most frequent cause was ascites (48%) followed by portal hypertensive bleeding (32%), bacterial infection (14%) and hepatic encephalopathy (5%). Over 50% of bacterial infections were from spontaneous bacterial peritonitis [17].

Prognosis

A number of studies have been reported since 2000 that

yield significant information about the prognosis of cirrhosis. One such study for patients with nonalcoholic fatty liver disease has shown that the mortality rate among community-based patients is higher than the general population [18]. Risk factors for death included increasing age, impaired fasting glucose, and the development of cirrhosis. In this study, liver disease was the third leading cause of death compared with the 13th leading cause of death in the general population.

Time trends in mortality from cirrhosis have also been reported. From a population-based study of inhabitants from northeastern Spain, the mortality rate from cirrhosis declined between 1987 and 1997. Liver-disease death rates were 2–3-fold greater for men compared with women and, in particular, individuals who are 45 years and younger with viral co-infection in the setting of human immunodeficiency virus [19]. From a cohort of 10 154 Danish patients with cirrhosis hospitalized between 1982 and 1993, the 10-year survival rate was significantly reduced in patients with alcoholic cirrhosis (34%) compared with patients with primary biliary cirrhosis (58%) or viral hepatitis (66%) [20]. From a defined population in southern England during 1968–1999, alcoholic liver disease was the principal hospitalization diagnosis in 34% of cases of cirrhosis [21]. At 30 days after admission, the case fatality rate was 15.9% with a standardized mortality ratio of 93. At one year, the overall case fatality rate was 33.6% with a standardized mortality ratio of 16.3. Unlike the other studies, there was no improvement in mortality rates over the time period.

National mortality trends for cirrhosis related to alcohol use in North America, southern and western Europe, Latin America and the Far East have declined over time. Reduced per capita consumption of alcohol has been cited as the dominant factor explaining these survival patterns. In the UK and Scotland, however, a reversed trend is observed, with significant increases in cirrhosis-related mortality since the 1980s and 1990s (Fig. 33.1) [7]. The most affected area is Scotland where mortality rates have tripled for both sexes and all age groups since 1990.

Studies have also been performed to examine the influence of race/ethnicity on mortality risk from cirrhosis. While African Americans did not appear to have a greater risk for liver-related hospitalization or death based on data from the NHANES survey [8,9], other studies suggest that in the USA, significant mortality differentials are found among high-risk groups such as American Indians and Hispanic Americans [22]. From 1991 to 1997, White Hispanic men in the USA incurred the highest mortality rates from cirrhosis followed by Black non-Hispanic men,

White non-Hispanic men, White Hispanic women, and non-Hispanic women [23]. Another study supports the figures demonstrating higher age-adjusted mortality rates from cirrhosis in Black people than in White people [24].

Based on improvements in therapy and intensive care medicine, the risk of death from acute variceal hemorrhage in the control groups of clinical trials has declined over the past four decades [25]. For Swedish patients within a population-based vicinity, an increase in 5-year survival rates was observed between 1969 and 1979 based on hospital discharge records [26]. Rates were observed to plateau (4 to 6 cases per 100 000 population) and remain stable between 1990 and 2002. In contemporary patients with cirrhosis from chronic hepatitis C and variceal hemorrhage as the first manifestation of decompensation, a 1-year survival rate of 90% and a 5-year rate of 80% are reported [17]. Among 216 patients admitted to the hospital for management of moderate- to large-volume ascites between 1980 and 1990, the probability of survival at 1 year was 59%, and at 5 years 27%. Median survival was estimated at 2 years with nearly 50% of patients dying of progressive liver failure [27]. Median survival with ascites as the initial manifestation of decompensated liver disease is 4 years, while the median survival with hepatic encephalopathy is 1–3 years in contemporary patients with cirrhosis [15,17].

Bacterial infection remains a major cause of morbidity and mortality in patients with cirrhosis. From the US National Hospital Discharge Survey, a dataset representing 1% of all hospital discharge records from non-federal hospitals, it appears that patients with cirrhosis are more likely to have and die from sepsis during hospitalization when compared with patients without cirrhosis [28]. In addition, patients with cirrhosis and respiratory failure were 2.6 times more likely to die than individuals without cirrhosis and respiratory failure.

Healthcare utilization

With an estimated 5.5 million people (2% of the US population) affected, cirrhosis is a significant cause of morbidity, resource utilization and death in the USA [50]. In the USA an estimated 1.7 million hospital discharges during 1995–1999 were associated with the diagnosis of cirrhosis [28]. The estimated 1-year cumulative incidence rate for repeat hospitalization to manage complications of cirrhosis is 45%. At 5 years, an estimated 83% of patients may be rehospitalized following an initial admission [17]. Ambulatory care data are noted for an annual total of 758 000 visits to physician offices for the management of chronic liver disease [30].

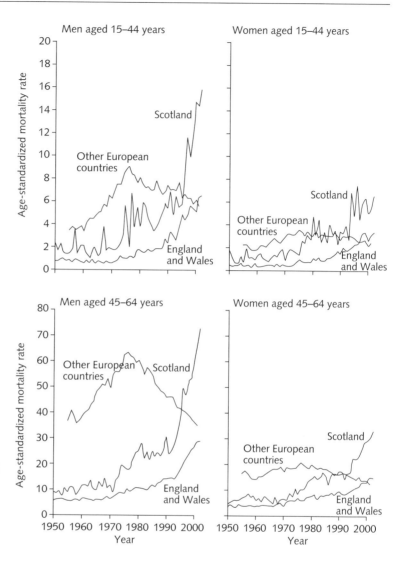

Fig. 33.1 Time trends in age-standardized mortality rates for liver cirrhosis per 100 000 by age group, gender and country between 1950 and 2002. (Reproduced from Leon and McCambridge [6], with permission from Elsevier.)

The vast majority of direct cost attributed to chronic liver disease stems in large part from hospitalization. These visits were responsible for an estimated $1.1 billion in costs during the year 1998. An additional $129 million from ambulatory care visits and $16.9 million for the cost of medications is also noted. Adjusting for inflation, an estimated $1.5 billion is spent annually for managing chronic liver disease and cirrhosis. Based on increased length of stays and missed work, an additional $230 million dollars per year are lost as indirect expenses [30].

Hepatocellular carcinoma (HCC)

Incidence and prevalence

The development of HCC is closely associated with cirrhosis and chronic viral hepatitis. The incidence and prevalence of HCC demonstrate marked geographic variability, largely due to the endemic nature of chronic viral hepatitis in Asia and sub-Saharan Africa (Fig. 33.2). Recent estimates from population-based cancer registries indicate that approximately 564 000 new cases of HCC de-

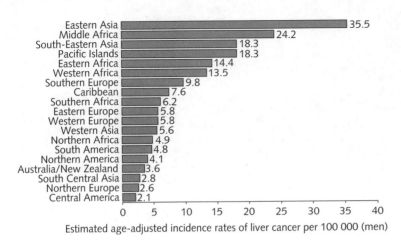

Fig. 33.2 Estimated age-adjusted incidence rates of liver cancer among men by geographic region. The incidence is highest in regions with endemic viral hepatitis. (From Bosch *et al.* [31], with permission from the American Gastroenterological Association.)

veloped worldwide in the year 2000. In the USA and western Europe, the vast majority of cases of HCC arise in the setting of cirrhosis (most commonly secondary to chronic hepatitis C). The incidence of HCC has nearly doubled in the USA over the past two decades, with 8500–11 500 new cases of HCC occurring each year (Fig. 33.3) [31].

Risk factors
Chronic viral hepatitis

Chronic infection with viral hepatitis is the major risk factor for HCC and is attributable for 75–80% of cases of HCC globally. Worldwide, hepatitis B virus accounts for 50–55% and hepatitis C virus accounts for 25–30% of

cases of HCC [31]. In the USA, hepatitis C virus accounts for 47% of cases of HCC [31]. Patients from endemic areas of the world frequently acquire infection with viral hepatitis perinatally or early in life and, therefore, have had a long period of exposure by early adulthood. Surveillance procedures are recommended for hepatitis B surface antigen (HBsAg)-positive patients from Asia (beginning at age 40 for men and 50 for women) and Africa (beginning at age 20) [42].

Gender

Male gender is a well-documented risk factor for HCC. In the year 2000 HCC occurred more frequently in men

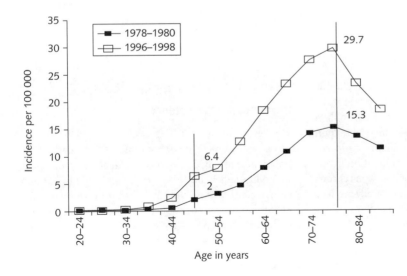

Fig. 33.3 Temporal trends in the age-specific incidence rates for hepatocellular carcinoma. There is a threefold increase for patients aged 45–49 years and two-fold increase in patients aged 75–79 years. (From El-Serag [30], with permission from the American Gastroenterological Association.)

(398 364 cases) than in women (165 972 cases) and was the fifth and eighth most common malignancy in men and women, respectively, around the world. Reported male-to-female incidence ratios range from 1.4 to 3.3 [31,32]. In the USA, over 70% of cases occur in men [31,33].

Race/ethnicity

In the USA, the incidence and mortality rate of HCC is higher among Black and Asian Americans than White Americans [33–35]. The increased disease burden among Asian Americans is largely related to immigration from regions with endemic hepatitis B viral infection [33]. Black people with HCC had higher rates of concurrent hepatitis B and diabetes mellitus than White people [35]. Increased mortality rates among Black Americans may be due in part to lower rates of therapy for HCC (Fig. 33.4) [36].

Geography

The epidemiology of HCC exhibits a pronounced geographic variability, with HCC being more prevalent in eastern and southeastern Asia and sub-Saharan Africa. HCC is the second most common cause of cancer-related death in Asia. In Japan, the annual death rate from HCC has steadily increased from 9.4 per 100 000 to 27.1 per 100 000 between 1960 and 2000 [31,37,38].

The incidence and mortality rates from HCC are also increasing in Western nations [37,39,40]. In the USA, approximately 50% of cases are secondary to chronic infection with the hepatitis C virus, and the incidence of HCC has risen steeply over the past two decades. Based on

published data from the National Cancer Institute Surveillance Epidemiology and End Results registry, the age-adjusted US incidence of HCC doubled between 1985 and 1998 [39,40]. Within the USA there are geographic variations in HCC incidence, with the higher rates in Hawaii, San Francisco-Oakland and New Mexico relative to Connecticut, Iowa and Utah. Multivariate analysis revealed that these regional differences were only partly explained by age, gender and race [41].

Environmental exposures

Dietary exposure to aflatoxin, a mycotoxin that contaminates crops such as peanuts, corn and soybeans, has been linked to an increased risk of HCC. While studies have suggested that the incidence of HCC is greater in patients with hepatitis B who are exposed to aflatoxin, no population-based studies are available to determine the effects of aflatoxin exposure independent of chronic viral hepatitis [31].

Obesity and diabetes mellitus

Obesity has been linked to an increased risk of HCC-related mortality. In a large, prospective, population-based cohort study, age-adjusted mortality rates for primary liver cancer increased from 4.53 per 100 000 in lean women (BMI 18.5–24.9) to 7.52 per 100 000 in obese women (BMI 35.0–39.9). The increased mortality was even more pronounced in men, where mortality rates increased from 9.24 per 100 000 in lean men to 47.80 in obese men [43].

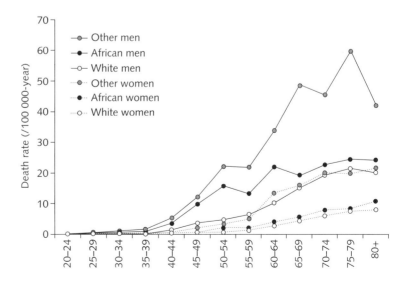

Fig. 33.4 Age-specific HCC mortality rate by age and race. Persons categorized as 'other' race are predominantly of Asian origin. (From Kim *et al.* [33], with permission from the American Gastroenterological Association.)

Recent data suggest that diabetes mellitus is a risk factor for the development of HCC. While much of the published data comes from hospital-based studies, at least one recent population-based study of 2061 cases has identified a three-fold increase in the risk of HCC among patients with diabetes [44,45]. While more research is required, diabetes may become a clinically significant risk factor given the epidemic of diabetes and obesity in the USA.

Natural history and prognosis

As medical care for patients with cirrhosis improves, an increasing proportion of cirrhotic patients die from HCC (Fig. 33.5) [37]. As HCC typically develops within a diseased liver, the prognosis of HCC is poor. The mortality of HCC approaches its incidence rate with more than half a million deaths attributable to HCC worldwide each year. Worldwide, HCC is the third most frequent cause of cancer-related death [46]. In the USA, the mortality rate of HCC has risen in conjunction with the incidence rate. Data from the National Center for Health Statistics and the Agency for Healthcare Research and Quality demonstrate a 67% increase in the mortality rate of HCC between 1980 and 1998 [34].

Healthcare utilization

The rising incidence of HCC in the USA has led to sig-

nificant increases in healthcare expenditures and mortality attributable to HCC [31,33,34]. Among Medicare recipients diagnosed with HCC between 1992 and 1999, the median age of diagnosis was 74. Only a minority of patients were treated with curative intent (13%), while most patients underwent palliative therapy (61%) or received no specific therapy (26%) [49]. A recent study of nationally representative databases revealed that hospital charges for HCC-related treatments doubled from 1988 to 2000, to exceed $500 million. An increasing proportion of treatment-related expenses are due to hospital-based care [34]. Given the increasing incidence of HCC in the USA, healthcare expenditures for HCC can be expected to continue to rise.

Prevention of cirrhosis and HCC

The major public health initiative for the prevention of cirrhosis is to continue efforts at reducing excessive alcohol consumption. In addition, strategies developed to reduce the burden of disease from obesity and diabetes mellitus will have a favorable impact on the epidemiology and prognosis of cirrhosis. Mass vaccination against hepatitis B should also reduce the chance of developing HCC in high-risk areas. While current guidelines recommend surveillance for at-risk populations, these measures are aimed at reducing HCC-related mortality and do not impact disease incidence.

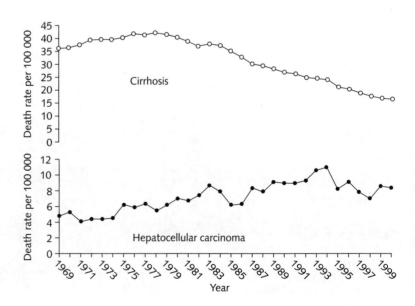

Fig. 33.5 Age-adjusted death rates for cirrhosis and HCC in Italy. (From Fattovich *et al.* [36], with permission from the American Gastroenterological Association.)

Issues/gaps in knowledge

Several crucial gaps in our epidemiologic knowledge concerning cirrhosis and HCC point to future research endeavors.

1 There is an absence of **population-based** epidemiologic investigations examining the potential role of environmental and genetic exposures that may be associated with the development of cirrhosis and HCC. Adequate sample sizes, consistent case definitions, and appropriate control group inclusion are required.

2 Also absent is information on health status associated with cirrhosis and HCC, including preferences for therapies among persons with cirrhosis. Considerable morbidity and impaired health-related quality of life have been observed for patients with cirrhosis in referral-based populations [29]. No community-based study of health-related quality of life has been reported to date. Likewise, evidence to date supports an incremental worsening in health-related quality of life for patients with cirrhosis and HCC when compared with patients with cirrhosis alone [47]. No population-based data, however, are available for comparative purposes.

3 There is absence of information on economic evaluations for management strategies for prevention and therapy of complications from cirrhosis.

Conclusions

Cirrhosis and its complications are associated with progressive liver failure and death in the absence of liver transplantation. As a result, this condition is responsible for significant medical and economic burdens on affected patients and healthcare delivery systems, respectively. The use of accepted methodologies for outcomes and health services research has identified emerging information on the epidemiology and natural history of the disease. Additional knowledge, including the cost-effectiveness of intervention strategies to reduce morbidity and mortality outside of liver transplantation, is required. This will enable disease management strategies in cirrhosis that require the allocation of scarce resources.

References

1. Ludviksdottir D *et al.* Epidemiology of liver cirrhosis morbidity and mortality in Iceland. *Eur J Gastroenterol Hepatol* 1997;**9**:61.

2. National Center for Health Statistics. Current estimates from the National Health Interview Survey. *Vital Health Stat* 1995;**10**:261.

3. Browning JD *et al.* Prevalence of hepatic steatosis in an urban population in the United States: impact of ethnicity. *Hepatology* 2004;**40**:1387.

4. Perez A *et al.* High frequency of chronic end-stage liver disease and hepatocellular carcinoma in a Hispanic population. *J Gastroenterol Hepatol* 2004;**19**:289.

5. Browning JD *et al.* Ethnic differences in the prevalence of cryptogenic cirrhosis. *Am J Gastroenterol* 2004;**99**:292.

6. Leon DA, McCambridge J. Liver cirrhosis mortality rates in Britain from 1950 to 2002: an analysis of routine data. *Lancet* 2006;**367**:52.

7. Ruhl CE, Everhart JE. Coffee and tea consumption are associated with a lower incidence of chronic liver disease in the United States. *Gastroenterology* 2005;**129**:1928.

8. Ioannou GN *et al.* Is obesity a risk factor for cirrhosis-related death or hospitalization? A population-based cohort study. *Gastroenterology* 2003;**125**:1053.

9. Ioannou GN *et al.* Is central obesity associated with cirrhosis-related death or hospitalization? A population-based, cohort study. *Clin Gastroenterol Hepatol* 2005;**3**:67.

10. Pessione F *et al.* Cigarette smoking and hepatic lesions in patients with chronic hepatitis C. *Hepatology* 2001;**34**:121.

11. Gallus S *et al.* Does coffee protect against liver cirrhosis? *Ann Epidemiol* 2002;**12**:202.

12. Tverdal A. Coffee intake and mortality from liver cirrhosis. *Ann Epidemiol* 2003;**13**:419.

13. Benvegnu L *et al.* Natural history of compensated viral cirrhosis: a prospective study on the incidence and hierarchy of major complications. *Gut* 2004;**53**:744.

14. Gheorghe L *et al.* Natural history of compensated viral B and D cirrhosis. *Rom J Gastroenterol* 2005;**14**:329.

15. Sola R *et al.* Probability of liver cancer and survival in HCV-related or alcoholic-decompensated cirrhosis. A study of 377 patients. *Liver Int* 2006;**26**:62.

16. Planas R *et al.* Natural history of decompensated hepatitis C virus-related cirrhosis. A study of 200 patients. *J Hepatol* 2004;**40**:823.

17. Adams LA *et al.* The natural history of nonalcoholic fatty liver disease: a population-based cohort study. *Gastroenterology* 2005;**129**:113.

18. Ribes J *et al.* Time trends in incidence and mortality for chronic liver disease and liver cancer in the interval 1980–1997 in Catalonia, Spain. *Eur J Gastroenterol Hepatol* 2004;**16**:865.

19. Sorensen HT *et al.* Long-term survival and cause-specific mortality in patients with cirrhosis of the liver: a nationwide cohort study in Denmark. *J Clin Epidemiol* 2003;**56**:88.

20. Roberts SE *et al.* Trends in mortality after hospital admission for liver cirrhosis in an English population from 1968 to 1999. *Gut* 2005;**54**:1615.

21. Singh GK, Hoyert DL. Social epidemiology of chronic liver disease and cirrhosis mortality in the United States, 1935–

1997: trends and differentials by ethnicity, socioeconomic status, and alcohol consumption. *Hum Biol* 2000;**72**:801.

22. Stinson FS *et al.* The critical dimension of ethnicity in liver cirrhosis mortality statistics. *Alcohol Clin Exp Res* 2001;**25**:1181.

23. Stranges S *et al.* Greater hepatic vulnerability after alcohol intake in African Americans compared with Caucasians: a population-based study. *J Natl Med Assoc* 2004;**96**:1185.

24. McCormick PA, O'Keefe C. Improving prognosis following a first variceal haemorrhage over four decades. *Gut* 2001;**49**:682.

25. Stokkeland K *et al.* Improved prognosis for patients hospitalized with esophageal varices in Sweden 1969–2002. *Hepatology* 2006;**43**:500.

26. Fernandez-Esparrach G *et al.* A prognostic model for predicting survival in cirrhosis with ascites. *J Hepatol* 2001;**34**:46.

27. Foreman MG *et al.* Cirrhosis as a risk factor for sepsis and death: analysis of the National Hospital Discharge Survey. *Chest* 2003;**124**:1016.

28. Marchesini G *et al.* Factors associated with poor health-related quality of life of patients with cirrhosis. *Gastroenterology* 2001;**120**:170.

29. AGA. *The Burden of Gastrointestinal Diseases.* Technical Report. Bethesda, MD: American Gastroenterological Association, 2001:8.

30. El-Serag HB. Hepatocellular carcinoma: recent trends in the United States. *Gastroenterology* 2004;**127**:S27.

31. Bosch FX *et al.* Primary liver cancer: worldwide incidence and trends. *Gastroenterology* 2004;**127**:S5.

32. El-Serag HB *et al.* The continuing increase in the incidence of hepatocellular carcinoma in the United States: an update. *Ann Intern Med* 2003;**139**:817.

33. Kim WR *et al.* Mortality and hospital utilization for hepatocellular carcinoma in the United States. *Gastroenterology* 2005;**129**:486.

34. Yu L *et al.* Risk factors for primary hepatocellular carcinoma in black and white Americans in 2000. *Clin Gastroenterol*

Hepatol 2006;**4**:355.

35. Davila JA, El-Serag HB. Racial differences in survival of hepatocellular carcinoma in the United States: a population-based study. *Clin Gastroenterol Hepatol* 2006;**4**:104; quiz 104.

36. Fattovich G *et al.* Hepatocellular carcinoma in cirrhosis: incidence and risk factors. *Gastroenterology* 2004;**127**:S35.

37. Kiyosawa K *et al.* Hepatocellular carcinoma: recent trends in Japan. *Gastroenterology* 2004;**127**:S17.

38. El-Serag HB, Mason AC. Rising incidence of hepatocellular carcinoma in the United States. *N Engl J Med* 1999;**340**:745.

39. El-Serag HB *et al.* The continuing increase in the incidence of hepatocellular carcinoma in the United States: an update. *Ann Intern Med* 2003;**139**:817.

40. Davila JA *et al.* Geographic variation within the United States in the incidence of hepatocellular carcinoma. *J Clin Epidemiol* 2003;**56**:487.

41. Bruix J, Sherman M. Management of hepatocellular carcinoma. *Hepatology* 2005;**42**:1208.

42. Calle EE *et al.* Overweight, obesity, and mortality from cancer in a prospectively studied cohort of U.S. adults. *N Engl J Med* 2003;**348**:1625.

43. Davila JA *et al.* Diabetes increases the risk of hepatocellular carcinoma in the United States: a population based case control study. *Gut* 2005;**54**:533.

44. El-Serag HB *et al.* The association between diabetes and hepatocellular carcinoma: a systematic review of epidemiologic evidence. *Clin Gastroenterol Hepatol* 2006;**4**:369.

45. Gish RG. Hepatocellular carcinoma: overcoming challenges in disease management. *Clin Gastroenterol Hepatol* 2006;**4**:252.

46. Bianchi G *et al.* Reduced quality of life of patients with hepatocellular carcinoma. *Dig Liver Dis* 2003;**35**:46.

47. Hoyert DL *et al.* Deaths: preliminary data for 2003. *National Vital Statistics Reports* 2005;**53**:1.

48. El-Serag HB *et al.* Treatment and outcomes of treating of hepatocellular carcinoma among Medicare recipients in the United States: a population-based study. *J Hepatol* 2006;**44**:158.

Nonalcoholic Fatty Liver Disease

Paul Angulo

Key points

- Nonalcoholic fatty liver disease (NAFLD) comprises a spectrum of liver pathology including bland steatosis, steatohepatitis, cirrhosis and hepatocellular carcinoma.
- NAFLD affects a substantial proportion of the general population from several countries.
- The prevalence and incidence of NAFLD is expected to increase worldwide as the global obesity epidemic grows, and with the trend in developing countries toward a Western lifestyle.
- Insulin resistance is almost a universal finding in patients with NAFLD, and NAFLD is considered the hepatic manifestation of the metabolic syndrome, which includes central obesity, hyperglycemia, low HDL (high-density lipoprotein) cholesterol, hypertension and hypertriglyceridemia.
- Improvement of insulin resistance with lifestyle intervention constitutes an essential step in both the treatment and prevention of nonalcoholic fatty liver disease. Medications that increase insulin sensitivity and the antioxidant defenses in the liver hold promise for the treatment of NAFLD.

Clinical summary

Patients may complain of fatigue or malaise and a sensation of fullness or discomfort in the right upper abdomen. Health-related quality of life is significantly diminished due to insulin resistance-associated comorbidities. Hepatomegaly and acanthosis nigricans in children are common physical findings. Patients with "cryptogenic" cirrhosis share many clinical features of patients with NAFLD suggesting that their cryptogenic cirrhosis is in fact the cirrhotic stage of unrecognized NAFLD. Insulin resistance and oxidative stress play a key role in the development and progression of NAFLD. Mild to moderate elevation of serum aminotransferases is the most common and often the only laboratory abnormality found in patients with NAFLD. The aspartate transaminase/alanine transaminase (AST/ALT) ratio is usually less than one, but this ratio increases as fibrosis advances.

Imaging studies, including ultrasonography, computed tomography (CT) scan and magnetic resonance (MR) imaging are sensitive in detecting steatosis, but the grade and stage of disease can be determined only with a liver biopsy. Histological features include steatosis alone or in combination with mixed inflammatory cell infiltration, hepatocyte ballooning and necrosis, Mallory's hyaline and fibrosis. These histological features are mostly seen in acinar zone 3, although portal-based injury is commonly seen in children.

The diagnosis of NAFLD requires the exclusion of alcohol abuse and other etiologies as the cause of the liver disease. Treatment of patients with NAFLD should focus on the management of associated conditions including obesity, and glucose and lipid abnormalities (Fig. 34.1). Lifestyle intervention with change of diet and increased physical activity is the cornerstone in the management of NAFLD. Medications, including insulin sensitizers and antioxidants, are being evaluated in placebo-controlled trials. Patients with NAFLD with simple steatosis seem to follow a relatively benign course, whereas in others, NAFLD progresses to advanced fibrosis and cirrhosis with its consequent complications of portal hypertension and liver failure. Cirrhotic stage NAFLD constitutes a common indication for liver transplantation to date. As in other types of cirrhosis, cirrhotic-stage NAFLD may be complicated by hepatocellular carcinoma (HCC) [1,2].

Disease definition

NAFLD refers to the accumulation of fat, mainly triglycerides, in hepatocytes so that it exceeds 5% of the liver weight. Primary NAFLD results from insulin resistance

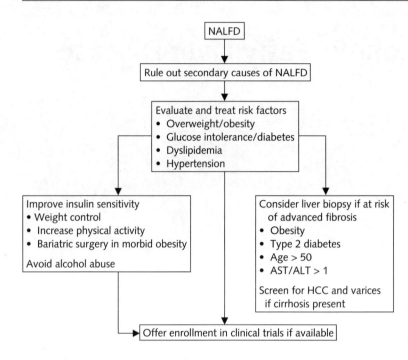

Fig. 34.1 Diagnosis and treatment algorithm for nonalcoholic fatty liver disease (NAFLD).

and thus frequently occurs as part of the metabolic changes that accompany obesity, type 2 diabetes and dyslipidemia. However, it is important to exclude secondary causes of steatosis (Table 34.1). The histological damage in NAFLD is very similar to that seen in patients with alcoholic liver disease, but NAFLD is by definition not alcohol-induced. Alcohol abuse, hepatotoxic medications and other liver conditions should be ruled out. However, given the high prevalence of obesity, diabetes and dyslipidemia in the general population, NAFLD often coexists with liver diseases of other etiology [3].

Incidence and prevalence

The incidence of NAFLD remains unknown because no prospective studies have been conducted. The true prevalence of NAFLD and its different stages remains incompletely defined. The reported prevalence of NAFLD varies based on the information available in a given population and the diagnostic criteria used. Table 34.2 summarizes the results of several studies on the prevalence of NAFLD. Population-based studies provide more accurate figures, but few such studies have been reported to date. Using proton MR spectroscopy, the Dallas Heart Study (a population-based cohort study performed in an ethnically diverse community in the USA) reported that one in three adult Americans have steatosis [3]. The finding indicates that over 70 million adult Americans suffer from NAFLD. In that study [3], 79% of patients with NAFLD had normal aminotransferase levels, and thus, studies using liver enzymes as a surrogate for NAFLD underestimate the prevalence of NAFLD. A high prevalence rate of NAFLD has been reported from other countries. Using liver ultra-

Table 34.1 Causes of nonalcoholic fatty liver disease (NAFLD)

Primary	Obesity, glucose intolerance, type 2 diabetes, hypertriglyceridemia, low HDL (high-density lipoprotein) cholesterol, hypertension
Nutritional	Protein-calorie malnutrition, rapid weight loss, gastrointestinal bypass surgery, total parenteral nutrition
Drugs	Glucocorticoids, estrogens, tamoxifen, amiodarone, methotrexate, diltiazem, zidovudine, valproate, aspirin, tetracycline, cocaine
Metabolic	Lipodystrophy, hypopituitarism, dysbetalipoproteinemia, Weber–Christian disease
Toxins	*Amanita phalloides* mushroom, phosphorus poisoning, petrochemicals, *Bacillus cereus* toxin
Infections	Human immunodeficiency virus, hepatitis C, small bowel diverticulosis with bacterial overgrowth

Table 34.2 Selected studies on prevalence of nonalcoholic fatty liver disease (NAFLD) and nonalcoholic steatohepatitis (NASH)

Author (year)	Study	Diagnostic method	Country	No. of individuals screened	Prevalence of NAFLD (%)	Prevalence of NASH (%)
Browning (2004)	Population-based	MR spectroscopy	USA	2 287	31	ND
Bedogni (2005)	Population-based	Ultrasonography	Italy	598	23	ND
Fan (2005)	Population-based	Ultrasonography	China	3 175	15	ND
Nomura (1988)	Population-based	Ultrasonography	Japan	2 574	14	ND
Clark (2003)	Population-based	Aminotransferases	USA	15 676	5.4	ND
Ruhl (2003)	Population-based	Aminotransferases	USA	5 724	2.8	ND
Jimba (2005)	Health evaluation	Ultrasonography	Japan	1 950	29	ND
Hamaguchi (2005)	Health evaluation	Ultrasonography	Japan	4 401	18	ND
Park (2006)	Health evaluation	Ultrasonography	South Korea	6 648	16	ND
Hultcrantz (1986)	Hospital series	Liver biopsy	Sweden	149	39	ND
Lee (1989)	Hospital series	Liver biopsy	USA	543	ND	9
Nonomura (1992)	Hospital series	Liver biopsy	Japan	561	ND	1
Byron (1996)	Hospital series	Liver biopsy	USA	1 226	ND	11
Daniel (1999)	Hospital series	Liver biopsy	USA	81	51	32
Berasain (2000)	Hospital series	Liver biopsy	Spain	1 075	ND	16
Hilden (1977)	Autopsy series	Liver biopsy	Sweden	503	24	ND
Ground (1982)	Autopsy series	Liver biopsy	USA	423	16	ND
Wanless (1990)	Autopsy series	Liver biopsy	Canada	207	29	6
El-Hassan (1992)	Outpatients	Ultrasonography, CT	Saudi Arabia	1 425	10	ND
Lonardo (1997)	Outpatients	Ultrasonography	Italy	363	20	ND
Araujo (1998)	Outpatients	Ultrasonography	Brazil	217	33.5	ND
Omagari (2002)	Outpatients	Ultrasonography	Japan	3 432	9	ND
Luyckx (1998)	Bariatric surgery	Liver biopsy	Belgium	528	74	ND
Silverman (1990)	Bariatric surgery	Liver biopsy	USA	100	86	36
Dixon (2001)	Bariatric surgery	Liver biopsy	Australia	105	71	25
Beymer (2003)	Bariatric surgery	Liver biopsy	USA	48	85	33
Spaulding (2003)	Bariatric surgery	Liver biopsy	USA	48	88	56
Mathurin (2006)	Bariatric surgery	Liver biopsy	France	167	ND	14.4
Franzese (1997)[a,b]	Outpatients	Ultrasonography	Italy	72	53	ND
Tominaga (1995)[a]	Health evaluation	Ultrasonography	Japan	810	3	ND
Schwimmer (2006)[a]	Autopsy series	Liver biopsy	USA	742	9.6 (38 among obese)	3

[a]Pediatric series. [b]Obese children. ND, not determined.

sonography, a recent population-based cohort study performed in Italy found that one in four or five adults in that country suffer from NAFLD [4]. NAFLD has also reached epidemic proportions among populations typically considered at "low risk" for this liver condition, with a prevalence in China and Japan of 15% and 14%, respectively, among adults. The clinical implications of this alarming prevalence of NAFLD are derived from the fact that this liver condition may progress to end-stage liver disease and liver cancer [5,6].

Population-based studies provide better estimates of the prevalence of NAFLD in the general population compared with autopsy studies, hospital series or studies performed exclusively in obese populations (Table 34.2). The prevalence of NAFLD among children is unknown, but some data indicate that 2.6–9.6% of children have NAFLD, increasing up to 38–53% among obese children (Table 34.2).

Risk factors for disease

NAFLD may affect any age and ethnic group. The prevalence of NAFLD among adults in the USA seems to be different among different ethnic groups, affecting 45% of Hispanic people, 33% of White people and 24% of Black people. The prevalence is significantly higher in White men (42%) than in White women (24%). There is no gender difference in prevalence among Hispanic people or Black people [7]. In children and teens, the prevalence of NAFLD again seems to be different among the different ethnic groups, with the highest prevalence among Hispanic people and the lowest among Black children [8]. Differences in body fat distribution and body composition among the different ethnic groups may partially explain the racial differences in prevalence. For instance, Hispanic people have a higher proportion of body fat and higher waist to hip ratio than their taller counterparts [9]. Similarly, Asian people have a higher proportion of visceral fat and a lower proportion of lean body mass than White subjects with the same body mass index (BMI) [10].

The central (or upper body) obesity phenotype is associated with increased intra-abdominal (or visceral) fat. Visceral adipose tissue has greater lipolytic potential than subcutaneous adipose tissue, and the release of free fatty acids (FFA) from visceral fat directly into the portal circulation creates a "first-pass" effect [11]. Increased FFA concentrations, in turn, are considered a major mediator of insulin resistance. In contrast, FFA flux and concentrations in individuals with predominantly lower body obesity tend to be normal, regardless of BMI [11]. Therefore, patients with central obesity are characteristically insulin resistant, and more commonly present with NAFLD compared with patients having lower body obesity [12].

Besides central obesity, type 2 diabetes, dyslipidemia and hypertension are risk factors for the development of NAFLD. NAFLD, however, can also precede the development of these other comorbidities [5].

Environmental factors and lifestyle-related factors such as reduced physical activity and high-fat diets are well-known influences for the development of insulin resistance-associated comorbidities and NAFLD. The genetic predisposition for the development of central obesity and type 2 diabetes undoubtedly plays a role in the development of NAFLD, although family studies and studies specifically addressing the genetic susceptibility for NAFLD development are lacking.

Natural history and mortality

Changes in fibrosis stage have been specifically evaluated in four independent series (Table 34.3). Overall, fibrosis progresses over time, but it remains stable for a number of years in many cases and it may actually improve spontaneously in some cases [6,13–15]. Higher BMI and greater insulin resistance or the presence of type 2 diabetes are risk factors for a higher rate of fibrosis progression [6,15]. As fibrosis develops and progresses over time, other features of NAFLD, including steatosis, inflammation and ballooning of hepatocytes, significantly improve or disappear [15]; thus, liver biopsy features other than fibrosis severity may not be useful to predict the long-term prognosis in an individual patient with NAFLD. Furthermore, the histological features of NAFLD that create the basis for the histological diagnosis of nonalcoholic steatohepatitis (NASH) (i.e., inflammation and hepatocyte ballooning) are unequally distributed throughout the liver parenchyma, with liver biopsy resulting in misdiagnosis in some patients [16]. Also, aminotransferases, when elevated, improve or normalize spontaneously over time despite fibrosis progression [15].

Studies evaluating the long-term prognosis of patients with NAFLD are summarized in Table 34.4. Overall, the disease progresses slowly over many years or decades, but the prognosis is different across the different stages of NAFLD. Patients with simple, bland steatosis appear to have a more benign prognosis. For instance, a Danish study of a cohort of 109 predominantly morbidly obese subjects followed for nearly 17 years found the incidence of cirrhosis to be <1% [17]. During follow-up, a quarter of patients died but the survival curve of the general population fell within the 95% confidence interval of the survival curve of patients with bland steatosis. In that study [17], the patient who developed cirrhosis was the only one who died from liver-related causes. Conversely, patients with cirrhotic stage NASH have a worse prognosis, as demonstrated in three recent studies [18–20]. In those studies, 9–26% of patients died within 4–10 years of follow-up, with most causes of death related to end-stage liver disease.

Table 34.3 Changes in fibrosis stage evaluated in studies with sequential liver biopsy in nonalcoholic fatty liver disease (NAFLD)

Author (year)	No. of patients	Average time interval (years) between biopsies (range)	Progressed n (%)	Stable n (%)	Improved n (%)
Harrison (2003)	22	5.7 (1.4–15.7)	7 (32)	11 (50)	4 (18)
Fassio (2004)	22	4.3 (3–14.3)	7 (32)	11 (50)	4 (18)
Adams (2005)	103	3.2 (0.7–21.3)	38 (37)	35 (34)	30 (29)
Ekstedt (2006)	70	13.8 (10.3–16.3)	29 (41)	30 (43)	11 (16)

Table 34.4 Studies on long-term prognosis of nonalcoholic fatty liver disease (NAFLD)

Author (year)	Diagnosis[a]	n	Cirrhosis prevalence (%)[b]	No. of liver-related deaths (%)	No. of deaths overall (%)	Average follow-up (years)
Teli (1995)	Bland steatosis	40	0	0	14 (35)	9.6
Dam-Larsen (2004)	Bland steatosis	109	1	1 (0.9)	27 (24.8)	16.7
Matteoni (1999)	NAFLD	98	20	9 (9)	48 (49)	8.3
Adams (2005)	NAFLD	420	5	7 (1.7)	53 (12.6)	7.6
Ekstedt (2006)	NAFLD	129	7.8	2 (1.6)	26 (20.2)	13.7
Lee (1989)	NASH	39	16.3	1 (3)	10 (26)	3.8
Powell (1990)	NASH	42	7	1 (2)	2 (5)	4.5
Evans (2002)	NASH	26	4	0	4 (15)	8.7
Hui (2004)	Cirrhotic-stage NASH	23	100	5 (21)	6 (26)	5.0
Hashimoto (2005)	NASH with septal fibrosis or cirrhosis	89	48	6 (6.7)	8 (9)	3.7
Sanyal (2006)	Cirrhotic-stage NASH	152	100	22 (14.5)	29 (19.1)	10

[a]NAFLD denotes the inclusion of both patients with simple steatosis and patients with nonalcoholic steatohepatitis (NASH).
[b]Cirrhosis prevalence includes all patients diagnosed with cirrhosis at both baseline and during follow-up.

Overall, a diagnosis of NAFLD is associated with a shorter survival than expected for the general population of the same age and gender, as recently demonstrated in two independent studies [5,6]. A community-based study performed in the USA included 420 patients with NAFLD and found liver-related complications to be the third most common cause of death among NAFLD patients compared with the 13th most common cause of death in the general population [5]. This indicates that complications of end-stage liver disease contribute importantly to mortality in patients with NAFLD. Patients dying from liver-related causes were those with more advanced NAFLD [5], confirming observations of smaller studies [17–20]. Impaired fasting glucose or diabetes, older age and presence of cirrhosis are risk factors independently associated with a higher mortality in NAFLD [5].

Interestingly, a recent Swedish study of 129 patients presenting with abnormal liver enzymes found a significantly higher mortality among patients with NAFLD compared with the general population of the same age and gender after almost 14 years of follow-up [6]. Again, liver-related complications were the third most common cause of death among NAFLD patients, with cardiovascular disease and extrahepatic malignancy being the first and second most common causes of death, respectively.

The potential for NAFLD to result in end-stage liver disease is further highlighted by some data suggesting that NAFLD underlies a substantial proportion of cases of cryptogenic cirrhosis [21]. Of patients with cryptogenic cirrhosis, 50–73% have a BMI in the obese category or suffer from diabetes. The prevalence of NAFLD as an un-

recognized cause of cryptogenic cirrhosis is probably underestimated because some nondiabetic, nonobese (i.e., BMI <30) patients may suffer from central obesity and/or dyslipidemia, which may be the only risk factor(s) for NAFLD and have not been consistently measured in series of cryptogenic cirrhosis. Further, the presence of NAFLD increases disease severity and progression in other liver diseases including chronic hepatitis C infection, alcoholic liver disease and hemochromatosis [3].

Quality of life

The impact of NAFLD on health-related quality of life is currently being evaluated. Several studies have found a significant detrimental impact on health-related quality of life of the several comorbidities that conform the metabolic syndrome and that often cluster with NAFLD.

Prevention

There are no studies of measures aimed at preventing NAFLD development. However, preventing the development of insulin resistance and its clinical manifestations (i.e., the metabolic syndrome) is expected to prevent NAFLD development. Weight gain and obesity resulting from a more sedentary lifestyle and high-fat diets seem to be key factors in the development of insulin resistance and NAFLD [1]. Thus, achieving and maintaining appropriate weight control would be expected to prevent the development of NAFLD, as would the treatment of glucose and lipid abnormalities. This is further supported by data from the diabetes prevention program in the USA [22], demonstrating that both lifestyle intervention and the insulin-sensitizing drug, metformin, significantly reduce the development of the metabolic syndrome, which, intuitively, would prevent the development of NAFLD.

Issues in epidemiology knowledge

There is a relative scarcity of NAFLD prevalence data available from population-based studies. There are no data on the change in prevalence of NAFLD within a population over time, and there are no data on incidence of NAFLD. The lack of a diagnostic test or combination of tests with 100% accuracy precludes firm conclusions about the incidence and prevalence of NAFLD, and its different stages, in the general population. Liver enzymes are insensitive and nonspecific for chronic liver disease. Imaging techniques such as ultrasonography and CT scan may provide false negatives. More sensitive techniques, including MR imaging and spectroscopy, are hindered by expense and lack of feasibility in large populations. Liver biopsy has been considered as the gold standard, but is limited by sampling and interpretation error besides its cost and impractical applicability in population-based studies. Furthermore, unless uniform data become available, estimates of the prevalence and incidence of NAFLD over a given time period will probably be affected by increased awareness of the disease.

Recommendations for future studies

Further population-based studies are necessary to determine the true prevalence and the impact on health-related quality of life of NAFLD. Prospective studies with long-term follow-up will better define the natural history of NAFLD and its incidence in specific populations. Genetic studies are necessary to determine to what extent the genetic background predisposes to NAFLD development and progression to advanced liver disease. Carefully controlled clinical trials will better define the impact of lifestyle intervention and pharmacotherapy on NAFLD [23].

Conclusions

With the increasing prevalence of obesity, type 2 diabetes and the metabolic syndrome in the general population, NAFLD has become a common diagnosis in clinical practice of several medical specialties. Bland steatosis remains stable for a number of years and will probably never progress in many cases, with most liver-related morbidity and mortality observed in those patients whose disease progresses to advanced fibrosis and cirrhosis. Further studies are necessary to determine the impact of NAFLD on health-related quality of life and resources utilization as well as the extent to which preventing the development of the metabolic syndrome would prevent NAFLD development and reduce liver-related morbidity and mortality.

References

1. Farrell GC *et al.* Nonalcoholic fatty liver disease: from steatosis to cirrhosis. *Hepatology* 2006;**43**(2 Suppl. 1):S99.
2. Nobili V *et al.* NAFLD in children: a prospective clinical-pathological study and effect of lifestyle advice. *Hepatology* 2006;**44**:458.
3. Powell EE *et al.* Steatosis: co-factor in other liver diseases. *Hepatology* 2005;**42**:5.
4. Bedogni G *et al.* Prevalence of and risk factors for nonalcoholic fatty liver disease: The Dionysos nutrition and liver study. *Hepatology* 2005;**42**:44.
5. Adams LA *et al.* The natural history of nonalcoholic fatty liver disease: a population-based cohort study. *Gastroenterology* 2005;**129**:113.
6. Ekstedt M *et al.* Long-term follow-up of patients with NAFLD and elevated liver enzymes. *Hepatology* 2006;**44**:865.
7. Browning JD *et al.* Prevalence of hepatic steatosis in an urban population in the United States: impact of ethnicity. *Hepatology* 2004;**40**:1387.
8. Schwimmer J *et al.* Prevalence of fatty liver in children and adolescents. *Pediatrics* 2006;**118**:1388.
9. Lopez-Alvarenga JC *et al.* Short stature is related to high body fat composition despite body mass index in a Mexican population. *Arch Med Res* 2003;**34**:137.
10. Dudeja V *et al.* BMI does not accurately predict overweight in Asian Indians in northern India. *Br J Nutr* 2001;**86**:105.
11. Angulo P. NAFLD, obesity and bariatric surgery. *Gastroenterology* 2006;**130**:1848.
12. Stranges S *et al.* Body fat distribution, relative weight, and liver enzyme levels: a population based study. *Hepatology* 2004;**39**:754.
13. Harrison SA *et al.* The natural history of nonalcoholic fatty liver disease: a clinical histopathological study. *Am J Gastroenterol.* 2003;**98**:2042.
14. Fassio E *et al.* Natural history of nonalcoholic steatohepatitis: a longitudinal study of repeat liver biopsies. *Hepatology* 2004;**40**:820.
15. Adams LA *et al.* The histological course of nonalcoholic

fatty liver disease: a longitudinal study of 103 patients with sequential liver biopsies. *J Hepatol* 2005;**42**:132.

16. Ratziu V *et al.* Sampling variability of liver biopsy in nonalcoholic fatty liver disease. *Gastroenterology* 2005;**128**:1898.

17. Dam-Larsen S *et al.* Long term prognosis of fatty liver: risk of chronic liver disease and death. *Gut* 2004;**53**:750.

18. Hui J *et al.* Long term outcomes of cirrhosis in nonalcoholic steatohepatitis compared with hepatitis C. *Hepatology* 2003;**38**:420.

19. Hashimoto E *et al.* The characteristics and natural history of Japanese patients with nonalcoholic fatty liver disease. *Hepatol Res* 2005;**33**:72.

20. Sanyal AJ *et al.* Similarities and differences in outcomes of cirrhosis due to nonalcoholic steatohepatitis and hepatitis C. *Hepatology* 2006;**43**:682.

21. Clark JM *et al.* Nonalcoholic fatty liver disease: an underrecognized cause of cryptogenic cirrhosis. *JAMA* 2003;**289**:3000.

22. Orchard TJ *et al.* The effect of metformin and intensive lifestyle intervention on the metabolic syndrome: The diabetes prevention program randomized trial. *Ann Intern Med* 2005;**142**:611.

23. Adams LA, Angulo P. Treatment of nonalcoholic fatty liver disease. *Postgrad Med J* 2006;**82**:315.

35 Hepatitis B and C

W. Ray Kim

Key points

- Both hepatitis B and C viruses (HBV and HCV) are transmitted parenterally via infected blood or body fluids and may be commonly transmitted by contaminated needles and unprotected sexual contacts. Perinatal exposure is also an important means of transmission, especially for hepatitis B in endemic populations.
- In the USA the incidence of new infections with HBV and HCV has been decreasing in the past two decades, largely due to safer needle-using practices and universal precautions in healthcare as well as exclusion of blood donors with infection. For hepatitis B, widespread vaccination programs have been effective in reducing its incidence in children.
- Despite these decreases in acute infections, the prevalence and burden of chronic HBV and HCV infection remain substantial in the USA. Population-based prevalence estimates for chronic HBV and HCV infection are 1.3% and 0.4%, indicating nearly 2% of the US general population has chronic viral hepatitis.
- The burden of liver disease related to chronic HBV is disproportionately high among Americans of Asian/Pacific Islander descent. The burden of chronic hepatitis C has been increasing particularly among people born in the 1950s, among African and Mexican Americans, and those who are homeless or incarcerated.

Introduction

Hepatitis B virus (HBV)

HBV is a DNA virus belonging to the hepadnavirus family. Infected hepatocytes produce at least three types of viral proteins that are utilized in the diagnosis of HBV infection (Table 35.1). The S protein constitutes the viral envelope and is detected as HBV surface antigen (HBsAg) in the serum. The C protein, a component of the viral nucleocapsid, remains within hepatocytes and is not detectable in the serum. However, antibodies against this protein, namely, anti-HBc, are a marker of exposure to the virus. Hepatitis B e antigen (HBeAg) consists of the C protein and pre-C protein. Presence of HBeAg connotes active replication of the virus. Patients who lack HBeAg usually have detectable antibodies against it in the serum (anti-HBe), which indicates either suppression of viral replication by the host immune system or presence of the so-called pre-core mutation, which allows active replication of the virus while not producing the pre-C protein. The most accurate marker of HBV replication, however, is the serum level of HBV DNA. Classically, serum levels $>10^5$ copies/mL have been understood to represent active viral replication, although more recent data indicate that liver damage occurs at lower levels.

Table 35.1 Diagnostic testing for HBV and HCV infection

Test	Interpretation
HBsAg	Active infection (acute or chronic)
Anti-HBs	Immunity to HBV infection
Anti-HBc (total)	Exposure to HBV
HBeAg	Evidence of active HBV replication
Anti-HBe	Low replication or pre-core mutant
HBV DNA	Amount of virus in the blood (correlates with degree of replication)

Test	Interpretation
HCV antibody (EIA)	Screening
HCV RNA (qualitative)	Confirmatory test
HCV RNA (quantitative)	Pre- and intra-treatment test to assess response to therapy
Genotype	Pre-treatment test to determine Treatment regimen
RIBA	Confirmation of positive anti-HCV antibody (rarely used clinically)

EIA, enzyme immunoassay; HBc, hepatitis B C (core) protein; HBeAg, hepatitis B e antigen; HBsAg, hepatitis B surface antigen; HBV, hepatitis B virus; HCV, hepatitis C virus; RIBA, radioimmunoblot assay.

Hepatitis C virus (HCV)

HCV is an RNA virus that belongs in the flavivirus family, along with the dengue fever virus and yellow fever virus. The proteins generated by HCV may be structural (envelope and core) or nonstructural (polymerase, protease, etc.). The initial test in the detection of HCV infection utilizes anti-HCV antibodies directed against the core and nonstructural proteins. Currently used anti-HCV testing is highly sensitive and specific for these antibodies. Detection of HCV RNA is the hallmark of the infection with HCV. In population-based studies, 20–35% of subjects who have anti-HCV do not have detectable HCV RNA in the serum, which indicates previous exposure to HCV and recovery therefrom. These individuals test positive to RIBA (radioimmunoblot assays), as opposed to individuals in whom the anti-HCV test is false positive.

Transmission of HBV and HCV

Both HBV and HCV are transmitted parenterally, that is, by exposure to blood, blood products and tissue. The incubation period of hepatitis B is 6–24 weeks (average 16 weeks) and that of HCV 3–12 weeks (average 7 weeks) [1,2].

HBV is transmitted by percutaneous and mucous membrane exposures to infectious body fluids, such as serum, semen and saliva. Perinatal transmission is thought to be a major route by which HBV infection perpetuates in endemic countries. The risk of transmission in general correlates with the HBV DNA level in the maternal serum [3,4]. The risk is greatest for infants born to women who are HBeAg-positive with high levels of HBV DNA (often >100 million copies/mL); 70–90% of such children are HBsAg-positive at 6 months of age. The risk in infants born to mothers with negative HBeAg (and low levels of HBV DNA) ranges from 10 to 40%. Fortunately, the risk of perinatal HBV transmission can be significantly reduced by passive and active immunizations. Although HBsAg has been found in breast milk, breastfeeding by a HBsAg-positive mother has not been shown to pose an additional risk for the acquisition of HBV.

Children born to HBsAg-positive mothers who do not become infected during the perinatal period remain at risk of infection during early childhood [5]. Up to 40% of infants born to HBeAg-negative mothers may become infected by 5 years of age. In this setting, "horizontal" transmission of HBV is known to occur during early childhood, in addition to the potential mother-to-child transmission.

Although the exact mechanism by which this occurs is unknown, frequent interpersonal contacts of nonintact skin or mucous membranes with blood-containing secretions or saliva is probably the route of transmission. Because the concentration of virus in the blood is often extremely high in children and because HBV remains infectious on surfaces in the environment for long periods of time (>1 week) under ambient conditions, indirect inoculation of HBV through inanimate objects may occur among children relatively efficiently.

Among adults, high-risk sexual activity is one of the most frequent routes of transmission for HBV [6]. Although homosexual men were historically one of the groups at the greatest risk for HBV infection, heterosexual transmission is the most common cause of acute HBV infection in adults. Factors associated with an increased risk of HBV infection among heterosexual men and women include number of sexual partners, number of years of sexual activity, and history of other sexually transmitted diseases. Thus, transmission of HBV from persons with acute or chronic hepatitis B to their homosexual or heterosexual partners is an important source of infection, because most persons with chronic HBV infection remain asymptomatic.

Transmission of HBV via transfusion of blood and plasma-derived products has been all but eliminated in most countries through donor screening for HBsAg and viral inactivation procedures. However, transmission of HBV may continue to occur in other healthcare settings. For example, transmission of HBV among chronic hemodialysis patients may occur when appropriate isolation guidelines are not followed, which includes using dedicated equipment and staff in a separate room for patients with chronic HBV infection. In addition to contamination of instruments and equipment, direct person-to-person exposure may transmit HBV [7]. Finally, nonsexual interpersonal transmission of HBV can occur, such as long-term household (or institutional) contacts of a chronically infected person over a long period of time. The precise mechanisms of transmission are unknown, but it may mirror the spread of HBV among children as described above.

With regard to HCV, blood transfusion before 1992 and injection drug use have historically been the two most important risk factors in the USA. Presently, however, injection drug use is by far the most common route of transmission for HCV. In a recent report based on the National Health and Nutrition Examination Survey, 58% of participants aged 20–59 years who had used illicit drugs (excluding marijuana) were positive for anti-HCV (149 times more likely to have positive anti-HCV compared with those with drug use history) [8]. Respondents with 20 lifetime sexual partners were five times more likely to be anti-HCV-positive compared with those with 0–1 partners. Other factors associated with positive anti-HCV included age at first sexual encounter, lower family income and education, a positive antibody to herpes simplex virus 2 (HSV-2), as well as a history of blood transfusion before 1992. Among persons aged 20 to 59 with HCV infection, 99% had one of the following risk factors: (i) a history of illicit drug use (other than marijuana); (ii) transfusion prior to 1992; (iii) 20 lifetime sexual partners; or (iv) abnormal levels of serum alanine transaminase (ALT) [8].

Like HBV, HCV may be transmitted in the perinatal period from infected mother to the newborn. The risk of transmission is lower for HCV than HBV: less than 6% of babies born to infected mothers have been reported to acquire the infection [9]. Co-infection with HIV increases the risk of perinatal HCV transmission. Limited data suggest that HCV is not transmitted from mother to baby by breastfeeding. Unfortunately, there is no known means to reduce the risk of transmission.

Incidence of HBV and HCV in the USA

HBV and HCV are reportable infectious diseases in the USA, and the Centers for Disease Control and Prevention (CDC) has put in place mechanisms to capture incident cases of HCV infection. These include passive surveillance programs such as the National Notifiable Disease Surveillance System and hepatitis-specific active surveillance programs such as the Sentinel Counties Study of Acute Viral Hepatitis.

According to CDC, the **incidence of acute hepatitis B** has declined steadily since the late 1980s (Fig. 35.1) [10]. Between 1990 and 2002, the incidence of acute hepatitis B declined by 67%, from 8.5 per 100 000 population (21 102 total cases reported) to 2.8 per 100 000 population (8064 total cases reported) [6]. By age, the most significant decline occurred among persons aged 0–19 years, from 3.0 in 1990 to 0.3 in 2002. Among persons aged 20–39 and >40 years, acute hepatitis B incidence declined by 67% and 39%, respectively, with the majority of this decline occurring during 1990–1998. The incidence of acute hepatitis B among men has been consistently higher than among women.

The reduction in HBV incidence in the USA may be attributed to several measures implemented in 1991, which include universal infant vaccination, universal screening of pregnant women and postexposure prophylaxis of infants born to infected mothers [2]. Between 1995 and 1999, the immunization strategy was expanded to include vaccination of all persons aged 0–18 years who have not been vaccinated previously. While these achievements in children are encouraging, recent data indicate that the incidence of HBV infection among men over 19 and women over 40 years may have increased. The most common risk

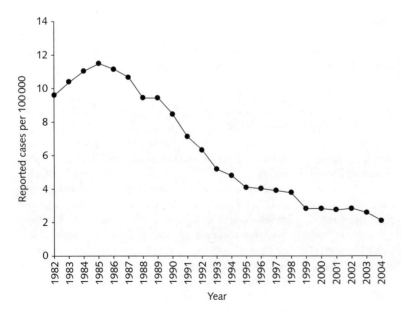

Fig. 35.1 Incidence of acute hepatitis B in the USA. (Reproduced from Anonymous [10], permission waived by CDC.)

factors reported among adults with acute hepatitis B continue to be multiple sexual partners, homosexual activity and injection-drug use.

The **incidence of new HCV infection** is very difficult to estimate accurately. This is because many patients with acute HCV infection are asymptomatic and thus do not present themselves for diagnosis. Underreporting by healthcare providers of diagnosed cases is also thought to be common. Furthermore, individuals at high risk of infection may not have ready access to healthcare, decreasing the likelihood of timely diagnosis of newly acquired HCV infection. Because of these limitations, enumerating reported cases of acute hepatitis C significantly underestimates the true incidence of hepatitis C infection [11].

Given these limitations, CDC has undertaken mathematical modeling studies to estimate the past incidence of HCV. The model indicated that the annual incidence of acute HCV infection in the USA decreased from an average of approximately 230 000 new cases per year in the 1980s to 38 000 cases per year in the 1990s (Fig. 35.2) [12]. The number of persons with transfusion-associated HCV infection decreased significantly since the introduction in 1985 of guidelines for selecting safer blood donors. It declined further with the institution of screening of blood donors for anti-HCV, beginning in 1989 with the first-generation test, and followed in July 1992 with the second-generation assay. Much of the recent decline in incidence can be accounted for by a decline in cases among injecting drug users, which can be related to safer needle-using practices. Trends in other risk factors, including sexual, household exposure and occupational exposures, have remained relatively stable over time.

Prevalence of HBV and HCV

On a global scale, HBV is vastly more common than HCV. More than 2 billion people in the world have been infected with HBV, with active infection present in over 350 million [13]. This compares with an estimated 170 million people currently infected with HCV [14]. The geographic distribution of HBV and HCV is not uniform. HBV is most common in the Far East and Southeast Asia, sub-Saharan Africa, the Amazon basin and Eastern Europe. HCV is more evenly distributed throughout the world than HBV, with a significant number of people from North America and Europe having the infection [14].

The NHANES have been a valuable tool in estimating the prevalence of hepatitis B and C in the USA. The NHANES are a series of cross-sectional national surveys designed to provide representative prevalence estimates for a variety of health measures and conditions. Each survey is designed to be representative of the US civilian non-institutionalized population. In studying the epidemiology of viral hepatitis, NHANES conducted in three periods have been used. The first was conducted between 1976 and 1980 ($n = 28 000$), the second between 1988 and 1994 ($n = 40 000$), and the most recent between 1999 and 2002 ($n = 21 500$) [15].

The **prevalence of chronic HBV infection** was studied in the first two NHANES surveys, which reported similar estimates of HBsAg-positive individuals (0.33% and 0.42%) [16]. In both surveys, the prevalence of HBV infection was low until 12 years of age, when it increased in all racial groups. While the NHANES data are useful in the estimation of HBV prevalence in the USA in general, the surveys did not include statistically valid samples

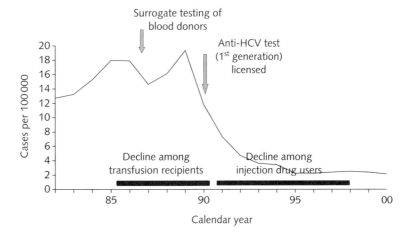

Fig. 35.2 Estimated incidence of acute HCV infection in the USA. (Reproduced from Anonymous [10], permission waived by CDC.)

from populations in which HBV is most common, such as Asians, Pacific Islander and Alaskan Natives [6,17]. Thus, NHANES probably represents an underestimate of the true prevalence of HBV in the USA. In Asian and western Pacific countries where HBV is endemic, the estimated prevalence of chronic HBV infection ranges from 2.4% to 16%.

A recent survey assessed the prevalence of chronic HBV infection among Asian/Pacific Islander (A/PI) populations living in New York City [18]. Of 925 survey participants who reported not having been tested previously for HBV infection, 137 (14.8%) were HBsAg-positive, whereas another 496 (53.6%) had evidence of resolved HBV infection. The prevalence of chronic HBV infection was higher among males (19.7%) compared with females (8.7%) and among persons aged 20–39 years (23.2%) compared with those aged >40 years (9.6%). Prevalence of chronic HBV infection varied by country of birth, from 21.4% among those born in China, to 4.6% among those born in South Korea, to 4.3% among those born in other Asian countries. Although this study was limited to New York City, screening programs in Atlanta, Chicago, New York City, Philadelphia and California have reported similar prevalences of chronic HBV infection (10–15%) among A/PI immigrants to the USA, pointing to a disproportionate burden of chronic HBV infection among A/PI and other immigrant populations.

NHANES data have also been used to estimate **the prevalence of chronic HCV infection** in the USA. NHANES (1988–94) estimated 1.8% of Americans, or 3.9 million people, to be anti-HCV-positive, of whom an estimated 2.7 million were HCV-RNA-positive (chronic HCV infection) (Fig. 35.3) [19]. A recently published study utilized the subsequent NHANES data (1999–2002) and estimated

that 1.6% of the US population (4.1 million) was anti-HCV-positive. Of those, 1.3% (3.2 million) had chronic HCV infection [8]. The comparison between the two estimates reveals that little change occurred in the prevalence of chronic HCV during the 1990s. While it lends support to the data indicating a low incidence of new HCV infection, it also indicates that advances in HCV therapy have not made a demonstrable impact in reducing the burden of chronic HCV infection at the population level.

According to the recent NHANES data, HCV prevalence is significantly higher in males and non-Hispanic Black people, and also increased linearly with age to a peak prevalence in the 40–49-year age group. Within this age group, non-Hispanic Black people had a higher prevalence, at 9.4%, compared with non-Hispanic White people, at 3.8% ($P < 0.001$). A birth cohort analysis indicated that the peak in age-specific prevalence moved from 30–39 years to 40–49 years between the two NHANES datasets.

The limitation of NHANES data with regard to HCV is that some of the population groups with high HCV prevalence have been excluded. For example, in a study on homeless veterans, the prevalence of anti-HCV was as high as 41.7%. Incarcerated persons also have a higher prevalence of HCV than the general population [20,21]. A recent study by Fox *et al.* [22] reported that the prevalence of anti-HCV among incarcerated persons in California was 34.3%. These data suggest that HCV prevalence estimates based upon the NHANES data probably represent an underestimate of the true prevalence.

Mortality from HBV and HCV

Most mortality statistics in the USA are typically based on death certificate data [23]. Mortality from HBV-related liver disease has been estimated to have increased in the past two decades [24]. The age-adjusted death rate for HBV increased fourfold from 0.1 per 100 000 in 1978 to 0.4 in 1998. The death rate was higher in men (0.5 for men, 0.2 for women) and in non-White people (0.3 for White people, 0.4 for Black people and 1.2 for other races). Although the increase in death rate over time was observed in all races and both genders, it was most pronounced in men of other (non-White, non-Black) race (Fig. 35.4).

Figure 35.5 describes the age-adjusted death rate classified as death from hepatitis C (non-A, non-B hepatitis prior to 1991) between 1982 and 1999 [11]. In 1982, 814 deaths were attributed to viral hepatitis, which increased sixfold by 1999 to 4853 deaths. There was a corresponding increase in the age-adjusted death rate from 0.4 to 1.8

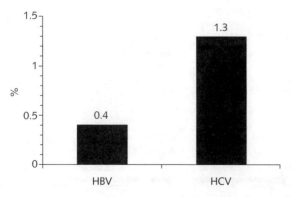

Fig. 35.3 Prevalence of chronic HBV and HCV in the US general population (NHANES 1988–1994).

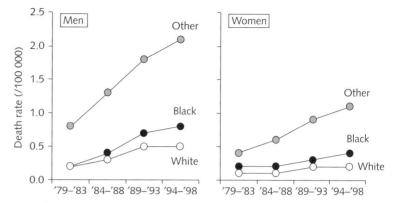

Fig. 35.4 Age- and race-specific mortality from HBV-related disease in the USA ("Other" includes all decedents that did not belong in the "White" or "Black" racial groups).

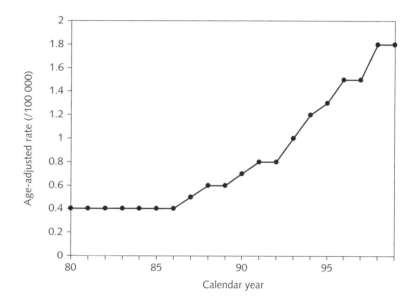

Fig. 35.5 Mortality from HCV-related causes in the USA.

deaths per 100 000 persons per year. Projection studies have suggested that the burden of liver disease secondary to chronic HCV infection will continue to rise throughout this decade [25].

Conclusions

Hepatitis B and C viruses are both parenterally transmitted and, thus, share some common epidemiologic features. Both viruses may be transmitted by contaminated needles, unprotected sexual contacts or perinatal exposure. Incidence of new infections with HBV and HCV has been generally decreasing in the USA thanks to safer needle-using practices and universal precaution

in healthcare as well as exclusion of blood donors with infection. In addition, vaccination programs in children have resulted in a profound decrease in acute HBV infection in adolescence and young adulthood. Despite these decreases in acute infections, the prevalence and burden of chronic HBV and HCV infection remain substantial. Chronic HBV is disproportionately high among Americans of Asian/Pacific Islander extractions. Chronic HCV infection is peculiarly prevalent among people born in the 1950s, especially among African and Mexican Americans and those who are homeless or incarcerated. In the USA as a whole, the burden of HBV and HCV (i.e., mortality) has been increasing in the recent past, and focused epidemiologic attention is urgently needed to screen, promptly diagnose and effectively treat those with existing chronic infection as well as to continue prevention measures in children and adolescents.

References

1. Hoofnagle JH. Course and outcome of hepatitis C. *Hepatology* 2002;**36**:s21.
2. Alter MJ. Epidemiology and prevention of hepatitis B. *Semin Liver Dis* 2003;**23**:39.
3. Shepard CW *et al.* Epidemiology of hepatitis B and hepatitis B virus infection in United States children. *Pediatr Infect Dis J* 2005;**24**:755.
4. Xu ZY *et al.* Prevention of perinatal acquisition of hepatitis B virus carriage using vaccine: preliminary report of a randomized, double-blind placebo-controlled and comparative trial. *Pediatrics* 1985;**76**:713.
5. Beasley RP, Hwang LY. Postnatal infectivity of hepatitis B surface antigen-carrier mothers. *J Infect Dis* 1983;**147**:185.
6. Anonymous. Incidence of acute hepatitis B – United States, 1990–2002. *MMWR Morb Mortal Wkly Rep* 2004;**52**:1252.
7. Harpaz R *et al.* Transmission of hepatitis B virus to multiple patients from a surgeon without evidence of inadequate infection control. *N Engl J Med* 1996;**334**:549.
8. Armstrong GL *et al.* The prevalence of hepatitis C virus infection in the United States, 1999 through 2002. *Ann Intern Med* 2006;**144**:705.
9. Anonymous. Recommendations for prevention and control of hepatitis C virus infection and HCV-related chronic disease. *MMWR* 1998, Atlanta, GA: Centers for Disease Control and Prevention (CDC): 1–9.
10. Anonymous. *Hepatitis Surveillance Report 61.* Atlanta, GA: Centers for Disease Control and Prevention, 2006:1.
11. Kim WR. The burden of hepatitis C in the United States. *Hepatology* 2002;**36**:S30.
12. Williams I. Epidemiology of hepatitis C in the United States. *Am J Med* 1999;**107**:2S.
13. Anonymous. *Hepatitis B.* World Health Organization, 2006.
14. Anonymous. Hepatitis C – global prevalence. *Wkly Epidemiol Rec* 2000;**75**:18.
15. Anonymous. *NHANES 2001–2002 Public Data General Release File Documentation.* Atlanta, GA: Centers for Disease Control and Prevention, 2004.
16. McQuillan G *et al.* Prevalence of hepatitis B virus infection in the United States: the National Health and Nutrition Examination Surveys, 1976 through 1994. *Am J Public Health* 1999;**89**:14.
17. Coleman P *et al.* Incidence of hepatitis B virus infection in the United States, 1976–1994: estimates from the National Health and Nutrition Examination Surveys. *J Infect Dis* 1998;**178**:954.
18. Anonymous. Screening for chronic hepatitis B among Asian/Pacific Islander populations – New York City, 2005. *MMWR Morb Mortal Wkly Rep* 2006;**55**:505.
19. Alter MJ *et al.* The prevalence of hepatitis C virus infection in the United States, 1988 through 1994. *N Engl J Med* 1999;**341**:556.
20. Cheung RC *et al.* Viral hepatitis and other infectious diseases in a homeless population. *J Clin Gastroenterol* 2002;**34**:476.
21. Briggs ME *et al.* Prevalence and risk factors for hepatitis C virus infection at an urban Veterans Administration medical center. *Hepatology* 2001;**34**:1200.
22. Fox RK *et al.* Hepatitis C virus infection among prisoners in the California state correctional system. *Clin Infect Dis* 2005;**41**:177.
23. Kim WR *et al.* Burden of liver disease in the United States: summary of a workshop. *Hepatology* 2002;**36**:227.
24. Kim WR *et al.* Rising burden of hepatitis B in the United States: Should the 'other' virus be forgotten? *Hepatology* 2002;**36**:222A.
25. Armstrong GL *et al.* The past incidence of hepatitis C virus infection: implications for the future burden of chronic liver disease in the United States. *Hepatology* 2000;**31**:777.

Index

Page numbers in *italics* refer to figures and those in **bold** to tables or boxes; note that figures, tables and boxes are only indicated when they are separated from their text references.

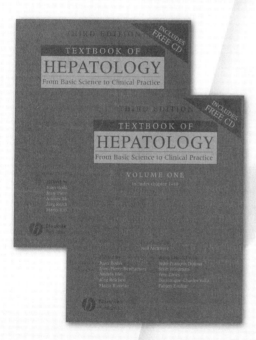
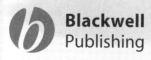